PSYCHIATRY FOR
SOCIAL WORKERS

PSYCHIATRY FOR
SOCIAL WORKERS

LAWSON G. LOWREY, M.D.

Second Edition

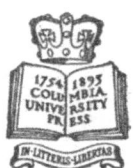

COLUMBIA UNIVERSITY PRESS

NEW YORK · MORNINGSIDE HEIGHTS

Published in Great Britain, Canada, and India by
Geoffrey Cumberlege, Oxford University Press
London, Toronto, and Bombay

First edition, 1946
Second edition, 1950

TO

MY ESTEEMED FORMER CHIEFS

CLARENCE MARTIN JACKSON

ELMER ERNEST SOUTHARD

WHOSE LIVES AND WORKS

HAVE BEEN A NEVER-FAILING

SOURCE OF INSPIRATION

OF ALL *the branches of medicine, psychiatry— by the very nature of the diseases with which it deals—requires both the highest degree of specialization and the broadest medical and cultural education. Mental diseases are apparently the only diseases which deserve the appellation of social diseases, not because they are caused by social factors alone but because a mentally sick individual functions with the totality of his endowments. A psychological conflict leading to disease cannot but use as its vehicle the sum total of the cultural conflicts which are characteristic of the individual's age. One cannot understand the disease without understanding its language, and its language is always the language of the primitive cultural past intimately interwoven with the cultural present.*—Gregory Zilboorg, A HISTORY OF MEDICAL PSYCHOLOGY, p. 523.

PREFACE TO THE FIRST EDITION

THE LIAISON between social work and psychiatry is a comparatively recent development. Social workers have been employed in state hospitals for only a little more than thirty years; training, leading to a diploma in psychiatric social work, has been going on for somewhat less than thirty years.

World War I gave great impetus to psychiatry, to social psychiatry, and to the evolution of clinics for the study and treatment of children's problems; i.e., preventive psychiatry. It may seem strange that the need for clinics for children should have been the result of a war, but the studies of psychotic, psychoneurotic, and delinquent soldiers all revealed signs of disturbances in childhood; hence the importance of these clinics.

It was following the war that the idea of the clinical team of psychiatrist, psychologist, and psychiatric social worker really became effectively operative. These services had been available in psychopathic hospitals, but it was not until child guidance clinics were organized that a really adequate union of techniques was secured. These were community clinics, and as such they came into intimate contact with all the organized agencies of the community.

The needs of social agencies in dealing with their clients had a great deal to do with drawing psychiatry out of its hospital isolation. The establishment of psychopathic hospitals and out-patient departments for psychiatric diagnosis and treatment contributed markedly to this development. Psychiatrists began to see the importance of environmental factors and interpersonal relationships in the development of the illnesses of their patients. Social workers found how personality difficulties in their clients operated to produce social maladjustments.

The rapid development of dynamic psychiatry and psychotherapy and the increasing absorption by social work of concepts derived from these fields have led to a situation in which a book such as this, dealing with clinical psychiatry specifically oriented toward social work, should be useful. For example, there are psychiatric conditions which are irreversible and untreatable, and it is essential that they be recognized. Other conditions are acute and reversible, demanding medical or surgical treatment. The social worker must know how to use hospitalization for cases of these types and must not be unwilling to do so.

Many cases of the so-called functional disorders are not accessible to psychotherapy, but in some a supportive type of social therapy may be extremely important. Environmental manipulation is still an important method of treatment. Group therapy may be acceptable to some patients who could not accept individual therapy, or the reverse may be true.

In this volume I have tried to present the data of psychiatry in a manner which will help the social worker to a greater awareness of the type of personal disturbance she is dealing with in her client. This in turn indicates where she may and where she may not be of help. It has been particularly difficult to make a differential selection of material; practically every chapter could be expanded into a book. There is some duplication of material in certain chapters. This is more or less inevitable, and where it occurs the material has been presented from different approaches. It has been necessary to present some statistics; they have been kept to a minimum and carefully selected to demonstrate points which could not otherwise be clarified.

I have proceeded on the assumption that every reader will at some time have had a course in social psychiatry and have read some textbook on psychiatry. It may be advisable to re-read or read one of the standard texts in connection with reading this volume, since it is not intended that this shall be a textbook. It is not a discussion of the origin and nature of human behavior, except incidentally in relation to its major content. Social psychiatry as such is not presented, though obviously it enters into the discussions.

Finally, there is no attempt to present psychoanalytic concepts and techniques, except as they are necessary for the interpretation of clinical phenomena.

The book aims to present the indicator symptoms of deviations in mental functioning, with special reference to differential symptom pictures which help the social worker in her task of reaching some conclusions with respect to the types of situations in which she needs expert advice, where special types of placement or treatment are necessary, or where she may safely undertake supervision or a treatment plan of her own. This involves a descriptive synthesis of the major types of the psychoses, neuroses, mental defects, epilepsies, psychopathic personalities, and behavior disorders. Included are data on causation (etiology), pathology (organic), psychopathology, course, the usual prognosis, and indicated treatment.

It is always impossible to acknowledge one's debt to teachers, colleagues and writers from whom one absorbs ideas, information, and ways of thinking. In my case, their number is legion.

I am particularly indebted to the staffs of the several organizations with which I have worked, to my patients, and more especially to my students in medicine, psychology and social work, whose inquiring minds have always proved a great stimulus.

My greatest debt is to Victoria Sloane for her painstaking editorial assistance, without which the volume could hardly have been completed.

LAWSON G. LOWREY

New York

PREFACE TO THE SECOND EDITION

IN PREPARING THIS EDITION I have carefully considered the questions, criticisms, and suggestions that have reached me from teachers and practitioners of psychiatry, psychology, and social work and have incorporated them in so far as possible. Critical analyses that appeared in reviews of the original edition have also been utilized.

Each chapter has been revised, and much new material added. General statistics have been brought forward to 1945 and 1947 wherever possible and desirable. In response to suggestions from several social workers, the worker is throughout referred to as "he" instead of the traditional "she." Chapter VII, which contains the material on psychosexual development, is retitled so that the heading is more indicative of the actual content.

A section on the psychosomatic conditions has been included in the chapter on the neuroses, although no attempt is made to present an exhaustive discussion. The section on psychological examinations in Chapter II is completely rewritten to emphasize the utilization of test results in evaluating the dynamics of personality functioning. Discussion of the traditional uses of tests for estimating capacities and abilities, with special reference to educability, has been retained, though largely rewritten. Chapter XVI has been retitled "Mental Disorders in the Young," which seems more exact in the light of the definition of mental disorders followed throughout the book.

The most important change, however, is the addition of Chapter XIX, "The Social Worker and Treatment." Having received numerous requests to elaborate on therapy, especially with neurotics, I reviewed the material on the treatment of individual disorders. It became clear that any attempt to expand these short sections would result in a considerable amount of repetition and yet provide no systematic and comparative statement of principles. It is outside the scope of this volume to attempt a detailed analysis of treatment methods and their applicability to varied situations. But it does seem essential to outline some of the basic principles of social casework treatment and of psychotherapy and to indicate at least some of the similarities and differences.

Psychotherapy is the subject of considerable controversy at present. Under discussion are questions of what constitutes psychotherapy, who should practice it, preliminary and definitive training, conditions to which it is applicable, and the safeguards that are necessary to insure a reasonable degree of effectiveness. Since there are so many unsettled issues, I have tried not to be dogmatic. The demarcations presented in this edition and the division of work and responsibility are based upon my own experience and express my best judgment at this time. Many professional groups are keenly interested in the alleviation of problems in personal and social adjustment. While each professional discipline has its own special approach, certain elements are common to all, and an attempt should be made to recognize them.

Since this is a book on clinical psychiatry, it must deal with specific data—the hard facts which form the core of psychiatric problems. Furthermore, these data must be brought into relationship with social work in many of its settings. It is impossible to interpret a symptom or a person or a situation without facts unless one is content to try to fit human beings and realistic social situations into some sort of theoretical construct. That would definitely not be good casework or clinical procedure. Description and delimitation can no more be avoided in psychiatry than in science, and the problem is to select and present the fundamental facts as a necessary basis for correlation and interpretation. One difficulty is our variable use of terms and concepts. To obviate this, at least to a slight degree, I have defined common terms and either used them interchangeably or given reasons for certain preferences.

The treatment of mental disorders is not as simple as is sometimes implied in popular formulae and dramatic stories. Much of the popular writing is effective at a relatively simple, conscious, educational or reeducational level. If sound, it may be excellent as mental hygiene, but it can hardly reach the level of therapy. Failure in the integration of the emotions and the instinctive drives is not the only important feature of mental disturbance. The tendency to overstress the emotional aspects, to the neglect of the biologically conditioned disorders, unfortunately leads to much wasted effort and is neither good mental hygiene nor adequate therapy.

I express thanks to my many friends who have given me suggestions and criticisms. They deserve mention by name, but the list is too long. I trust that each will recognize the effect of his contribution. I must, however, mention by name Victoria Sloane, whose assistance has been invaluable in this revision, as it was in the original.

L.G.L.

New York
April, 1950

CONTENTS

PSYCHIATRY FOR
SOCIAL WORKERS

CHAPTER I

INTRODUCTION

PUBLIC HEALTH AND SOCIAL IMPLICATIONS

MENTAL DISORDERS constitute one of the most formidable public health problems of modern times. Their ramifications pose serious questions to many public and private social agencies, to courts and to families, as well as to the afflicted individuals. The care and treatment of the multitude who present serious mental deviations, for example, the psychoses, feeblemindedness, and epilepsy, are responsible for large expenditures of public and, to a lesser extent, private funds. In addition, various types of social service are frequently necessary for the families involved because of economic and other problems. Delinquency is often a complication of mental disturbance, as are also educational failure and vocational instability. In short, psychiatric disorders present a series of grave and perplexing questions to several professions, to lay groups, and to individuals.

Social workers deal with people whose self-sufficiency has for some reason become impaired or, as in the case of children, has not developed. To effect the adjustment and readjustment of the individual client to himself, to the realities of his personal limitations and assets, and to his environmental setting, is perhaps the most important aspect of the worker's approach. Personality deviations of any type or degree may be present and can complicate the worker's efforts, sometimes to an insuperable extent. Some of the personality difficulties are so mild that they may be said to be normal, though perhaps exaggerated, reactions to a situation. At the other end of the scale are the grave and incurable forms of deviation, while between these two extremes are many gradations.

It is essential for the social worker to be able to *recognize* indicator symptoms of incipient or marked disturbances, to *know when* to call for psychiatric diagnosis and treatment, and to *understand the limitations* of psychiatric and case work treatment techniques.

The broad social and public implications of the mental disorders are sharply pointed up by hospital statistics, as a few illustrations will demonstrate. The American Medical Association reports that in 1947 there were 585 hospitals for nervous and mental diseases in this country, compared with 575 in 1943. The strictly mental hospitals are not segregated in these lists. The bed capacity was 681,000, a gain of approximately 30,000 over 1943. The number of such institutions had increased by only twenty-two since 1927, but beds had increased by some 330,000, to nearly double the 1927 capacity. Hospital beds for nervous and mental cases in 1947 exceeded by nearly 90,000 the number in somewhat more than 4,500 general hospitals. In fact, the American Medical Association reports that the nervous and mental institutions have 47.9 percent of all hospital beds, by contrast with 41.6 percent in general hospitals.

Hospitals for nervous and mental diseases have an average of 1,163 beds and a daily occupancy of almost 96 percent, while general hospitals average 130 beds with 77 percent occupancy. However, the neuropsychiatric institutions average only 500 admissions each per year, contrasting sharply with the average admission rate of 3,230 for general hospitals. This marked difference in turnover is related to the accumulation of cases, especially in the strictly mental hospitals, because of the chronicity and relative incurability of certain types of mental disorder.

The principle of state care for the mentally diseased and defective has been generally accepted for many years. Expenditures for the operation of state mental hospitals and training schools for defectives constitute a large and constantly increasing item for most states, amounting to 10, 15, or even 20 percent of their annual budgets. Many estimates of the costs to society of mental disorders have been made, and when the loss of productive effort is included,

the figures are staggering. U.S. Public Health Service * estimates
that it cost approximately $400,000,000 to operate mental hospitals
in 1947, an increase of nearly 65 percent over expenditures in 1945.
The 1948–49 appropriations for the Department of Mental Hygiene
in the State of New York alone † exceed $107,000,000, about
$35,000,000 more than in the previous year and more than two and
a half times the appropriation for 1942–43. The Public Health
Service figures show that state, county, and city hospitals, with
an average daily resident-patient population of 481,000, spent
$264,000,000 for maintenance in 1947, or $549 per capita. There

* Figures released in September, 1948, by Federal Security Agency, Public
Health Service, Mental Hygiene Division. In September, 1949, the National
Institute of Mental Health released additional statistics for 1947 (Mental
Health Statistics, *Current Reports:* Series MH-B50, No. 1). A total of 934
organizations, comprised of 628 mental hospitals, 103 psychiatric services of
general hospitals, and 203 institutions for mental defectives and epileptics,
reported approximately 1,140,000 patients on the books during 1947. This
large figure includes, in round numbers, 757,800 patients registered at the
beginning of the year, 276,000 first admissions, and 90,500 readmissions. The
number of patients on books at end of the year was 773,100, a net increase of
15,300 for the year. Of those on the books, only 675,000 were actually in hospital.
    The 195 state hospitals increased from 506,800 patients at the beginning
of the year to 514,000 at the end; they admitted some 119,000 cases. County
and city hospitals (93) showed the same census of 25,000 at beginning and
end of the year; 122 veterans' hospitals gained from 54,200 to 59,000, while
five other federal hospitals remained stationary at 9,000 patients. Psychopathic hospitals gained slightly more than 300 patients, to a total of 1,580 at
end of the year, while private hospitals (197) remained practically stationary
at 14,000, though they admitted 50,100 patients during the year.
    Institutions for mental defectives and epileptics showed an increase of
census from 141,800 to 143,900. An interesting point is that 94 public institutions had 137,300 patients at the year's end, while 109 private institutions had
only 6,600. These institutions admitted 13,300 cases during the year; 12,060
were first admissions.
    Of the overall total of 309,000 "separations" during the year, 254,400 were
discharged and 54,450 died.
    The psychiatric services of general hospitals, with approximately 6,000
beds occupied at beginning and end of the year, admitted somewhat more
than 106,000 patients, 85,100 for the first time. Nearly 36,000 of these cases
were transferred to other hospitals, chiefly public.
† Mental Hygiene News, N.Y. Department of Mental Hygiene, June, 1948.
Included are 18 state hospitals, 2 psychiatric institutes, 5 training schools for
defectives, Craig Colony for epileptics, and the preventive work and general
administration of the department.

were, on the average, 45,000 patients in the Veterans Administration hospitals, which spent $96,000,000, or $2,133 per capita. Private hospitals, having a census of 14,000 patients, expended $35,000,000; per capita cost, $2,500. The over-all picture then is: $395,000,000 expended for the maintenance of an average of 540,000 patients, or $731 per capita.

When these figures are compared with those given for 1945 in the same report, some rather striking points emerge. The average daily number of patients in all the hospitals increased 5.3 percent, but expenditures rose 65 percent, and per capita costs 31.4 percent. The number of patients remained practically stationary in private hospitals, while expenditures and per capita costs increased 25 percent. In the state, county, and city hospitals the resident daily population increased 4.6 percent, expenditures 46.7 percent, and per capita costs 50.4 percent. Figures for the veterans' hospitals are the most striking. The daily patient load increased 15.4 percent, but total expenditures nearly tripled, and the per capita costs increased one and a half times.

A tabulation of patients under care throughout the country at the end of 1945 * showed approximately 518,000 resident in permanent-care hospitals for mental diseases, and more than 119,000 in institutions for mental defectives and epileptics.† More than 2,000 patients were in family care, and 72,500 were in other extramural care. The grand total of "patients on the books" was in excess of 592,000. In addition, some 9,000 patients, nearly all in residence, were registered in temporary-care hospitals, including 9 psychopathic hospitals and the psychiatric wards of 114 general hospitals.

The permanent-care hospitals received as "first admissions" in

---

* These and subsequent statistics, except in Chapter XVII, are derived from: U.S. Bureau of the Census, *Patients in Mental Institutions*, 1945 and 1937 for the country as a whole; and N.Y. State Department of Mental Hygiene, *Annual Reports*, 1938, 1943, and 1945, covering the state.

† Reports from 190 state, 33 veteran, 95 city and county, and 192 private hospitals for mental diseases. Also 87 state, 1 city, and 92 private institutions for mental defectives and epileptics.

1945 nearly 142,000 people, or approximately 32,000 more than in 1937. Of the 1945 admissions, more than 114,500 were psychotic, and about 19,000 were not. Of the latter group, approximately half were alcoholics and drug addicts. Psychopathic personality, mental deficiency, and epilepsy, in that order, account for about 15 percent of the admissions without psychosis; about one fourth were unclassified at the time of reporting. In somewhat more than 8,000 cases, the mental disorder was "not reported."

State hospitals received about 65 percent of the psychotic admissions, but only 42 percent of the nonpsychotics. Veterans' hospitals received 17 percent of the psychotic and 26 percent of the nonpsychotic admissions. About 2 percent of the psychotic and less than 1 percent of the nonpsychotic cases were admitted to city and county hospitals. Private hospitals received about 16 percent of the psychotic and 30 percent of the nonpsychotic patients. Figures are not cited for the temporary-care institutions, because some two thirds of their 100,000 admissions during the year were returned to the community with or without a diagnosis of some type of personality disturbance after a period of observation.

More than 44,000 patients were readmitted to permanent-care hospitals in 1945, and some 10,000 were transferred from one hospital to another. Approximately 126,000 patients were discharged, 83 percent as recovered (26%) or improved (57%). Deaths numbered slightly more than 46,000.

The 180 institutions for mental defectives had approximately 138,000 patients on register at the end of 1945, of whom over 119,000 were resident. Some 115,000 were mental defectives and almost 21,000 were epileptic. About 14 percent of the defectives and 12 percent of the epileptics were nonresident. The number of patients actually present in the institutions increased from 99,343 at the end of 1936 to 119,232 at the end of 1945, or by 20 percent. About 95 percent of the cases were in public institutions. Approximately 7,300 patients were discharged, and 2,900 died within the year.

Admissions to these institutions in 1945 numbered slightly over

11,300, which is approximately equal to the average per year for ten years. For an average daily resident-patient population of 113,500, expenditures in round numbers amounted to $43,000,000. The average daily census had increased by about 5,500, or 5 percent, over 1943, while expenditures increased by $7,000,000, or nearly 20 percent.

These statistics are given in some detail to help visualize the magnitude of the problem and certain shifts in provisions for care. Over a ten-year period the number of resident patients in mental hospitals increased by 20 percent, and first admissions per year increased almost 34 percent. The death rate per thousand patients under treatment remained about the same (65–70), though the actual number of deaths was of course greater. It is important that there was a marked increase in the discharge rate, the 126,000 discharges in 1945 being 55 percent greater than in 1936. Expressed in ratio of discharges to 1,000 patients under treatment, the increase was from 147 to 183; in the state hospitals, from 109 to 115.

The admission rate per 100,000 of the general population increased from 82.8 in 1936 to 101.5 in 1945; for state hospitals the rise was from 59.6 to 67.0. The rate of resident patients in all types of hospitals increased from 337.5 per 100,000 of population to 371.1; in the state hospitals, from 284.6 to 344.5.

It is evident, therefore, that the morbidity rate for mental diseases, as measured by admissions to hospitals and the daily average number of resident patients, is increasing at a faster rate than is the general population. On the other hand, the rate for first admissions to institutions for mental defectives and epileptics has been practically stationary at 8–9 per 100,000, except for moderate jumps in years when new facilities become available. The total of resident patients in these institutions, however, does show an increased rate, from 77.6 per 100,000 in 1936 to 85.4 in 1945.

These statistics do not completely cover the public health aspects of mental disturbance, but they make it evident that there is a continuous march of people into and out of the institutions. They also demonstrate that there is a continuous accumulation of chronic cases. Patients actually remain in the hospitals for ten, twenty, and up to fifty or more years. There is no way to arrive at a reliable estimate of the number of people who require hospital care. Many mental disorders develop over a period of years, and there are other factors which make it entirely probable that more than a million people are mentally disabled to such an extent that they really need hospital care. It is certain that at all times there are seriously disturbed people in the community, many of whom are not under treatment of any kind.

Expansion of accommodations or new types of facilities always result in an increase of institutionalized patients. The public has gradually become more accepting of psychiatry and hospital care for the grossly deviate; hence there is less opposition to hospitalizing relatives. That the rate of admission to hospitals has increased faster than the population has grown is often cited as proof that mental disease is on the increase. This is, however, only a presumption, and other factors affecting hospital admissions must be considered. Among them are increased public recognition of mental illness, earlier identification of pathological conditions, more willingness to accept treatment, and improved, larger, more accessible facilities.

Preventive medicine, better prenatal and pediatric care, more efficient control of infectious and contagious diseases, and other life-saving techniques of modern medicine have extended the life span and also prolonged the lives of many into the ages of greatest vulnerability to mental disease. To these factors may be added the increased tempo and complexity of modern life and other causes often adduced to explain the increase in hospital patients.

So far as cases requiring treatment or training in institutions are concerned, state hospitals and training schools care for the great mass of patients (85%) as well as the bulk of readmissions and transfers from other hospitals. Interestingly enough, the admissions to private hospitals are very much higher than would be expected in view of the number of beds available in them. This means that the stay is shorter. The admissions also show a higher rate of patients transferred *to* than *from* other hospitals.

There are other points to be considered, even with regard to hospitalized patients. Patients develop illnesses outside the hospital and may be ill for long periods before hospital care becomes necessary. The same general observation holds true for mental defectives, that is, they first become problems in the home and in the community. Furthermore, there are many more defectives than any institutional program so far developed could care for. It is recognized that stable, high-grade defectives, if properly trained and supervised, make adequate social adjustments within their limitations; hence the importance of "special class" programs in the public schools, with emphasis on motor-manual training. Such training makes it possible for many defectives to be self-maintaining and thereby avoids institutionalization. The cost per pupil is much higher than for regular classes, but is less than the cost of maintenance in an institution. Costs, however, are unimportant in comparison with the benefits to the individual and to the community from programs of this type.

Patients who are discharged from institutions must make some sort of adaptation to the community and may need social service for variable periods. The usual practice is to "parole" patients, most commonly for a year. Many hospitals supervise or follow these patients through extramural clinics during the parole period. While social workers are attached to such clinics, 184 state hospitals in 1945 reported only 410 social workers actually employed, an average of one to approximately 1,050 patients. Twelve states reported no social workers, and only 10 states had more than 10 workers. To say the least, it is difficult to see how one social worker can function for 19,000 patients, as reported from one state. The best ratio found in any state was one worker to 395 patients. The reports available for 1937 and 1945 show considerable increases in the number of social workers employed by state hospitals and in the number of states with 10 or more workers. There was a more favorable average worker-patient ratio in 1945, but the smallest and largest ratios were distinctly worse than they had been in 1937. While it is apparent that progress is being made within hospital organizations, it remains true that social service needs for extramural psychiatric patients must, in general, be provided by community agencies and workers.

The case load of all social agencies invariably includes some psychiatric problems, from serious to mild. It has been estimated that at least a quarter of the cases of social failure present psychiatric problems. This figure is too small when the less marked types of personality deviation are included, as they must be to complete the picture of psychiatric complications in social work.

In addition to the psychotic, the feebleminded, and the epileptic who live within and outside of hospitals and schools, there is a much larger group of mentally disturbed, yet in ordinary parlance they are not regarded as "mental" cases. These are the neurotics (or psychoneurotics), the "nervous invalids," the sufferers from "functional" disorders of heart, stomach, and other organs of the body —the psychosomatic disturbances. In general and special medical practice physicians have reported (in the literature and in personal communications) that from 40 to 70 percent of their patients were in need of psychotherapy in relation to their physical medical problems.

It is estimated that from 10 to 15 percent of our adult population are neurotic, in contrast to approximately .3 percent who are psychotic and perhaps one percent mentally defective. Especially when the neuroses find expression in somatic symptomatology, they may be quite incapacitating. These neurotic patients constitute a great load for social agencies and clinics. All too often they receive little help because the true nature of their problems is not recognized. When this is true, they easily become the especial prey of charlatans and quacks.

Finally, both as a social and a public health problem there is the large group of psychopathic personalities. Some of these abnormal personality types are characterized by antisocial behavior and are recidivist delinquents. In general, psychopaths are troublesome, maladjusted individuals, unstable socially, vocationally, and in personality reactions.

The questions a social worker faces in dealing with the maladjusted individual client are best presented in terms of the nature of psychiatric conditions, their origin or causation, their natural history or course, methods of investigation, and methods of treatment. These points, in the main, make up the content of this volume.

It is unfortunate that there are people who still have resistance to psychiatrists and psychiatric concepts. While this is not true of some sections of the public, resistances do appear in the most unexpected places. For instance, an intelligent woman called my office for an appointment to bring her enuretic son for treatment. She said she had been thinking of bringing him to a psychiatrist for the past five years, but had delayed because she feared something else might be "spoiled" if the enuresis were stopped. In reply to questions during the interview concerning what might be "spoiled," she squirmed uncomfortably and finally blurted out, "Well, he is such a nice boy now." What she actually feared was loss of the dependent, overattached mother-son relationship.

A young married woman who called for an appointment for her thirty-year-old single sister also feared psychiatrists because they might "spoil" something. Further discussion with her brought out the fact that she feared her sister's naïve virginal mind might be corrupted. "You know," she said, "we girls were brought up very refined morally." Still another objection to going to a psychiatrist, as many of my patients put it, is that their friends could understand a broken leg, or a fever, or appendicitis, but they do not see why anyone should need treatment for a psychological conflict or why behavior problems in children should require psychiatric attention. "Will power" and "discipline" should, in their opinion, solve these problems. Despite all the effort expended in the field of mental hygiene education, there is much general ignorance yet to be dispelled. In this area the efforts of social workers are invaluable and should certainly be extended.

Great impetus was given to psychiatry by the fact that so many men were found to be psychoneurotic in the induction examinations and among those discharged in the Second World War. The First World War gave to psychiatry and to psychiatric social work both tremendous stimulation and general recognition. That American draft army was the first in the history of the world to be "screened" by psychiatrists and psychologists. Many men were excluded for neuropsychiatric reasons, but under conditions of combat and even in service not exposed to combat many developed mental conditions necessitating care and treatment. At the end of 1937 Veterans Administration hospitals were caring for approximately 26,000 patients. In that year they admitted nearly 4,500 for the first time. By the end of 1946 these hospitals, now numbering 33, were caring for more than 48,000 patients, and received over 30,000 first admissions that year. The further development of veterans' facilities will tend to alter somewhat the pattern of services in state hospitals, but not the over-all picture of incidence of mental disorders and hospitalization.

In the Second World War there was great emphasis on treatment, especially in the early stages of psychiatric breakdown. No completely new methods were evolved, but several combined procedures were extensively utilized, with generally excellent results. This was particularly true of psychotherapy combined with narcosis or hypnosis and of group-therapy methods. Especial emphasis on various aspects of rehabilitation has developed during the postwar years, along with the marked increase of interest in psychological problems.

DEVELOPMENT OF HOSPITAL CARE FOR MENTAL CASES

Mental disorders were recognized in very early times, and valid ideas concerning these disorders are to be found in some of the earliest medical writing. In fact, Hippocrates used descriptive terms which are still in use. Yet for many centuries these disorders were regarded as in some way manifestations of the supernatural. Persons afflicted mentally were likely to be worshiped or damned, in accordance with the type of demoniacal possession they were supposed to have. While asylums are reported to have been established more than two thousand years ago, special institutions for the mentally sick were developed with comparative slowness, and it was not until the eighteenth century that institutions were widespread. In this country the first institution to receive such cases was the Pennsylvania Hospital, opened in 1752. The first asylum devoted exclusively to mental cases was opened in Williamsburg, Va., in 1773. Until the end of the eighteenth century the mad or insane or lunatics, as they were variously known, were regarded with suspicion and classed with criminals. These unfortunates were confined in dungeons, were chained, whipped, starved, violated, and even put to death. During colonial days in this country many such patients were kept chained in their own homes, as some old New England houses still bear evidence.

Most of the early American asylums were under the direction of a warden or steward, and medical attention was not provided on a continuous basis. Gradually, however, medical superintendence became the rule, so that in 1844 thirteen men formed the "Association of Medical Superintendents of American Institutions for the Insane," functioning today as the American Psychiatric Association. At present practically all institutions for the mentally ill are directed by physicians, usually psychiatrists. In a few states, however, the superintendencies of state hospitals are "political plums," and each changing state administration brings a change in superintendents. Such appointees are rarely psychiatrists. On the other hand, training schools for defectives are frequently headed by nonmedical officers, although early developments in the training of the feebleminded (in France, *ca.* 1800) were due to the efforts of physicians.

What may be called the modern and more strictly medical approach to the problems of treatment for mental disorders dates back only to the end of the eighteenth century. In the 1790's Pinel in France, Tuke in England, and Rush in America were emphasizing "moral treatment" of inmates, that is, the reduction or abolition of restraint and punishment. It must be admitted that this continues to be a problem in hospitals, which, after all, care for the most disturbed cases, often with insufficient personnel.

In the 1840's came the campaign of Dorothea Dix against the abuses she discovered in her visits to jails, almshouses, and asylums throughout the country. Resulting reforms were tremendous, but this is a never-ending problem. The issues are revealed in Clifford Beers' book (*The Mind That Found Itself*), and in his life work, exemplified in the National Committee for Mental Hygiene which was organized in 1909. State care for mental cases was gradually developed, although in some states it is not yet completely accepted and county and city care of chronic cases still obtains.

Institutions for mental diseases, especially the state hospitals, have been under great criticism in the past few years. Intolerable, inhumane, and grotesquely bestial conditions were properly exposed. It seems incredible that such mishandling of mental patients could occur in this country. Nevertheless, there were the facts, a sharp indictment of our society as a whole. As a result of the exposé, public interest was aroused, the National Foundation for Mental Health was formed, and local societies for mental hygiene were stimulated. There was a considerable increase in expenditures for state and receiving hospitals. It remains true, however, that mental hygiene educational efforts must be continuous if we are to secure the necessary citizen participation in keeping hospital and other vital programs at maximum efficiency.

Psychopathic hospitals or institutes are the latest developments in the field of hospital care and their number has rapidly increased during the last few years. They fill a great need in making psychiatric hospital care less formidable and more available to incipient and borderline cases.

It is important for a social worker to know the hospital facilities available in the community and state and what steps are necessary to secure treatment for clients who need hospital care. The social worker must not let any personal qualms stand in the way of securing adequate hospital care for clients.

Up to about 1890 the chief emphasis in the care of the mentally disordered was on the humanitarian aspects—removal from jails and the abandonment of other treatment usually reserved for criminals, the organization of hospitals, the abolition of restraint and punishment. Then came a period characterized by the development of clinically descriptive classifications of mental disorders and intensive laboratory studies, especially of pathological anatomy. In the first decade of the twentieth century these efforts began to be really effective. Great changes in psychiatric theory and practice occurred in the period from 1905 to 1915. It was during this period that more precise laboratory tests came into general use. Examples of diagnostic tools developed at that time are: (1) the Wassermann test for syphilis; (2) examination of the spinal fluid; (3) tests of intelligence. Within this period also were begun: (1) outpatient examination and treatment for psychiatric patients; (2) the addition of social workers to state hospital staffs; (3) the establishment of "psychopathic" hospitals; (4) new methods for treatment of neurosyphilis; (5) greater utilization of psychiatry by social agencies; (6) an almost complete reorganization of diagnostic categories, with emphasis on prognosis (Kraeplin's contribution); (7) the organization of the first state society for mental hygiene followed by the organization of the National Committee; (8) the appearance of psychoanalysis as a method of treatment; (9) the development of other "dynamic" approaches related to controversies over theory and practice of psychoanalysis.

Wide evolution of social psychiatry followed the war of 1914–18. Emphasis in the 1920's and 1930's was especially on work with children, a trend which still continues. In essence, this is a program of preventive therapy, that is, treatment of the present problems is designed to prevent the development of more serious behavior and personality difficulties. The child guidance clinics effectively co-ordinate the efforts of psychiatrist, psychologist, and psychiatric social worker, operating as a clinical team. Special emphasis is laid on the fourfold approach through social, physical, psychological, and psychiatric examinations. This point deserves emphasis, since such an approach is or may be essential to the understanding of all types of psychiatric problem. Such a team approach characterized most of the psychiatric work in the armed services during this last war. It is being continued in Federal and other hospitals and clinics which care for veterans, and has spread to various types of organization which deal with personality problems.

Psychiatry has also been called into industry, into education, and into many other fields unheard of at the turn of this century. At that time psychiatry was for the most part isolated in hospitals; even contact with the medical profession as a whole was comparatively slight, and with general social problems it was almost nonexistent.

Psychiatry has always suffered a dearth of treatment methods. Those which were best developed in the first years of this century were hydrotherapy, occupational therapy, medication, surgery on occasion, and endocrinological approaches. Much depended, and still does depend, on the organized regimen of the hospitals. Psychotherapy, except in terms of persuasion and suggestion, was conspicuous by its absence. Even today the amount of psychotherapy available to hospitalized patients is limited both by the nature of the disorders treated in the hospitals and by the pressures of routine on the medical staff.

Intensive treatment of neurosyphilitic disorders (begun *ca.* 1914) marked the first great advance. Up to that point, general paresis had been resistant to all types of therapy. The early efforts were through the intensive use of the newly developed arsenical drugs. Since the middle 1920's chemotherapy has largely been replaced or supplemented by fever therapy, the fever at first being induced by malaria and later by electrical means. More recently, penicillin has been added to the therapeutic regimen. The results have been startlingly good.

Numerically and in terms of total effects general paresis presents no such problems, human and financial, as does schizophrenia. Methods of treatment for schizophrenia never resulted in much success. In fact, the psychotic reactions of the schizophrenic are such that they may best be regarded as a cure for otherwise insoluble conflicts. However, about 10 to 15 percent of hospitalized cases of schizophrenia made spontaneous *social* recoveries; they were able to leave the hospital and more or less successfully maintain themselves, even though some mental symptoms might still have been present.

The development of methods of insulin, metrazol, and electric shock treatment brought about considerable improvement in the outlook for schizophrenic patients, especially when treatment is begun early in the course of the disease. Similarly in the case of anxious depressions of the involution period, metrazol and electric shock have both proved of great value in shortening the attack and restoring the individual to useful social life.

Types of intensive psychotherapy have been developed chiefly in private practice, in child guidance clinics, a few clinics in general hospitals, and in clinical services related to various social agencies, special schools, and the public educational systems of a few cities. Psychoanalysis, beginning with the second decade of this century, is the best known and most widely used of these techniques, though a number of shorter methods have been evolved. These include "attitude" and "relationship" therapy (especially used by social workers in consultation with psychiatrists), the "individual psychology" of Alfred Adler, and, more recently, what is called "short contact psychotherapy."

It is obvious that the past thirty years represent the period during which there was major emphasis on treatment. The greatest activity ever shown in therapy of all types, both in the mental hospitals and outside them, is going on at present. The essential feature of child guidance therapy is the simultaneous attack upon the problems of both the child and his parents, and this approach has been adapted to other situations. As a result, we find treatment efforts more planfully directed to the milieu of older individuals as well as to the patient's personality disturbance.

Among newer developments are the utilization of play methods in therapy and group therapy of several types for children and parents, for neurotics and psychotics. There is also narcoanalysis, a combination of narcosis by drugs and analysis of the background of symptom formation. Hypnosis has come to the fore again, as it did in the First World War, including a new method for its use, called hypnoanalysis.

The emphasis on psychotherapy alone or in conjunction with other methods is noteworthy. A word of caution is necessary: not all conditions are amenable to psychotherapy. Unless this is borne in mind, some very discouraging waste of effort may result from the improper selection of cases.

Psychiatry, social work, clinical psychology, and other disciplines have, each in its own way, contributed to the evolution of social psychiatry. It has sometimes happened that progress has been impeded by professional jealousy or useless striving for supremacy. The problems are so great that social work and psychiatry each has its particular province and still must pool resources and techniques to deal adequately with many situations. One of the purposes of this book is the promotion of harmonious, progressive collaboration between these two disciplines.

CHAPTER II

THE DATA OF PSYCHIATRY

PSYCHIATRIC STUDY involves securing two major sets of data: (1) those derived from the history (longitudinal section), and (2) those derived from examinations for present signs and symptoms (cross section). It is usual to develop fairly detailed outlines for history taking, mental examination, and so forth. These are essential for training purposes, and help to build an orderly record of maximum usefulness with a minimum of wasted effort in searching records for data. The drawback to their use lies in the tendency to use them rigidly and so produce a stereotyped approach to patients and to recording, which, in the end, becomes sterile. Such a procedure fails completely to give a picture of the patient as a living, functioning individual. Where the work of studying and treating patients is departmentalized, as is necessary in a hospital or a clinic, it is obviously desirable to use various record devices, such as specially printed forms, paper of different colors for different departments, and so forth, and to group similar data together.

In general, professional workers are taught during training to make complete and detailed studies of their cases, so that important but obscure leads will not be missed to the detriment of the understanding and treatment of the client and his problems. Without doubt, this is a valuable and necessary procedure in training, but it must never be allowed to become an end in itself. That is, the object must not be to use methods of observation, examination, and recording according to rule, but to use them so as best to obtain a proper understanding of the problems with which one is confronted.

In social work the most pertinent data, at least those of greatest value in understanding the dynamics of a situation, are derived from interviews with the client. These may be checked in various ways, and there may also be other principal informants. It is important always to remember that in such interviews an outline may be a useful guide, but it is, after all, a guide only to desired information, and not to the ordering of the interview or the sequence of topics.

Record writing procedures vary a great deal. The most useful, from the standpoint of developing orderly processes of thinking about the client and his situation, is to record topically the data secured in an entirely different order by informal procedures. But the outline for recording is not the outline for interviewing; indeed, it is doubtful whether there can ever be a complete outline for interviewing.

Actually, all data required for a complete mental examination can be obtained by observation of the patient's behavior and by securing his own version of his life history, if he can give it, supplemented, of course, by careful questioning regarding specific details. Psychiatric cases vary greatly in spontaneity, continuity of thought processes, ability to verbalize, span of attention, degree of comprehension, emotional stability, and so forth. At one extreme are the mute, inaccessible states of the schizophrenic, the retarded production of the depressed, the disoriented babbling of the delirious, the inaccessibility of coma, and the disjointed mutterings of the deteriorated who are still able to verbalize. At the other extreme are the flight-of-ideas type of production of the hypomanic and the well-connected, pseudo-logical, often profuse, verbalizations of the paranoid. For patients who for any reason are inaccessible to a verbal approach, reliance must be placed upon history obtained from others, observations of behavior, and physical and laboratory examinations.

Perhaps the most important point to bear in mind is the need to be alert to the possible significance of minor variations in the spontaneous production or in the responses to questions. These may give leads for questioning along lines possessing value in differential diagnosis, uncovering the truth from resistive patients, or easing the situation with tense, sensitive ones. The ability to recognize the possible significance of minor changes in tempo, expression, speech, and general behavior is also an important index of skill in interviewing.

The processes of interviewing and recording should be kept entirely separate, even though the interview must provide the material for a complete record according to any outline used. Formal outlines exist to make sure of (*a*) adequate and complete examinations, (*b*) orderly presentation of data, and (*c*) a reasonable interpretation of data in the interests of adequate and differentially correct treatment. If these points are borne in mind, a systematic analysis of the data of psychiatry and their utilization in understanding the client and his problems may be undertaken. This analysis is intended to be suggestive rather than exhaustive, since all hospitals, clinics, and agencies have their own outlines for securing and recording data in accordance with their individual needs.

Two particular considerations influence the nature of the data that are desirable and useful in what is here termed the "social" examination. First, is the general classification of the problems the patient presents; the second relates to the use to which the collected material is to be put. Taken together, these two points may be designated as the frame of reference for history taking, as well as for other examination procedures. The amount and type of information necessary for differential diagnosis of the psychoses will differ from that which is required for determining the cause and degree of feeblemindedness, the cause and extent of disability in the convulsive disorders, or the nature and treatability of a neurotic disorder. Similarly, there will be a difference in the material that is most useful to social agencies, according to their functions. The more obvious the psychiatric disability, the more circumscribed will be the nature of the information needed for differential diagnosis. The questions at issue may be of a more general nature, such as social dependency, delinquency, domestic disharmony, vocational adjustment, rehabilitation, and the like. In such cases, the type of information, the methods used in study, and the manner of recording will necessarily be quite different. The following sections are specifically oriented for psychiatric problems of all types.

DATA FROM THE SOCIAL EXAMINATION

History (Anamnesis)

It is customary to begin the record of the history with data regarding the family. These may be viewed in two ways. First, there are data which illuminate the problems of heredity. In general, it has been found that heredity is not an important factor in mental disease, except in the cyclothymic (manic depressive) psychoses, which do very definitely tend to occur in families, in perhaps one third of the cases of feeblemindedness and in a few relatively uncommon types of familial disorders, of which Huntington's chorea is an example.

Nevertheless, it is important to know the family history at least as far back as the grandparents. The health history, with age and cause of death for those not living, may reveal important factors regarding the biological stability of the family group and so throw some light on that of the client. Since this is especially true regarding chronic diseases, inquiry should be made for any evidence of nervous and mental disease and defect among the immediate ancestors and collaterals. Queries should not be too pointed and should be reserved until a spontaneous account of the family history has been obtained. People are frequently very protective regarding questions which indicate the possibility of mental disorder in themselves or members of their family. A surprising number of people who will vigorously deny having mental trouble of any sort will admit being "nervous" or having a "nervous breakdown." This part of the history should be secured in any terms acceptable to the informant or the client. Usually the informant will offer some explanation for any admitted difficulties. These ideas of the etiology should be recorded and treated seriously at the time, even when they are obviously inadequate or patently absurd.

Longevity in a family may or may not be important. Tendencies to particular types of physical disease may appear in the family, and vary according to ages. Thus, heart disease, arteriosclerosis, several endocrine and metabolic disorders, such as thyroid disturbances and diabetes mellitus, chronic kidney disease, some chronic infections, and various other physical disorders do tend to appear recurrently in families. This does not, of course, mean that these disorders are hereditary in the ordinary sense of that term. There may be a constitutional predisposition to the development of certain diseases, or the conditions of life may be similar, or disease in the mother may unfavorably affect the developing fetus. Thus, *hyper*thyroidism in a mother during pregnancy occasionally produces a *hypo*thyroid condition in the fetus and infant. If the mother is syphilitic and bears a live child, the infant may have congenital, but not hereditary, syphilis.

For our present purpose the social history of the family and its interpersonal relationships is of greater importance than is the medical history. In the social history will be found the details of behavior, social and economic position, living situations, and the interaction of personalities which in combination create the "emotional climate" in which the client was reared. Early environmental influences are, as is well recognized, of great importance in shaping personality, determining the direction of development and the manner in which the instinctive drives are integrated into a smoothly functioning whole. Therefore the history of the immediate family, its organization and status, is very important. The attitudes of the members of the family group toward each other and toward the outside world in all its combinations are of especial significance.

The general status of the family is to be judged by occupation, area of residence, educational level achieved by the various members of the family, income, race, religion, social or cultural standards, records of delinquency, divorce, and the like. Changes in status of family or of individuals in it, especially if sudden or profound, should be carefully studied for their effects upon family relationships. Such changes are sometimes due to the introduction of a transmissible disease, such as syphilis, which affects physical and mental development; alcoholism and various other causative factors may be discovered.

Racial Origin

There are some differences in the types of mental disorder according to racial origin, but the precise significance of these is obscure. The New York State Department of Mental Hygiene in its reports lists seven racial origins and a "mixed" group. These are all the races with over 2 percent each of more than 22,000 first admissions for institutional treatment.

The largest is the "mixed group," representing a trifle more than one fourth of the admissions, followed by Hebrew (13%), Irish (10.5%), Italian (9.5%), African (9%), German (7.7%), Slavonic (5.6%). Six major groups of psychoses are analyzed to show the relationship of race to mental diseases.

1. Senile: Germans and the Irish lead; Africans and Slavs are most infrequently represented.
2. Arteriosclerotic: the same relative standings pertain as in the senile group.
3. General paresis: Africans and Italians lead; Hebrews and Irish are the smallest minority.
4. Alcoholic group: Irish and Africans are most numerous; Italians and Hebrews are least numerous.
5. Cyclothymic (manic depressive): Hebrews, Germans, and "mixed" are most numerous; Slavonic, Irish, and African least frequent.
6. Schizophrenia: Slavs and Hebrews lead; Germans and Irish are least numerous.

If the cyclothymic and schizophrenic groups are combined, the Slavonic, Hebrew, and Italian peoples lead, while "mixed," German, and Irish stand fifth, sixth, and seventh, respectively. Those of mixed descent, although the largest group numerically, stand about halfway between the two extremes with regard to frequency in these several psychoses. Incidentally, it may be noted that the six psychoses analyzed represent approximately 80 percent of first admissions to the state hospitals.

If the admission rates by race for the six types of psychoses given above are compared with the total admission rates in percentages for the same psychoses, certain racial differences are emphasized. This is especially true with regard to the relatively high rate of schizophrenia in patients of Slavonic and Hebrew descent, and the low rate among the Irish; the high rate of general paresis among Africans, and the low rate among Hebrew patients; the high rate of arteriosclerotics and seniles among the Irish, and the low rate among the Slavs; the high alcoholic rate among the Irish, and the low rate among the Hebrews; the low rate of cyclothymics among the Africans, and the somewhat high rate among the Hebrews.

Nativity

The questions of race and of nativity enter into such problems as social and cultural standards, organization of the family, and so forth. A familiar factor here is the conflict which arises between foreign born parents and their standards, and native (U.S.) born children and the standards which interest them.

In New York, which has a large foreign born population (approximately 18 percent for the state and 28 percent for New York City), 34.7 percent of more than 22,000 first admissions to the state hospitals were foreign born. Approximately 60 percent of them were naturalized citizens, and about 85 percent had been living in this country fifteen years or more. The largest group (21%) consisted of persons seventy years of age and over.

As in the case of racial descent, it is not at all clear that being foreign born or native born has any particular influence on (*a*) the incidence of mental disorders that require hospital care, or (*b*) the type of psychosis or other disorder leading to admission to hospitals.

Sex Difference

Some differences according to sex appear to be significant in the incidence of a few of the psychoses. Thus, psychoses due to syphilis and alcohol are much more frequent among males (by 3 and 6 to 1, respectively), and involution and cyclothymic psychoses among females (by 3 and 1.5 to 1, respectively). Incidence of the other psychoses is about equal for males and females. When we consider the psychoneuroses and psychosomatic disorders, which are not covered by hospital statistics, there is a general impression that they occur considerably more frequently in females than in males, but this may be doubted.

It is true that the admission rate for males is disproportionately higher than for females, whether we consider all first admissions or only those with psychosis. Males constituted 58 percent of all first admissions and 55 percent of first admissions with psychosis, although the ratio of males to females fourteen years of age and over in the population as a whole was about 100 to 107 in 1945. However, both discharge and death rates are substantially higher for males, so that patient population at the end of any hospital year is regularly about 52 percent male and 48 percent female.

Age Factor

So far as psychotic conditions are concerned, it has already been indicated that there are some differences in what may be expected according to the ages attained by members of a family group. A few disorders, such as epilepsy, mental deficiency, tics, speech defects, and various organically determined deficiences may appear or be diagnosed for the first time at any age. In the very young (under ten years) who present marked symptoms of a psychiatric disturbance, the chief things to be expected are mental deficiency, organic defect states, and epilepsy. Of the organic defect states the outstanding conditions are: birth injuries, encephalitis, juvenile paresis, meningitis, and other infectious diseases of the nervous system. On the other hand, children in this age range most frequently present problems in social behavior and in personality formation which are not related to any specific type of internal pathology, especially not of the nature of a psychosis. There may have been a specifically pathological milieu, and from the alteration in the stimuli to normal development there may have developed some internalized psychopathology. This in turn may express itself in neurotic symptoms or psychopathic-appearing behavior. Yet it must not be forgotten that in studying an educational problem, for example, there may be actual gross disease processes which represent the essential features to be treated.

Among those over age fifty there is greater likelihood of organic conditions associated with arteriosclerosis and brain tumor, the presenile involution changes, and senile atrophic conditions. Syphilis, alcoholic disorders, and infections may also occur. And, of course, cyclothymic, schizophrenic, neurotic, and psychopathic conditions are also encountered, sometimes being clearly recognized for the first time only at these later ages.

Alcoholic and syphilitic disorders, schizophrenia, cyclothymia, neuroses, and psychopathic states may be recognized at almost any age, but their greatest incidence is in adult life. Similar comments may be made regarding general disease incidence; there are some variations in types according to age. Whatever is learned by the social worker in interviews should be recorded in relation to the ages of the individual members of the family group.

Educational, Vocational, and Economic Status

Aside from the obvious facts of occupation, earning, and educational level attained by the several members of the family, there are important points regarding the way in which these levels have been reached and maintained. In school, for instance, the *ease* with which a given grade level was reached may be of much more significance than is the level itself. It is therefore necessary to ascertain the grade reached and the age of leaving school, together with reasons for leaving. If these points indicate the possibility of special difficulty, it should be tactfully ascertained whether the individual failed to be promoted, which subjects were particularly difficult for him, and which were especially easy, whether there had been conduct problems in school, truancy, special placements, and so on.

Much can be gathered regarding educational and to some extent cultural background from the language of the client, by observation of accent, articulation, vocabulary, literacy, idiomatic phraseology, slurring, elisions, and so forth. Also, there are specific ways in which speech and language may indicate types of mental disorder, as shown in another section.

As regards occupations, it is particularly important to ascertain the type of employment and frequency of and reasons for changes of position. Is the occupation satisfying? And if not, why does the individual stay in it? How was the choice of occupation made, and, particularly, was it a voluntary or enforced choice? How successful is the client?

To a considerable extent the occupation determines the income and thus in many ways determines the individual's opportunities. However, in many instances people do not earn as high an income or achieve as much recognition as is possible in their occupation or profession. The reasons for this may lie in personality maladjustment, even though environmental and extraneous factors may be held responsible for the lack of success. Irregularity of employment or of demands for paid services may be related to personality instability. On the other hand, stability in poorly paid employment or in positions socially unimportant or actually disapproved may be an index of defective personality make-up, such as low-grade intelligence or emotional dependence. However, some apparently simple, routine, unpleasant types of employment are much more remunerative than is commonly thought, and the superior economic return serves to keep some men steadily in them.

The factual data required in recording such information are important in themselves for purposes of identification and determination of needs and the capacity for self-maintenance of the client; but their evaluation from the standpoint of the dynamics of the situation is even more important. They have much to do with revealing the attitudes of the client, his relationships to his family, to himself, and to the world at large.

The material discussed in this section has its greatest value with reference to the client's life and, as such, properly belongs with the personal history. It has been given in detail at this point because of the fact that variations in status within the family do occur, and may be helpful in understanding the patient and his problems. A changing educational, vocational, and economic status in a family group may have a great deal to do with interpersonal relationships, and so influence personality development or general status of the client.

Social Standards (Cultural)

Cultural standards may be understood in terms of the societal, educational, vocational, and economic background of the family (or individual). For this reason it is usually necessary to be familiar with the client's race, nativity, education, occupation, religion, marital status, reputation, social standing, and other items. Again, perhaps the most important point is to ascertain how the client deviates from the accepted standards of family and neighborhood and his attitudes toward family standards and his own deviations. As examples, we may use religion and divorce to illustrate the dynamics involved.

With respect to religion, it is not enough to know the patient's religious affiliation. It is much more important to know his attitudes toward religion in general, his church organization in particular, and to what extent he participates in religious activities. Religious fanaticism must be interpreted, as must denial of religion, apostasy, and other unusual attitudes.

So far as cultural standards are concerned, divorce may be regarded as quite au fait, or it may be considered a delinquency or a definitely forbidden act. It is also important to know the assigned causes for divorce, how culpable the client feels about it, what his attitude is toward the past and the future with relation to the divorce, and what changes are caused by the divorce in relationships to the family and others. In case the client is the child of divorced parents, his attitudes toward each of them, to the divorce, and to the family relationships should be ascertained. The pathological effects of the broken home upon the development of personality and attitudes are well known.

Personal Data

In securing the history it is best to begin with the present illness or difficulty. It is this which has brought the client, or the interested person who refers the client, to the social worker for treatment or service. Once a reasonably clear picture of the present situation is obtained, background data of personal and family history may easily be secured, since their relevance to the origin and development of the immediate difficulties will have become more or less clear to the informant, or to the client if the case is self-referred.

It must be emphasized that at this early stage of investigation the primary issue is to clear up a number of diagnostic points, which will generally vary in accordance with the nature of the problems. In thinking psychiatrically about a problem presented by an adult, we should first consider whether there is some type of gross mental deviation—psychosis, feeblemindedness, or epilepsy. The next thing to be considered is whether we are dealing with a typical form of psychoneurosis, a psychopathic personality, or with a reactive state. Obviously we do not think in watertight compartments or in the exact sequence in which these conditions are mentioned. Nor is there a particular sequence of questions or other examination procedures that must be followed in order to permit a differential diagnostic analysis of the data. On the contrary, all the possibilities listed above must be borne in mind until the clinical picture is clarified by the addition of facts derived from the different fields of examination.

In recording personal history, the usual procedure is to arrange the material in several divisions, namely, developmental, health, school progress, intellectual development, economic and vocational, emotional reactions, and social relations. Present illness or difficulty is customarily described in a separate section.

The record of developmental history is usually limited to the prenatal period and the first two years of life. It includes such items as: any difficulties of the mother during pregnancy; length and severity of labor, use of forceps, evidence of any type of birth injury; age of teething, sitting up, creeping, walking, talking; circumstances of breast and bottle feeding, digestive difficulties, ease of weaning, and age when solid food was first taken; when toilet training was begun and problems connected therewith; when bowel and bladder control were established; when enuresis ceased. Naturally, a more detailed developmental history is sought in the case of children than in the case of adults or older adolescents. Delays or irregularities in the developmental changes are also significant with reference to feeblemindedness in adults and may be important in relation to later neuroses or psychopathic personality. Ordinarily these data cannot be obtained from the client, unless by association in the process of psychoanalysis or because the events were so important that the client had frequently been told of them by his family. Indeed, it may be difficult to obtain much in the way of a developmental history from anyone in the individual's milieu, and in many adult cases this lack is not particularly important.

The health history includes the record of all past illnesses. Detailed inquiry should be made into those which are ordinarily chronic or crippling, with specific questions regarding the allergies, reaction to fever, delirious states from whatever cause, convulsions or spasms, and symptoms of epidemic encephalitis such as lethargic drowsiness, etc. Data regarding onset, course, and outcome of all serious illnesses should be obtained, along with any available information regarding the patient's emotional reactions to the illness and its later effects, if any. Prolonged illnesses in childhood may operate to produce an overdependent attitude or demanding or aggressive or withdrawing social behavior.

The school history includes such items as grade attained, failure to be promoted, skipping grades, quality of achievement, special abilities and disabilities revealed, and behavior problems centered in the school. These give some index of the level of intellectual ability and preparation for work.

The economic and vocational record of types of work, what changes were made in type, frequency, and reasons for such changes, earnings, progress or retrogression in responsibility, and so forth, will indicate the use the individual has made of his capacities and training. It also shows what the adjustment to colleagues and superiors has been.

The emotional inventory has to do with the general temperament, degree of instability and of irritability, temper tantrums, self-control, and such items. One should have a general picture of the temperamental make-up, particularly of any changes which may have occurred either at previous times or in relation to the present difficulties.

Under "social relations" are included all items which indicate how the individual has conducted himself with others. Inquiry should be made regarding his reactions in the family, with children and adults, and in the successive stages of his development. Love affairs, marriage and subsequent relationships and any data on sexual interests and activities should be included here. Evidence of aggressiveness and hostility in social relationships and of timidity and withdrawal should be fully brought out.

Present Illness or Difficulty

The illness should be described in detail, including time of onset, nature of the first manifestations, how they developed, and ways in which the picture is changed. Anything in the external situation which seems to be important either as a remote or a precipitating causative factor must be completely recorded. With regard to the psychoses, environmental situations may have some importance as contributing or precipitating factors, but in general much more weight is usually ascribed to them than is actually justified from what we know of the natural history of the psychoses. However, the earliest sign of a psychosis is generally a change in the social behavior. In fact, treatment is usually not sought until changes in behavior necessitate some action.

Factors in the external situation and the individual's reaction to them are especially important in producing behavior problems and minor personality disorders. Hence the necessity for detailed information about such items in order to understand and interpret them.

A careful history of the present illness and its development is essential for the study and diagnosis of psychosomatic disorders. In many cases with a diagnosis of gastric or duodenal ulcer, spastic colitis, several types of cardiac condition, and certain other organic conditions, a careful history of the nature of specific attacks and the development of the disorder will reveal that emotional factors have played an important part in their production or elaboration. The relationships involved here are discussed in another section.

DATA FROM EXAMINATION OF THE PATIENT

Physical Examination

Two aspects of the physical status of the patient are of immediate concern. The first is what the social worker may observe and record. These observations may be helpful to the physical examiner, who sees the patient at a different time and under different circumstances, to other observers, and to the social worker at another time. The second aspect is the utilization of the report of the physical examination itself, understanding its implications and making sure that recommended special examinations, re-examinations, and treatment procedures are carried out.

The first element in a good physical examination is *inspection*, which, taking into account age, sex, color, and race, by systematic observation seeks to determine any ways in which the individual obviously departs from the normal or the average. Wherever possible, of course, such observations are reduced to exact measurement, such as height, weight, circumference of the head, and various other measurements which may be of importance. Especially with children it is important not to trust too much to "the eye" in estimating that a child is undersized, average, "large for his age," obese, emaciated, or otherwise physically deviant.

In the social work interview it is possible to make these observations and a great many more. Facial expressions, such as the appearance of tenseness, sorrow, dullness, weariness, or, on the contrary, relaxation, elation, brightness, self-confidence, or "openness" may all be noted. It is fair to say that these should not be overinterpreted, but, so far as is possible, they should be reported in terms of what is actually seen. Needless to say, character cannot be read by the physiognomy.

Are the usual facial lines present? Remember that their presence and the depth to which they are marked is to some extent determined by age. Does the patient smile or laugh? If so, at what? Is there weeping; if so, in what connection? Is anger shown; if so, how and about what? Is the "complexion" healthy? If not, in what way does it deviate? When the face is at rest, or the patient speaks, are there tremors or tics?

While for many of these points judgments are based on relative standards and therefore subject to a wide margin of error, nevertheless, noting them as accurately as possible will often be of value in the light of other data.

Is the speech clear? If it is not, what is the nature of the difficulty? Is there stuttering and stammering, lisping, defective enunciation, an accent, mispronunciation, or any other speech problem? Is speech coherent and controlled? Slow or rapid? Is there evidence that when speaking attention wanders, or that the patient goes from topic to topic apparently without being aware of the shift (flight of ideas)? Are irrelevant sounds or sights woven into the talk (distractibility)? Is there a strong urge to talk? Can the conversation be diverted from the topic which occupies the center of the patient's attention? Once started, must all the gory details be given, even though the subject is not especially important (circumstantiality)? To some extent these questions are within the mental field, but that is more or less inevitable when dealing with speech, the most important avenue of expression and communication between people.

How does the patient enter the room? Is there any peculiarity in the gait, such as a limp, straining or twisting of the body or any part of it in locomotion? Are the arms and hands freely used? Are there tremors of hands or fingers? What is the character of the handshake? Is it overeffusive, is the grip free or is it limp—perhaps cold and clammy? In this connection there are other points which more properly belong with the mental examination.

Does the patient flush and pale easily? Does this seem to be related to the topics of the interview, or is it apparently determined from within? Is the patient quiet and at ease, or restless and perhaps very changeable in outward manifestations of mood? Is there a tendency to "doodle," much hand-mouth behavior, or picking at some part of the body?

It will be seen that these are all matters of behavior and activity which can be directly observed in the course of an interview and may be important in understanding the verbal content.

As an example of the ease with which the presence of many disorders can be recognized, the common cold and signs of respiratory infections may be cited. Again, if the neck is exposed so that its base is visible, any fullness which might indicate enlargement of the thyroid gland may be observed. Extreme obesity, emaciation, gigantism and dwarfism are also readily recognizable. All visible defects of teeth or lack of teeth and missing limbs, fingers, or other physical losses should be recorded.

Many disease processes are not observable as obvious and simple disturbances of function. No one has yet seen or heard a headache, a gastric pain, or a spell of dizziness, though changes in expression or posture associated with these may be visible. Hence the need for general and special physical examinations.

The acute infectious processes, with localization primarily elsewhere in the body, may affect the functioning of the nervous system in any or all of three ways. Fever is one of the defensive reactions of the body to infection, such as diphtheria, pneumonia, scarlet fever, and typhoid fever, to mention only a few disorders. Fever, especially if high, may affect mental functioning, with resulting delirium or even coma. People vary in their resistance to fever; some become delirious with only slight elevations of temperature, 101–102 degrees, and later remember nothing (amnesia) about the period of delirium. Others will show no such symptoms until the temperature reaches, let us say, 105–106 degrees. The former have nervous systems that are regarded as thermo-labile, that is, unusually susceptible to inner temperature change, while the latter are thermo-stable. Little is known beyond these facts as to the relationship between instability to temperature change and the development of a psychosis other than a temporary delirium. It is true, as will be discussed later, that some acute physical disturbances may set off a chronic psychotic reaction, but such cases are not very common.

A second way in which mental processes are affected by an acute (nonnervous) infection is that of *toxemia*. It is characteristic of the infections, such as those already mentioned, that poisons are produced at the site of the infection and circulate throughout the body. This may result in a localized paralysis, one of the unfortunate sequelae of diphtheria, or in a generalized toxic reaction in the central nervous system. This may result in delirium or comatose reactions, even in the absence of excessive fever.

The third way in which acute infectious diseases in the body interfere with mental functions is that of direct, though secondary, infection of the meninges and perhaps also the brain, an encephalitis. In such cases, severe typhoid fever and pneumonia being examples, the causative organisms circulating in the blood stream (septicemia) lodge in the brain and its coverings, which then become secondary loci of infection. In addition to the delirium and coma previously mentioned, permanent defects may result because of actual destruction of brain tissue in these cases.

While the central nervous system has a large margin of safety from infection, toxemia, starvation, and other processes which lead to wasting or destruction of bodily tissues, it has no reserve capacity for replacement of its essential elements—the nerve cells —once they are destroyed. Under optimum conditions a healthy nerve cell can replace destroyed processes (the nerve fibers), but there is no reserve supply of partially developed or dormant cells to grow into an area where the cells have been lost. This function of filling in is taken over by the neuroglia, the connective tissue of the nervous system, and scarring (gliosis) with hardening of the area involved is the result.

It should be noted that *severe cases* of the exanthemata (contagious diseases with eruptions on skin and mucous membranes), of which measles, scarlet fever, and smallpox are outstanding examples, are probably always complicated by eruptions in and on the meninges. Both clinical and autopsy experience indicates that in some cases which survive the immediate attack there is permanent damage to the nervous system, with resulting mental dysfunction.

The *chronic* infectious diseases, especially tuberculosis, may show few obvious signs to the observer, but the mental state may be affected in one of several ways. There may be a morbid mood of elation or depression, with or without some vague ideas of persecution. There may be a mild chronic toxic state, or an acute type of paranoid reaction which tends to run a very rapid course and ends in death. Finally, tuberculosis may lodge in the nervous system and produce neurological or mental symptoms, or both. If there is a single tubercle, symptoms of brain tumor may appear, and operation may be successful. But if there is a disseminated meningitis, the prognosis is very poor.

Tuberculosis has a rather high rate of incidence among patients in mental hospitals and is given as the cause of death in 8–10 percent of deaths there. While some rather remarkable theories about organ inferiority and the vegetative nervous system have been propounded to account for this, it seems much more reasonable to account for the relatively high incidence by the type of life the patients perforce lead and the greater chances of infection.

Some cases of endocrine disturbance are recognizable on sight, and in others the physical make-up is often strongly suggestive of imbalance. Acromegaly, due to the development of hyperpituitarism in adult life, hyperthyroidism, hypothyroidism, cretinism (due to early deficiency of thyroid), and obesity of the pituitary type are among the conditions in which inspection alone may establish the diagnosis or arouse enough suspicion to indicate the need for detailed physical examination and laboratory tests.

The major indices which the social worker may use are several. Body build; height, with special reference to the extremes (the dwarf and the giant); weight, especially the extremes of emaciation and marked obesity; any marked disproportions in length of trunk and legs and the comparative size of trunk and extremities should be noted in a few descriptive terms. Only the extremes are at all reliable as indicating underlying pathological states. Even when such states are present, there is often no known treatment, but that is a matter for medical decision. Some of the conditions, for example, the pituitary types of dwarfs and giants, are due to dysfunction of glands during the early developmental period, and the results are frequently irreparable by the time the condition is recognized for what it really is. Furthermore, it is only within comparatively recent years that replacement therapy for deficient secretion has been effectively developed. Thus, thyroid medication, the first to be successfully used, has been in existence for only about sixty years, and the active principle was identified and isolated chemically only some thirty years ago. Pituitrin and adrenalin were brought out between 1895 and 1900, while insulin and the various gonadal hormone preparations were developed in the period 1920–1940. Precision determinations of the rate of metabolism have been clinically possible for only about thirty years. These points are mentioned merely to emphasize the fact that knowledge of the endocrine glands, their function and the measurement of it, and treatment in states of disorder are very recent and that knowledge is still incomplete.

Only in the case of the thyroid gland is there a laboratory test which may be regarded as directly diagnostic. This is the well-known basal metabolism rate (BMR), which is markedly increased in the hyperthyroid states and markedly diminished in the hypothyroid conditions.

A number of other laboratory procedures are important in the differential diagnosis of endocrine dyscrasias. Included among these are x-rays, chemical studies of the blood and other body fluids, tests of functional capacity of several organs or systems, and some anatomical studies. These are highly technical processes, and their description and interpretation is not essential for present purposes.

Replacement therapy can work wonders in conditions for which proper preparations are available and treatment is begun early. This is true in cretinism, myxedema (hypothyroidism in the adult), and hypopituitarism, in which obesity and underdevelopment of the sexual organs may be outstanding signs (hence the name *adiposogenital dystrophy* for this particular type). In ovarian deficiency in the young and during the menopause, supplementary ovarian substance may be of great benefit. Similar results may be obtained with male gonadal substance when genitals fail to develop (eunuchoidism) and in the male climacteric.

In states of overactivity of the thyroid and the pituitary, surgical removal, with or without subsequent replacement therapy, usually offers the most hope. X-ray therapy is sometimes used.

The following brief review of observable physical signs which may lead to positive identification or the suspicion of disorder may be helpful in indicating cases which should be immediately referred to a physician or a clinic for study and treatment.

Thyroid.—Protruding eyeballs, flushing, sweating, fine tremors, visible pulsations, thinness, rapid, forceful heartbeat, and "nervousness" are signs of hyperthyroidism. Thick, waxen, dry skin, dry coarse hair, slowness physically and mentally, and gain in weight are signs of hypothyroidism (myxedema). Goiter occurs in both the hyper- and the hypo-states, as well as in conditions known as "simple goiter," which may produce no other symptoms. The presence of a goiter demands study by a physician. Obesity alone may be a sign. In children, stunted physical growth, marked mental retardation, and some of the signs of myxedema given above for adults, may indicate cretinism (mentally defective dwarf type, with no or very little thyroid gland).

Pituitary.—Acromegaly may develop in giants or in other adults previously of normal stature. The condition is characterized by enlargement of the bones. The hands and feet are large and appear somewhat puffy. The prominences over the eyes become much more marked, the lower jaw elongates and is pushed out forward of the upper jaw (prognathism). Since the bones also become softer, the tendency is for legs and back to become bowed. The nose enlarges, and the nares (nasal openings) seem to become more pronounced. Most of the circus giants show marked signs of acromegaly sooner or later. In the later stages of the disorder the victims are sometimes exhibited as "ape men."

These are all indications of pituitary overactivity. The gland itself may be enlarged, and often this is only evidenced by an x-ray of the head. If the tumor is large enough, however, symptoms of brain tumor with localizing symptoms for the pituitary area may appear.

Gigantism is due to excessive pituitary secretion (growth factor) prior to puberty. If the excess is curbed during the pubertal period, the result may be only an excessive height of, let us say, six feet four or more. In gigantism, not only does the growth in height continue, but there are frequently signs of muscular weakness, defective vision, and other indications that the state is truly pathological.

Gonadal.—Insufficiency of gonadal internal secretion may be suspected (with or without obvious signs of pituitary dysfunction) when the onset of puberty is markedly delayed, when the adult individual shows physical characteristics of the opposite sex, and when the physical signs belonging to the postclimacteric (involutional) period of life appear early. Replacement therapy has made great strides in recent years and is especially valuable for women who are showing disturbances during the menopause.

Excess of gonadal secretion (in most cases apparently due to lesions in some other gland in the chain) is definitely recognizable only in the period of life which is ordinarily prepubertal. In these cases sexual maturation occurs early, and the condition is called *pubertas praecox*. Cases are on record of the occurrence of puberty as early as in the fourth year. In my personal experience the earliest instance of puberty observed in a girl was that of a seven-year-old. She had well-developed breasts, typical distribution of pubic hair, and menstruated. Since the menses usually develop in the period from twelve to fourteen years of age, it is clear that acceleration was marked. One boy, age forty-two months, had a deep voice, a beard, axillary and pubic hair, and adult-sized genitals.

Venereal diseases.—Two issues confront the social worker whose client has a venereal disease. The first is the necessity for adequate treatment and obedience to quarantine regulations (in effect in some areas). The second is the necessity for dealing with the emotional reactions of the infected individual. A social worker may be disturbed by his own reactions to the "immoral" act which resulted in the venereal disease. It must, however, be remembered that many "innocent" infections are acquired through legitimate sexual or other contacts, as when a spouse is infected or in the rare instances when transmission is indirect. In any case, the syphilitic must be treated as a sick person, and the worker should not allow the moral aspect to stand in the way of securing proper treatment for the client.

Use of reports.—Usually reports of physical and laboratory examinations from a clinic or the private physician are sufficiently explicit so that the worker's role in relation to the treatment of any physical disorders is clear. Should this not be true in a specific case, a few questions put to the physician or writer of the report will usually suffice to clear up matters.

Patient's reactions to disease or defect.—To elicit the patient's true reactions may require a great deal of tact. Aside from any shame he may feel because of the nature of his disorder or the way in which it was acquired, there may also be resentment because of the limitations imposed upon him because of the disease or defect, or there may be a mild reactive depression. The patient may over-compensate psychologically and be defiantly overactive or more optimistic than he should be in view of the difficulty. In cases with visible maiming, expressions of sympathy or too-open curiosity on the part of the social worker may be deeply resented by the client. On the other hand, he will also resent indifference which seems callous.

Sensitive patients sometimes show marked tendencies to with-draw from social and other contacts because of their conflict over difference. For such patients the "health classes" operated in many clinics are of great value in reducing the feeling of isolation and uniqueness. This group therapy factor is also of great importance in occupational therapy and in the special or sheltered workshops, which exist chiefly for people with permanent and marked handi-caps, as the blind, for example.

Mental Examination

As already stated, the most satisfactory way to secure a picture of a patient's mental status is to lead him through an account of his past life. Of course, a patient is occasionally so full of his present situation that the past seems to him unimportant. Whatever he tells spontaneously is, naturally, to be noted and made part of the record. Questions may be injected relevant to the spontaneous production which will give a better-rounded picture of the pa-tient's present difficulties. More than in any other type of ex-amination, the attention of the psychiatric worker is focused on the evolution of the situation. So the eternal psychiatric question is— *why?* What is the sequence of events leading up to the present situation, with all its complications, personal and social? In any psychiatric examination or attempt to understand an individual, questioning will inevitably be necessary.

Broadly speaking, there are two major types of psychiatric patient. It must be borne in mind that the approach to the patient varies according to the type into which the case falls. Essentially this division into two groups is in terms of *insight*.

In the first group belong the patients who themselves have enough insight to seek treatment or will accept it when need and opportunity are pointed out. It is true that they often seek treatment for something other than their nuclear difficulties. Since insight may not be perfect and some particular symptom or group of symptoms may be distressingly prominent, the attention of the patient (and often of the doctor) may be distracted, perhaps only temporarily, from the true neurotic conflict. For these patients, formal history taking or formal mental examination is rarely necessary or desirable. The patient is usually loaded with symptoms and history and needs only an opportunity to talk freely and frankly. The mere fact that this is true should not mislead the examiner into closing his mind to possibilities other than the obvious. In fact, it is a good rule in differential psychiatric diagnosis to bear in mind the *most serious* and *least common* possibilities and exclude them first and as soon as possible. Another good rule is that the simplest explanation which covers all the facts is likely, in the long run, to be the best. A third precept is that the simplest treatment procedure which will actually meet the issues presented is by all means to be preferred.

A neurotic-sounding story may, in fact, result from or be a complication of an organic condition; or the reverse may be true. Because enuresis is a common childhood problem, it is sometimes overlooked that it also occurs with nocturnal attacks of epilepsy. Gastric pain and vomiting, especially if occurring at the same time daily with associated emotional stress and strain, may be neurotic in origin, or associated with gastric pathology, or symptomatic of such a crippling neurological disorder as tabes dorsalis.

One problem with many patients in this first group is that they are so full of explanations for their discomforts and symptoms that it is difficult for them to consider other possibilities or to give an adequate account of past and present experiences, especially their emotional reactions and other responses. Yet these reactions are important in understanding and treating the patient's condition. Only such persistent exploration as the unfolding of his story permits will serve to set the patient off on the trail of the origin of the conflicts. In many instances, of course, the patient has actually developed some real understanding of his problems, but has not been able to work them through completely.

In general, difficulties in this first group of cases are of neurotic origin. Some are epileptic, and some are recovered cases of psychoses. Many of them admit "nervousness" or a "nervous breakdown," but will not see it as a mental or even an emotional problem.

In the second group of cases the patients have no insight into either the nature of their illness or the fact that an illness, or even a difference, exists. In this group, patients with somatic delusions will complain bitterly about their symptoms—the heart is missing a beat occasionally, or the circulation has stopped, food does not reach the stomach or is not digested, the bowels are completely stopped up—but they will deny vigorously that there is anything wrong with the mind and the way it functions. The fact that there are no physical signs and symptoms to go with the complaints—no temperature, no pain, no loss of appetite or irregularity of the bowels—makes no impression whatever.

In other cases, without somatic delusions but with many types of psychotic symptoms, the patient is unable or unwilling to admit the presence of any illness or abnormality and emphatically denies mental disturbance of any sort. Even the most extravagant and bizarre ideas or the oddest and most anti-social behavior will be vigorously defended (if the patient verbalizes) as entirely right and proper. Because of these factors, lack of insight with denial of illness or abnormality, such patients must be placed under treatment despite themselves and kept under treatment even against their will and in the face of attempts to escape confinement. Some patients, even with a marked psychosis, may be persuaded to enter mental hospitals voluntarily. After a period of residence in the hospital many patients adjust to the situation and become reliable, trusted, working members of the hospital community. Because of the nature of their illness, there are still other patients who must be constantly watched or kept in semi-seclusion or in bed in the infirmary.

Since it is one of the tenets of American democracy that no one may be deprived of liberty without due process of law, it follows that legal procedures are prescribed in every state and territory for the proper judicial commitment of patients to state and private hospitals for mental disease and epilepsy, to training schools for mental defectives, and to institutions for the criminal insane and for the defective delinquent. These matters are discussed in another section.

In the interview situation the psychotic person may be under no less pressure to talk than is the neurotic, in spite of or even because of his lack of insight. The neurotic, because of inner fears or shame at his "weakness," may be very reserved about revealing his inner thoughts and conflicts. The psychotic, however, because of pressure of thought, generalized overactivity, or reaction to delusions of persecution or grandeur, may be extremely talkative. The great difference will be that the neurotic wants or tries to utilize treatment, advice, interpretations, and other aids offered by the interviewer, while the psychotic neither wants nor is inclined to accept any suggestions, not even for assistance with his own pet projects.

It is characteristic that neurotics have insight in varying degrees, and the psychotic does not. There are certain exceptions to the last statement, since some psychotics do have partial insight in the early stages of evolution of the psychosis. Also, it is an index of recovery from a psychotic attack, notably seen in the manic depressive reactions, that complete insight into the fact of having had a mental disturbance develops. Many such patients will seek help in the clear interval in the effort to forestall another attack. Furthermore, many patients come to recognize the premonitory symptoms of further difficulties and will either go to a physician for help or voluntarily enter a hospital for treatment.

The neurotic and the psychotic may come to the social worker or the psychiatrist of his own accord, or he may be brought by someone else. This is an important factor in determining the approach to the individual. If the client recognizes an inner problem and seeks help, the way is open to institute a treatment regime designed to reach and uproot the basic conflicts. There may be limiting factors in the total picture as it is revealed which make this undesirable or impossible, but there is no barrier in terms of the initial approach. It is the patient's basic recognition of the existence of an illness which makes psychotherapy possible. He may see one or more parts of his illness as the most important, and the therapist may see another. And, of course, the patient may be treated by methods other than psychotherapy without his recognizing the need for treatment of any type.

If the patient is brought to the social worker or the psychiatrist by another person, it may indicate that he does not have insight into his condition and his need for help. Or, and this is commonly true of the "problem" child, he may see very different problems for which he wants help than does the person who brings him. Psychiatrist and social worker in turn may see a central or nuclear problem which is quite different from the problems seen by any of the others involved.

When the patient has no insight into the fact of his illness, it is usually because he has a psychosis. The psychotic is likely to be resistive to any type of examination and to suggestions that he needs treatment or any kind of care. Or he may respond very well to a mental examination, not, of course, labeled as such, perhaps because of a need to share his unusual experiences with someone. Mental defectives very commonly lack insight, as is true of many epileptics. Or if they do have some insight, they minimize the extent or significance of their handicap.

Patients with delusions of grandeur or of persecution will, as a rule, talk freely about their ideas, though they may be secretive about their actual history or about many details of the delusions. The manic patient also talks freely, but the production is rambling and circumlocutory—typically the "flight of ideas," showing marked distractibility, rhyming and "clang" associations. Although these patients start to reply to a question, their attention is diverted by associated ideas or noises and sights, so that not only do they wander away from the original train of thought, but they do not spontaneously return to it.

Cases with senile and arteriosclerotic disorders may be quite garrulous, but the production is often incoherent and displays evidence of the amnesias characteristic of these disturbances. Thus, in senile dementia the amnesia is for recent events, and the memory loss tends gradually to recede farther and farther, so that the patient may literally be living in childhood. In many cases, especially in the early stages, the memory will be found to be reasonably accurate for that part of life which is recalled. A patient in the seventies may claim to be thirty-seven and give the year correctly if the premise of age is granted. So dates of marriage and of birth of children may be correctly stated. At the same time, the patient cannot recall what he had for breakfast, name the place he is in, give the time of day correctly, give month or even the season, date, or day of the week. In other words, there is disorientation for time and place and lack of memory dependent on failure of impressibility for current happenings, as well as a blotting out of recent weeks, months, or years. What is recalled may be circumstantially told with a great wealth of unnecessary detail.

The amnesia of the arteriosclerotic, on the other hand, is usually patchy and circumscribed. It will, in general, have to do with particular periods of time, which represent periods of confusion related to vascular episodes of one sort or another, such as temporary closure of one or more arteries, or a hemorrhage. Or the memory may fail with respect to certain types of experience, or certain classes of objects or symbols.

Logical, coherent verbalization may be slowed or completely inhibited in several types of disorder. In depressive states there is marked initial retardation in speech, and once production is started, it is slow and halting, although the patient gives evidence of a desire to co-operate and do what is required of him. In stupors and in coma speech is absent, although there may be some incoherent muttering. In delirium there may be much or little speech; anything from confused ravings to what seems to be a clear and coherent account of what is going on. In stuporous states, such as occur in the catatonic type of schizophrenia, periods of muteness may alternate with short periods when there is a great deal of repetitive speech, sometimes so confused that the term "word salad" applies very aptly. The speech may be merely a repetition of words the patient hears (echolalia), or it may consist of a monotonous reiteration of a series of words, phrases, or sentences (stereotypy).

When stuporous cases do become accessible, it will ordinarily be found that they do not have amnesia for the period of the stupor. They are aware of their surroundings and reasonably well oriented for time, place, and person. But thinking and feeling during the period are withdrawn into the self (autistic). Characteristically, stuporous patients externalize very little behavior, so they must be fed and cared for as one would tend a baby. Stupors, as here defined, occur in the functional or psychogenic disorders, notably in cyclothymic depressions and in schizophrenia.

In comatose states, on the other hand, there are always organic or toxic causes; consciousness is clouded and then suppressed; if the patient recovers, there will be amnesia for the period of the coma and perhaps for some time before it began.

In certain conditions, of which Korsakow's syndrome, an alcoholic disorder, is an excellent example, there is a fabricating or confabulating amnesia (pseudologia fantastica). In these cases the patient fills in his memory loss with stories made up to suit the occasion. The stories are usually so bizarre that they may be recognized for what they are, fabrications. Also, the story does not progress from day to day as it would if the patient were actually incorporating each day's experience into his consciousness and so into memory. Thus, for weeks on end a patient may say each day that he had just come into the hospital that morning, and repeat the same story of his experiences in getting there that he had told the first morning. Another characteristic of this sort of reaction is that the patient is open to suggestion of topics for his elaboration into a story. A favorite device is to ask if he saw "the bad accident" that morning. Even though he may have been bedridden for weeks, he will usually rise to this bait and tell an elaborate story, with all the gory details.

The whole question of speech production is bound up with factors of attention, perception, association, reasoning, judgment, recall (memory), emotions, intelligence level, the state of psychomotor activity, as well as general and special physical states. Impairment of any one of these or any combination of them may interfere with logical, coherent speech production. It is clear that this occurs in several ways: (1) speech is diminished, retarded, or suppressed; (2) the stream of speech is accelerated, and varies from a coherent train of thought with pathological content of delusions to incoherent or, perhaps, only repetitive jargon; (3) the speech forms may be distorted, as in stuttering and stammering; (4) there is evidence in the speech of distortion in the train of thought. Aside from hyperlogia or logorrhea (flight of ideas), hypologia (paucity), echolalia (repetition of words spoken by others), extravagant romancing (pseudologia fantastica), "word salad," and endless repetition of the same word or phrase (stereotypy or verbigeration), a characteristic type of interference with speech is blocking. This occurs especially in schizophrenics who retain some degree of verbal accessibility. The patient starts to give a relevant answer to a question or starts to make a remark, stops after a longer or shorter speech, and cannot finish the remark. Careful investigation shows that another train of thought intruded and cut off or blocked the thought that was being verbalized. Sometimes the blocking thought can be expressed but sometimes this is not possible.

With respect to speech production, one final caution is necessary. The ability to verbalize freely and easily is not an adequate index of treatability. It is not even a safe index to intelligence level. Volubility is often a defense reaction, and there are morons who have enough facility with words to mislead the uncritical into believing they are extremely bright. The converse is equally true; slow-spoken people of few words may be accessible to psychotherapy and be of superior intelligence. By and large, however, the ability to verbalize easily and fully a controlled, logical, and coherent train of thought does facilitate psychotherapy. Most communication between adults is verbal, though the accessories of speech, such as gestures, smiles, other facial expressions, posture, and the like, are important in the totality of communication.

A mental examination involves not only what the patient says and how he says it, but also observations of his general and specific behavior in the interview setting. For descriptive purposes we may use the customary division of deviations: *hyperkinesis*, generalized overactivity; *hypokinesis*, generalized underactivity; *akinesis*, absence of activity; *parakinesis*, activity having no specific relation to visible or recognizable stimuli, that is, activity beside the point. For all phases of mental activity, a three- or four-fold division holds. For sensation there are: hyperesthesia, hypesthesia, anesthesia, and paresthesia. Similarly for memory: hyperamnesia, amnesia, paramnesia. Many writers use only three divisions: hyper-, a- or an-, and para-. Words made up with these prefixes always mean, respectively: overfunction, under or absent function, and function not clearly related to any stimulus; that is, beside the point or paradoxical.

Psychological Examinations

The first successful and generally applicable scale for the measurement of mental ability was developed in 1905 by the French psychologist Binet and his psychiatrist associate Simon. They were seeking means to determine the presence and extent of mental deficiency, with reference to special educational needs. Their test consisted of a series of problems or tasks, graded in difficulty according to the level of ability of average children for each year of age beginning at three and extending to sixteen. Several aspects of intellectual functioning were examined for each age level, the results being expressed as mental ages. The test was so constructed that it could be administered to people of any chronological age, and the mental age determined by the results.

Goddard translated the Binet-Simon test into English in 1908 and issued the Vineland Revision of the scale in 1911. Since then American genius for mass production has gone all out in the elaboration of bigger and better tests of more and more functions and their application to ever larger numbers of the population. The result is a truly bewildering array of scales of every conceivable type, one or more of which is supposed to measure just about everything a human being may be expected to be or to do. There are manifold tests for intelligence, for special abilities and disabilities, for manual skills, vocational aptitudes, interests, attitudes, personality characteristics, degree of neuroticism, and so forth ad infinitum. The number of tests is now so large that it is doubtful if anyone could even name them all, let alone define, describe, and be proficient in the technique of administration for each one. For example, *The 1940 Mental Measurements Yearbook*, of some five hundred pages, comments on all manner of tests and presents over five hundred test items, many of which contain several entries. Many tests have been developed, flourished for a few years, and then disappeared. Even now, new tests are constantly being promulgated, though very few seem to involve new principles.

Despite the multitude and wide variety of tests and the many functional areas subjected to examination, it is feasible to make some useful classifications by erecting certain natural groupings. This will also help to clarify the functions of mental tests, their relationship to other diagnostic data, their interpretation, certain dangers to be avoided, and other aspects of their use. No attempt will be made to describe the tests in detail or the precise techniques of administration and interpretation. Special training and supervised field work are required to develop the skills that are necessary to avoid errors in technique, to observe adequately the behavior related to test situations, and to interpret correctly both the test results and the associated reactions. Nor is any attempt made to define intelligence or just what it is that is measured in the tests. We all know in a general way what is meant by intelligence, but there seems to be no inclusive definition of the term universally accepted among psychologists. Intelligence test results are composites, based upon estimates of several types of ability. It is generally accepted that intelligence may be tested by the use of verbal symbols, either oral or written, through motor or manipulative skills, and in terms of social competence. Utilization of a battery of several types of test helps greatly in the evaluation of personal potentialities, even though particular tests may have certain limitations.

Within recent years there has been a pronounced change in the use of all forms of tests. Even those whose primary purpose is to give a quantitative rating are now evaluated through the same test data to secure a dynamic picture of personality functioning, which naturally includes intelligence. As an example, a standard intelligence test may yield an IQ of 100 in three different people. One individual might present average intelligence and a normal personality; a second could be a case of organic deterioration, which would be indicated in the responses; while the third might be a schizophrenic, and here again the nature of the test data could indicate the general character of the disturbance. With other types of test, those classed as projective in particular, the major purpose is to reveal personality dynamics. The net result is that the clinical psychologist is no longer so much interested in measurements or psychometrics that lead to some quantified estimate of ability, such as the IQ; instead, he now sees as the chief value of tests their contribution to clinical differentiation and to knowledge of personality structure and functioning.

Tests are given either individually or to groups. Apparently most of the group tests may also be given individually, but the reverse is usually not true. Experiments have been made to adapt the Rorschach and some other individual tests for group administration. In evaluating the report of results, the first need is to know whether it was a group or an individual test. In the individual test, valuable observations regarding the behavior of the client in the test situation may be made, but this is not possible with the usual group procedure.

Psychometric results are usually scored in one of two ways. The original Binet method was in terms of mental age, stated in years and months, but most tests result in a point score which represents the number of questions or problems that are correctly answered, or the number correct minus the number wrong. In some instances the answers are weighted, ten points for one, five for another, and so forth. In many scales the points are converted by means of a standardized table into equivalent mental ages, and the IQ is calculated in the usual fashion. In other instances, tables are erected which assign an IQ according to the chronological age and the point score. In connection with these variations in methods of scoring and interpretation, there are many technical questions concerning which psychologists are not completely in agreement. What is here said regarding the use and interpretation of tests is based solely upon practical clinical considerations.

The significance of a point score or a mental age derived from a test will vary in accordance with the actual or chronological age of the person being tested. For instance, the mental age may be ten, and the individual making this score might be five or ten or twenty years chronologically. The first individual would be extremely superior, the second average, and the third feebleminded, according to the ratings given below. In the early use of tests the results were expressed in terms of the number of years of retardation or acceleration in mental age. This form of calculating was confusing and cumbersome and led to a great deal of disagreement concerning interpretation of, for instance, what constituted a rating of feeblemindedness.

Accordingly, when Terman developed the Stanford revision of the Binet-Simon test in 1916, he proposed the calculation of an intelligence quotient, the now familiar IQ, which expresses mathematically the relationship between chronological age and mental age. The formula is $\frac{MA}{CA}$ in months, and the result is expressed in whole numbers, which really represent percentages. For example, if the mental age is 120 months and the chronological age 120 months, the quotient is 1.00, or 100 percent. After chronological age sixteen in the original scale, and from age fifteen in the last revisions (Forms L and M, published in 1937), these ages are used as divisors without reference to the actual age of the person being tested. It may be added that this difference in divisors, plus some changes in the upper end of the scales, have made a difference in the highest IQ an adult can obtain. In the first Stanford revision this was IQ 122, but on the later forms it is 152, a point that serves to emphasize the need to know which test has been used when quoting an IQ.

This formula, fixing age fifteen or sixteen (it is fourteen in some other scales) as the upper limit for the divisor, is based on findings which indicate that there is no demonstrable, or perhaps mensurable, increase in native intelligence above these ages. At best, the increments are so small that tests of sufficient refinement to reveal them adequately have not yet been devised. As a practical matter, we know that the accumulation of knowledge and the assimilation of experience continue beyond these ages. There are scales for testing adults, and some tests at adult levels are included in the Stanford revisions. The most comprehensive scale is the Wechsler-Bellevue Adult Intelligence Scale, devised by David Wechsler. This is a point scale and is scored for three IQ's: verbal, nonverbal or performance, and full scale. The last IQ is secured by combining the results of the first two. The scale is extensively used for adolescents and for adults of all ages.

Mental testing was given tremendous impetus by the First World War. Two group scales were devised for testing the men called in the craft. The Army Alpha involves, as do most intelligence tests in the upper ranges of chronological age, the ability to read and write; it is essentially a pencil-and-paper test. Since the Army had to test illiterates and those with general and specific reading disabilities, the Army Beta was developed, a performance test involving auditory directions and manual manipulations. These two were the first group tests used on a large scale. Revisions were popular for a number of years, but are rarely used today.

A variety of group intelligence tests are available, chiefly of the pencil-and-paper type, and time-limited either for the total test or for each section. A number of these are for use in schools, and some, such as the Otis, the Henmon-Nelson, and the Pintner-Cunningham, are standardized in three groups according to the educational level of the pupils. Such tests are especially arranged so that they can be administered by teachers and scored according to standard tables. Appraisals of this type do not measure intelligence in any strict sense, nor do they provide data which indicate the presence of interfering emotional or physical factors. They do yield scores which correlate very well with academic achievement and provide a quick method for determining which children require individual tests. It is common practice to give individual examinations to children who make unusually low or high ratings on the group tests. In scoring, equivalent mental ages and intelligence quotients are derived from tables calculated in relation to the point scores; therefore the IQ's do not have the same values as those established through individual test measures.

To evaluate intelligence test results and their meaning in a particular case, it is clearly necessary to know which tests have been used. The bare results are often entered in school and other records without noting which test was used, with the possibility of giving a false impression as to the validity of the entry. Tests differ in make-up and in the essential nature of what is being tested; they differ in scoring and in the value of scores, in standardization, and in the type of mathematical computations to which the scores may be subjected. Strictly speaking, an IQ is directly obtainable only from the 1916 Stanford revision of the Binet-Simon, or from the 1937 Terman-Merrill revision. For the other tests, conversion tables are necessary, and accessory mathematical calculations must be worked out. These and some other points may be clarified by a brief comparison of the Stanford-Binet and Wechsler-Bellevue scales.

The Stanford-Binet consists of six items, each with a value of two months, for every test year. The tasks are presented consecutively and those which are successfully accomplished are added together. The result is the mental age by years and months; the intelligence quotient is then calculated, as previously noted. In actual administration, a basal year is established, the earliest year in which all items are passed. The examination is continued until a year is reached in which all items are failed, or until the tests are exhausted. The spread between the basal and the highest test years is called the scatter. In a reliable or regular test the scatter is usually small, not more than four or five years. In an irregular test, with wide scatter, some tasks may be accomplished and some failed even through the highest test year, although the basal year may be fairly low. The greater the scatter, the greater the evidence of irregularities in mental functioning because of interfering factors other than those of intellectual ability *per se*.

The Wechsler-Bellevue, on the other hand, does not produce a mental age, but is a point scale composed of five verbal and five performance test groups, and a vocabulary range. The sum of the items passed in each subgroup gives the raw scores, which are converted through tables into weighted scores. Summation of the weighted scores provides the data for the verbal IQ and the performance IQ; total IQ is secured by adding the two weighted scores. In all instances, the IQ's are taken from tables which are statistically derived as to what is normal for certain age groups in relation to their general status. The vocabulary range is used independently and serves as a check on the other test items. This test takes into account the slowing down of intellectual processes as age advances, that is, the lessening of ability to acquire and associate new experiences and the speed of so doing.

The Stanford is best standardized for children of school age up to about age fifteen; the Wechsler for adolescents and adults. Both have a mixture of varied verbal and performance items, differently grouped; both were standardized on white people only. Definite patterns for many psychoses and neuroses are revealed by the Wechsler-Bellevue. The Stanford-Binet also yields material for inferences regarding organic defects, reading disability, and other factors which interfere with securing a valid test result. Each test, used with appropriate age groups, yields information both as to intelligence levels and certain factors which may be interfering with adequate utilization of intelligence, or indicative of a deteriorating process. These basic tests of intelligence give clues for special testing which may be urgently needed to evaluate abilities and disabilities and their relationship to the functioning of the personality as a whole.

Mental tests may be grouped in another way; in this instance, according to what is being tested. There are three major classes from this viewpoint: tests of general intelligence, of performance ability, and of educational achievement. In ordinary practice, when it is desirable to do any testing at all, it is essential to give tests from each of these three groups. There are also many special purpose tests, among them projective tests such as the Rorschach, the Thematic Apperception Test (TAT), Bender's Visual Motor Gestalt, The Mosaic Test, and fable completion. Several examinations have been devised to reveal the extent and nature of special abilities and disabilities, such as specific reading defects, musical talent, and vocational aptitudes. Finally, there are numerous neurotic, behavior, and other types of personality inventories of varied significance and applicability. A well-rounded examination may require the use of one or several special tests.

It has sometimes been stated that the major purpose of mental testing is to recognize the mentally defective. This, I hold, is an error. It is true that the first large developments in mental testing were in relation to early detection of the feebleminded and the arrangement of special programs for them. But it must be emphasized that the intelligence test level is only one of a number of factors to be considered in arriving at a diagnosis of feeblemindedness.

There are many factors which may interfere with an adequate rating, so that it appears to be lower than it actually is. For example, a specific reading disability, emotional disturbances, or developmental handicaps related to such situations as having been reared in an infant's home may operate to lower the results of the test and fail to give a valid rating. The widespread use of testing has resulted in much greater usefulness than merely to indicate who is feebleminded.

As a matter of fact, tests of general intelligence have their greatest value in the correlation they present with academic educability. Speaking in terms of averages, it requires a mental age of six to learn to read; or, in terms of intelligence quotients, it requires a superior rating to be successful in college, and of high average to make a good record in high school. Children develop unevenly, and the IQ tends to be stable provided there are no unusual inhibiting factors in the test situation and the results on each successive test are reliable. Superiority of intelligence level tends to show up early, as do inferiority and average development, but there is one point to be remembered here. The IQ *is* a quotient, the tests have limits beyond which scores cannot advance, and the divisor finally becomes stable. It follows that the highest IQ which an adult can secure on the usual individual test is limited by these factors. High mental ages may be attained very early, and young children can and do score IQ's as high as 200, although such cases are rare. On the other hand, there are children who develop at a slower rate and may not reach their maximum IQ until the teens.

Actually, the tests were developed in terms of the binomial theory of distribution. According to this theory, any mensurable attribute of the human being will be so distributed in terms of magnitude that half of the cases will present measurements falling within a certain range, while one quarter will present measurements below this average range, and one quarter will have larger measurements. What this means in the case of the distribution of the results of intelligence testing is that there is standardization in terms of IQ. Thus, the average group includes IQ 90–110 in one classification, or 85–115 in another. IQ's 70–90 or 65–85 are rated as borderline or inferior; those with IQ below 70 or 65 are classed as feebleminded, while those with IQ 110 or 115 to 125 or 130 are rated superior. An IQ above 130 is rated as very superior or exceptionally superior. In a perfect curve of distribution 25 percent of cases would be in the inferior (about 22%) and very inferior (3%), 50 percent would fall in the average group, divided into low average, average, and high average, and 25 percent would be superior (22%) and very superior (3%). Actually, even in large samplings it does not usually happen that the curve of distribution is quite so perfect as this; there is usually some skewing of the curve, related to imperfections in the tests or to special factors in the group tested.

Many writers use terms other than those here presented to designate intelligence levels. Thus, "subnormal" is used as equivalent to inferior; "dull normal" refers to borderline or low average; "normal" is used in place of average; "supernormal" refers to superior and very superior. There are two chief objections to the use of the word normal in this connection. Normal as applied to human qualities has many qualitative connotations and distinctly implies the absence of defect or disease. Also, normal does not so exactly indicate the variations in levels of intelligence as does average, especially since these differences are expressed mathematically. Average and its variations below and above can be defined and delimited according to calculated formulae, while it is quite impossible to define normal in any such manner. For these and other reasons the classification of intelligence levels in terms of averages is preferred.

It was stated above that superior intelligence is required to be successful in college, and high average intelligence to make a good record in high school. It is true, however, that some students succeed in high school or college despite the fact that their intelligence level is below that which is ordinarily required. In such cases factors of interest, drive, and persistence compensate for the inadequate intelligence level. As an example, it took one student nine years to graduate from a professional school despite his hard work and great interest, whereas students of adequate intelligence completed this work in six years. Careful testing revealed his IQ to be 95. It is of interest that this particular student became suspicious of his own situation and requested the testing. He then utilized the test results to guide him in his further professional career.

The occurrence of discrepancies between intelligence level and educational success or failure emphasizes the necessity for testing performance skills and educational achievement, as well as general intelligence. There are a number of types of performance tests, of which the Seguin and Ferguson Form Boards, Healy Picture Completion, Porteus Maze, Kohs Block Design, and Stenquist Mechanical Assembly tests are typical examples. Grace Arthur and Pintner-Patterson have standardized scales for several age groups. While it is generally true that performance tests tend to give the same sort of rating—superior, average, inferior—as the subject obtains on tests of general intelligence, there are frequently significant differences in details. Thus, a person may score very superior on a test of general intelligence and only superior or high average on performance tests. Those with a rating of feeblemindedness on a general intelligence test will ordinarily rate inferior on performance tests, or possibly as high as average. We do not commonly find a superior rating on performance tests if the general intelligence test result is markedly inferior. If marked discrepancies are found, it is necessary to test for special disabilities, particularly in reading, since the presence of certain specific deficiencies will artificially lower the result of a general intelligence test.

The performance tests may give valuable clues concerning not only further educational possibilities but also vocational fitness. Many specialized tests of vocational aptitudes have been developed and are of value in special cases. These, however, are ordinarily not sufficiently detailed to do more than indicate certain broad categories of vocations into which a given individual may fit.

With regard to school children, educational achievement tests will show what use has been made of the intelligence, how well grounded youngsters are in fundamentals, and how adequately the school grade placement matches both the mental age and the educational achievements.

Discrepancies in test results of general intelligence, performance skills, and of educational achievements naturally lead to further analysis of individual test results, correlation with other data, and supplementary testing. It may be found that school grade placement is substantially above or below that indicated by intelligence or educational achievement tests. Some reasons why achievement test results may be above or below those to be expected on the basis of the general intelligence tests have already been advanced. Other factors which may be in operation are personality disturbances, physical difficulties, and conflicts centering in relationships with the teacher, companions, or in the home.

If the discrepancies are stable and not due to emotional or environmental factors, their evaluation leads to practical recommendations regarding further educational procedures and vocational training or placement. A major mental hygiene problem often occurs in this connection, since many parents and others find it difficult to accept the idea of training for or placement in a mechanical job. They are intent on preparation for college or a "white collar" job, without regard to the individual's potentialities and particular interests.

Many tests have been designed to reveal aspects of personality other than the functions of intelligence. For example, the Porteus Maze reveals character traits such as impulsiveness, lack of concentration, and inability to profit by experience. The test results correlate well with social adaptability, more so than with intelligence alone. Personality inventory, neurotic index, vocational interest, and other tests already mentioned are widely used in special studies, but most of them have not become part of psychometric routines. Special combinations of tests are used to estimate certain aspects of personality; an example is social maturity, expressed as a social quotient in the Vineland Scale. Several attempts have been made to develop measurements of emotional maturity to be stated as an emotional quotient, without particular success to date.

Outstanding examples of personality tests in use at present are the Rorschach and the Thematic Apperception Tests. Both are of the projective type; that is, the personality is revealed by the projections of the person being tested. In the Rorschach the subject is asked to tell what he sees in each of ten cards bearing ink blots, half of which are black and white, the rest in color. The answers represent the person's subjective, projected, emotionally-tinged reactions. The technique of administration is comparatively simple, but the scoring and interpretation are time-consuming and intricate. Even more than other tests, the Rorschach requires expert handling. Best standardized for adults, its interpretation for children must be tentative. It is extremely useful in differential psychiatric diagnosis, especially in questionable cases of schizophrenia, manic depressive psychosis, psychopathic personality, and neurosis. One important value is the help the test gives in determining the potential effectiveness of treatment.

In the Thematic Apperception Test twenty pictures of dramatic scenes are shown to the patient. He is asked to relate a story about each one, give his idea of what is occurring, how it developed, and what the end result will be. The patient's identifications and rejections, feelings of frustration, and a variety of tensions which are likely to be revealed may be very helpful in psychotherapy.

Two other tests, Bender's Visual Motor Gestalt and the Goodenough free drawings require brief mention. The motor gestalt test is carried out by offering the patient cards containing nine patterns to copy. There is no time limit and the cards are not removed until the figures are reproduced. Proper administration of the test requires extensive clinical experience. It appears to be of special value in exploring retardation, organic brain defect states, and regression. It is an excellent complementary test when used with the Rorschach.

In the Goodenough test, the individual is asked to draw a man.

Evaluation of the drawings has been standardized so that a mental age may be assigned. Leads into personality dynamics usually appear, which may be explored by asking for a story about the man. The general usefulness and significance of the test has been increased by asking for a separate drawing of a woman. Overt or latent aggressiveness, submissiveness, fears, doubts, and other mechanisms may be clearly revealed.

One precaution to be observed in the use of projective tests, judging by reports that come to me in the regular course of my clinical practice, is to guard against overinterpretation of the test results. Frequently the interpretations made, when compared with other data in the case, seem to be highly impressionistic and without valid foundation even in the test material itself. Such overinterpretations may have serious results if they are erroneously offered as proof of a diagnosis of grave disorder which is not, in fact, present. There are marked differences in the reactions of children and adults to many of these tests, and interpretations cannot be carried over with impunity from one age group to the other.

It is important to remember for *all* tests that they must be weighted and interpreted in the light of all the other facts in the case. No one's fate should be determined by the results of a single test or even by any combination of tests. Absurdly enough, the fate of many a child has been settled by a few points in IQ. In fact, there has been a tendency to determine which children should have special educational programs by an arbitrary separation according to IQ. Children with IQ 70 and under are, often by state law, eligible for special class placement in public schools; those with IQ 71 and over are not so eligible. Granted that it is necessary to draw the line somewhere, any such ruling as this is too hard and fast; it presumes an infallibility which does not exist. There is an irreducible margin of variability in the tests, such that the IQ should be written 100 ± 6 or even 100 ± 10, and the margin of error is even greater in group than in individual tests. In addition, the possible error is greatly increased if the test is administered by an unskilled person—a teacher, perhaps, who may have had some sort of elementary course in testing. There are many factors which may interfere with securing a correct rating, especially emotional difficulties related to the test itself or generalized pre-existing disturbances carried over into the test situation. Fortunately, there is likely to be internal evidence of most types of interference with test results. All well-trained psychologists are alert to factors that interfere with an adequate rating and include such observations in their reports.

An especially important source of interference in attempting to secure a valid test result is the issue of foreign birth, or being reared in a bilingual home where a language other than English is the first acquired. In part, the difficulties are due to the fact that the tests are standardized on native born, English-speaking children. To a considerable extent, however, the lowering of test scores is attributable to problems inherent in the language handicap. To meet this situation adequately there would need to be a recasting of the curve of distribution, possibly for each language group, with new IQ limits for the inferior, average, and superior groups. There are elements, of which this may be one, which have led certain writers to claim that average intelligence should be rated somewhere between IQ 85–100 instead of 100.

A number of personality disturbances interfere with adequate testing and so produce an artificially lowered result. This is true, for example, of the psychoses, hysteria, and epilepsy, which usually present a wide scatter on the tests. Organic brain disease, blocking, depression, dementia and amnesia, absorption in neurotic conflicts, distraction of attention, irritability, and many other symptoms can interfere. It may even occur that a person simulates co-operation, while inwardly determined not to permit a true picture of his abilities to be revealed by the tests. In one interesting situation of this kind, a girl of twelve deliberately tried to lower her score, but gave herself away when she could not control her reaction to the challenge of more difficult tests of exactly the type she had missed in simpler form. One who is trained only in the mechanics of testing may assign the same significance to two IQ's of 60, whereas a trained psychologist, by analyzing the scatter and qualitative variations in test responses, may easily demonstrate that in one case the IQ reveals mental deficiency, and in the other, definite signs of organic or other disease that has nothing to do with primary defect.

It has already been indicated that the value of particular tests varies with the age of the individual being tested. This point can best be elucidated by noting some of the tests most commonly employed with different age groups. For infants under two, the most widely used test is probably the Gesell scale of diagnostic developmental levels. The Cattell test has recently come into use for the same age level and has the advantage of yielding an IQ. These tests are also useful for ages two to six, but the Merrill-Palmer, Minnesota Pre-school, Kuhlman-Anderson, and Stanford-Binet are more valuable. Toward the end of this age period, reading-readiness tests and the Vineland Social Maturity Scale provide information regarding preparedness for entering school.

From age six through fourteen, the Stanford-Binet is the most widely used, although the Kuhlman-Anderson and Wechsler-Bellevue are also employed. The Arthur point scale of performance tests is advantageous. The Stanford achievement tests are perhaps the most used of the several tests of this type. Special diagnostic tests for reading and arithmetic are also available, those for reading being especially important.

The Wechsler-Bellevue is the only satisfactory intelligence test for adults, and is one of the most valuable for the teen age group, though psychologists vary in their preferences for tests at this age level. Some rely on the last revision of the Stanford-Binet, occasionally in combination with the Army Alpha or Beta; others use the Wechsler-Bellevue; while a few psychologists rely on the Army Alpha for general indications as to more specific testing. Vocational tests, aptitude and interest tests, and personality inventories are especially useful for adolescents and adults. The results from one type of test cannot ordinarily be directly translated into the terms used to express the results from another type.

To sum up, adequate psychological testing requires the use of properly standardized tests best suited for the age and education of the individual. While no formal routine and sequence of tests is advisable, the psychometric examination must include tests of general intelligence, performance abilities, and educational achievements. Special tests for personality make-up, vocational adjustment, and special disabilities are frequently necessary. Discrepancies in results call for further testing, social study, psychiatric evaluation, or all three. Test results are utilized both quantitatively and for understanding personality dynamics. The measurement function of mental testing is valuable chiefly with reference to academic educability and vocational placement. In determining the diagnosis of feeblemindedness, mental test results constitute only one item among many required for an adequate evaluation of the person. The presence of mental deficiency may be correctly established without a psychological rating in many cases, but the diagnosis may not safely be based on the results of a single mental test without evaluation of other factors. On the other hand, the finer delimitation of educational possibilities is not possible without adequate testing.

CHAPTER III

SPECIFIC ETIOLOGICAL FACTORS

ABOUT ONE HALF of the psychoses * have definite and demonstrable
pathology in the nervous system, or in other areas of the body, or
in both. The same can be said of at least one half the cases of mental
deficiency. Associated with the pathological findings are definite
causative or etiological factors. In some instances these etiological
agents are infectious organisms, as in syphilis. Toxic substances
introduced from without (the exogenous poisons) or elaborated in
the body (the endogenous toxins) commonly from infections in
organs other than the nervous system, also produce neurological
and psychiatric difficulties. Metabolic disorders, disturbances of
endocrine gland functioning, vitamin deficiences, senile atrophy,
cerebral arteriosclerosis, and some acute and chronic organic
diseases of the nervous system may be the essential etiological
agents in the production of a psychosis.

From the standpoint of clinical psychiatry these organic and
toxic psychoses and defect states are extremely important, both
because of the number of patients involved and because of the
types of treatment required. Such cases particularly require medical
and surgical treatment, rather than psychotherapy, social supervision, or other forms of therapy. Many of these cases are chronic
and irremediable; others are acute and recoverable with proper
treatment. Some of the diseases and intoxications are distinctly pre-
ventable; in many, however, prevention would be possible only in
terms of the psychology of the individual. This is true, for example, of the alcoholic psychoses. These do not develop under
conditions over which the individual has no control as do the senile

* Cf. discussion of definitions and groupings of mental disturbances on p. 107.

and other conditions, and personal psychology must be taken into account in preventive efforts.

Syphilis

This disease, caused by a microscopic pathogenic parasite, is highly contagious in certain stages and not at all in others. It is transmitted almost entirely through direct personal contact. Occasionally it is transmitted through some intermediate object, such as an eating or drinking utensil, pipe or cigarette, or, extremely rarely, a toilet seat. For such indirect transmission to occur, however, it is necessary that the interval between contact of the infected individuals with the intermediary object be short and the infected object still be moist. *Treponema pallidum,* the infecting organism, is fragile and loses its infecting capacity rapidly with changes of temperature and moisture.

So long as syphilis is thought of only as a "social" disease and the result of sexual indiscretion, its treatment and particularly its prevention present many complicated problems in public attitudes regarding morals. Viewed strictly as a public health problem, there has long been sufficient information available, if freely utilized, to stamp out syphilis in a comparatively short time, at least in countries as advanced as ours.

It should be borne in mind that a large proportion of infections are "innocent," even many of those acquired in a sexual relationship. Thus, every infection of a connubial partner by the mate through sexual intercourse must be so classed. All cases of congenital syphilis are innocent; even though the child is illegitimate. Infection of doctors, dentists, and nurses does occur in the course of professional activities despite precautions, and occasionally other people also acquire accidental infections. Nevertheless, there is a definite social stigma attached to having or acquiring syphilis, at least among large groups of our people.

Among those who adhere to these standards there is considerable emotional reaction to such infection, innocent or otherwise, characterized by guilt, anxiety, and depression. The fear of infection appears to affect the "morals" of many individuals, acting as a deterrent to sexual experimentation. Sometimes this fear is erected into a phobia which has the general psychodynamics of any phobia and must be treated in the same way.

Many people, however, have no such reaction and accept syphilis merely as a hazard of life. Some disregard this hazard to a considerable extent, with the attitude that the acquisition of the several venereal diseases is to be expected. Not infrequently one is told by the ignorant and uninformed person that it is better to have syphilis than it is to have gonorrhoea, since syphilis may be had only once, while many attacks of gonorrhoea can be experienced. The same person is likely to say of syphilis that the cure is worse than the disease, and consequently can be kept under treatment only with the greatest difficulty, if at all. Furthermore, as will be shown, the late effects of the disease are so different from the early ones that the patient frequently does not connect a neuropsychiatric disorder with syphilis. In fact, until the advent of accurate laboratory tests the total extent of the ravages of late syphilis were not completely known, and the diagnosis could be and often was missed.

For our purpose it is only necessary to state that the disease has an incubation period of three to six weeks and that there is a sufficiently orderly sequence of symptoms so that the disease is descriptively divided into three stages; frequently there is added a fourth, commonly called meta- or para-syphilis.

Primary syphilis is the stage in which the initial lesion (chancre) occurs. While this lesion most commonly appears on the genitals, it may appear anywhere on the body. There is a distinct predilection for moist surfaces, such as the mucous membranes of the mouth and lips. Usually it is assumed that there must be a preexisting break in the tegumentary structure. Thus, finger infections occur in the area of a "hangnail," a cut, or an abrasion.

The chancre has distinctive characteristics, being typically a hard, painless, ulcerated lesion. It may be small, concealed, and overlooked. Associated with it is a painless swelling of the lymph nodes draining the area in which the chancre is located. These swellings are quite different from the painful, red, tender swelling which occurs with an ordinary pyogenic or pus-producing infection.

After an interval, usually several weeks, the *secondary* stage occurs. At this time a skin eruption develops, grayish white patches appear in the mouth, there is generalized painless enlargement of the lymph nodes, the nervous system may be and apparently usually is invaded, and heart and large blood vessels may be affected. The extent of the eruption and severity of symptoms in this stage vary greatly. There is little doubt that in some cases where infection is discovered only with the advent of symptoms of late syphilis, the patient passed through both the primary and the secondary stages without being aware of them. In other cases the "great pox" is extremely severe and may even cause death. There are historical records of great epidemics with high mortality rates. The introduction of syphilis and other contagious diseases less serious with us, such as measles and scarlet fever, into a population not previously exposed in any way results in very florid diseases with extremely high death rates.

In the usual course of events, signs of the secondary stage disappear. There is often no particular evidence of any effect on the patient's health, and there may be no further signs or symptoms for years. Then, in the typical case with insufficient treatment or none, the *tertiary* stage develops. The characteristic lesion of this stage is the gumma, a tumorous, destructive, necrotic growth which may occur in the skin, bones, brain, heart, or any organ. The surface lesions are indolent and unresponsive to any form of treatment except antisyphilitic. In this stage, an apoplectic stroke or some other sudden episodic phenomenon may result fatally.

Syphilis is apparently less frequent now than it was twenty-five years ago. When the Wassermann reaction came into general use as a routine measure in examining all hospital admissions, around 1910–1912, in both general and mental hospitals about 16 percent of positive reactions in the blood were found. This did not mean the presence of neurosyphilis in everyone admitted to mental hospitals, and positive reactions were found in practically all types of psychotic cases. The incidence of syphilis in the population at large was then believed to be about 5 or 6 percent. The much more accurate figures of the present day indicate an incidence of about 1 to 2 percent, and it appears that the incidence among mental cases, as measured by positive tests, is also somewhat less. There has been some decrease in the percentage of cases of neurosyphilis among first admissions to state hospitals. In many cases neurosyphilis can only be proven with certainty by spinal fluid tests. In other words, a positive Wassermann in the blood merely proves the existence of systemic syphilis, which may or may not be producing symptoms of somatic disease. It sometimes occurs that spinal fluid tests are positive and the blood Wassermann is negative. It must also be borne in mind that laboratory syphilis, or neurosyphilis, does not tell the full story of the disease process in the patient; to do so requires clinical study. The following situations may therefore occur: (1) clinical signs of active syphilis, with negative blood Wassermann (primary stage; some tertiary and quarternary cases; some cases of congenital syphilis); (2) positive blood Wassermann, with no clinical signs of systemic disease or neurosyphilis (a few cases are "Wassermann fast"—i.e., no amount of treatment seems to bring about a negative reaction); (3) positive blood Wassermann, spinal fluid tests negative, with or without clinical signs and symptoms of neurosyphilis; (4) negative blood Wassermann, spinal fluid tests positive, with or without clinical signs and symptoms of neurosyphilis; (5) all tests positive —usually with clinical signs and symptoms of syphilis of the nervous system.

It is known that invasion of the nervous system, as judged by spinal fluid tests, may occur long in advance of the appearance of clinical signs and symptoms of neurosyphilis. On the other hand, stormy symptoms of sudden invasion of the nervous system may occur in the secondary stage.

In addition to syphilophobia and the depressive guilt reactions already mentioned, syphilis produces various clinical syndromes when it invades the nervous system, including the meninges. Acute and fulminating pictures may occur when the invasion occurs in the secondary stage, or there may be few or no symptoms.

Only a comparatively small percentage of syphilitics—some 10–15 percent—develop clinical neurosyphilis of any type. In the largest number of cases this occurs only several years after the infection, often from ten to twenty years later. There may have been no clinical signs or symptoms of syphilis of any type in the interim. Usually during this interval the cases are not infectious, though there is evidence that the spirochete may be ejaculated with the semen and thus infect a fertilized ovum and the mother as well. However, it was because of the long asymptomatic period between infection and the development of such clinical pictures as general paresis, tabes dorsalis, and primary optic atrophy that there was much debate over an extended period of time as to the syphilitic nature of these disorders. In addition to this long latent period was the fact that these quaternary cases did not yield to the usual types of antisyphilitic treatment, contrary to the rule for tertiary syphilis, which yielded readily to mercury and iodides.

There is good reason to doubt that syphilis was ever completely cured until the recent use of penicillin. Treatment was a matter of months or years and the most that might have been claimed was that the disease was rendered inactive. It is true that syphilitic men and women had healthy, nonsyphilitic children. On the other hand, men and women equally symptom-free had syphilitic off-spring. The more remote the time of infection, the more likely it is that the child will not have congenital syphilis.

When patients became free from symptoms, it was difficult to persuade many of them to continue treatment, which was inconvenient, sometimes painful, and expensive. For these reasons, among others, the rapid treatment methods and new preparations now in use are of great importance. Of even greater importance are measures to prevent infection, since no methods have yet been devised to halt illicit sexual relationships and prostitution. This involves both individual precautions and social measures. The inclusion of the venereal diseases in the list of reportable, communicable diseases has brought their control within the police power of the public health authorities. This means that all infectious cases may be forced, if necessary, to have treatment in quarantine. The Army and the Navy reduced the venereal disease rate very sharply by the use of prophylactic measures. Abstinence from illicit sexual relationships would, of course, be the best preventive, but no moral or religious or other code has yet been able to accomplish this.

Finally, it is believed that one reason why syphilis (as well as some other contagious diseases) is so much milder now in its manifestations in western European stocks than it was in the fifteenth and sixteenth centuries is that the race has acquired a limited immunity in the course of generations. A theory of this nature has also been offered to explain the fact that quaternary neurosyphilis develops in a small percentage of syphilitics. That is, immunity elsewhere in the body is greater than it is in the nervous system, which then becomes the host, though a long period is required for the organisms to become really active.

Alcohol, Drugs, and Other Exogenous Poisons

Among these etiological factors, alcohol holds first place. Because it is readily available, its use is the most widespread. It is worth noting that in many groups in which alcoholic liquors are forbidden for religious or ritualistic reasons, some other drug may be used which has the characteristic of producing states of exhilaration. Opium and its derivatives, hashish, betel, mescal, cocoa leaves, marijuana, and other stimulant preparations are used by rather large populations which eschew liquor of all types. Some religions, as do the Mormons, class coffee and tea with liquors and drugs and ban them.

Groups which habitually use alcohol may or may not also use habit-forming drugs which have serious consequences for the individual. The commonest drugs of this type in this country have been the opium derivatives, heroin and morphine in particular, cocaine, bromides, to a lesser extent hashish, and latterly marijuana.

Barbiturate habituation, sometimes with marked personality disturbances, has become a problem in recent years. Not many years ago all cigarettes or cigarette papers were popularly supposed to be "doped," and this presumably explained the "evil habit."

By the development of drugs which achieve the desired effect, but are not habit forming, and by restrictive legislation the use of the more harmful drugs to the extent of addiction has been reduced. This has in turn increased smuggling and illicit sale of drugs, although there has always been traffic of this sort because of large profits, availability of supplies, social disapproval, and other factors.

Aside from alcohol and some of the heavy metals which occasionally cause neuropsychiatric disorders, the drugs which produce addiction are those which relieve pain or produce sleep or both. A variety of euphoric, grandiose, and semi- or completely hallucinatory states have been described as the characteristic mental states induced by these drugs. Sleep, often comatose in character, follows, and on awakening there is likely to be some confusion, dullness, tremor, and other signs of a "hangover." These symptoms are most easily relieved by more of the same drug, and thus a vicious circle is set up. Deterioration and a variety of serious mental symptoms eventually occur in some cases. Tolerance to these drugs tends to be built up fairly easily, so that larger and larger doses are required as time passes. Food habits are disturbed, and symptoms now recognized as vitamin and mineral deficiencies are common.

Laws now require many somnifacient and analgesic drugs to be labeled "Warning—may be habit forming." Since it is indisputable that they are habit forming, many physicians are reluctant to prescribe sedatives except in extreme cases and then only for short periods under rigorous control. It is astonishingly easy for what should be normal bodily rhythms, such as appetite, sleep, and excretions to become altered so that an artificial corrective is necessary to keep them functioning. As a result, tonics, sedatives, and laxatives are widely used for self-medication. Fortunately, although they are habit forming in the broad sense of the term, resulting disturbances are usually limited and do not as a rule produce particular effects on the personality as a whole. The sedatives are the most likely to cause disturbances of personality, even to the extent of psychoses. It has been truly said that it is not so much their use as their abuse that causes trouble. It is believed, with considerable justification, that abuse of these drugs is usually related to an underlying instability of the personality. Certainly millions of people use sedatives and analgesics of all types, from aspirin and bromoseltzer to codeine, heroin, and morphine, without disturbance in personal or social functioning. The number of drug addicts is unknown, but it is known that they appear only rarely in mental hospitals and do not constitute a large proportion of private psychiatric patients. One estimate places the number of addicts in this country at 100,000.

In many cases habituation and addiction follow legitimate use in physical diseases or to relieve excessive fatigue resulting in insomnia, loss of appetite, depression, and other symptoms. Availability of drugs has also been asserted to be the cause of addiction among doctors and nurses.

Drug addiction, especially to the opium series and cocaine, is credited with bringing about the degradation and deterioration of large cultural groups. The use of opium by the Chinese is usually cited in support of this. It is certain that drug addiction does bring about deterioration and blunting of moral and social sensibilities. When deprived of the drug, an addict often resorts to crime to obtain supplies. In the euphoric phases, crime may seem to the addict to be negligible at the moment.

With regard to alcohol, the evidence again seems to be that abuse rather than use creates the greatest problem. Its manufacture presents no difficulties, since fermentation is a natural and universal phenomenon, requiring only some type of carbohydrate and wild or cultivated yeast.

The alcoholic habits of different cultural groups vary widely. So far, no particular personality factors have been demonstrated to account for these variations. They were probably accidentally determined in the beginning and have gradually evolved into social customs. It has been noted that tribes of "primitives" show particularly marked reactions to alcohol and tend to develop violent thirsts. In animal experiments it has been shown that the continuous use of alcohol results at first in the procreation of monsters and affects the birth rate. But as succeeding generations are alcoholized, abnormalities disappear and offspring are apparently not affected. There would seem, therefore, to be some sort of biological habituation in the course of generations, and this probably also applies to man, at least to some degree.

Drinking and drinking habits constitute important social, economic, and psychological issues for which no large-scale solution has yet been found. The general psychology of drinking may be expressed by the concept of escape. Small quantities of alcohol relax tension, release some inhibitions, and promote a feeling of well-being. Quantities large enough to produce a state of intoxication will produce overactivity, such as volubility, boisterousness, and lack of ordinary social restraint. Eventually inco-ordination of thought processes, of speech, and of motor activity develops. Such stages will be followed by coma, light or deep according to the amount imbibed.

In states of intoxication basic personality patterns may be revealed which are ordinarily obscured by inhibiting or compensating mechanisms. Activity may continue and even seem to be fairly normal, yet there may be amnesia after sleeping it off. Or inco-ordination may appear early, with or without subsequent amnesia. Belligerence, depression, paranoid trends, phobias, doubts, and other reactions often occur.

The greatest problem, however, is that of habitual drinking to excess, or chronic alcoholism. Here, again, all sorts of explanations have been advanced, but the problem is still imperfectly understood. Several types of habitual drinking are distinguishable, such as social drinking, spree, and chronic drinking. Particularly with regard to the spree drinker and the chronic alcoholic, emotional conflicts and instability have been assigned as causes. That is to say, unresolved neurotic conflicts and defective personality structure are regarded as underlying factors. Secondary effects on personality occur, which in turn tend to intensify the drinking. Extreme cases show a tremendous degree of dilapidation of personal and social behavior, the so-called Bowery bum being a typical example. To what extent allergy to alcohol or vitamin deficiency enter into the increased need for alcohol and into its effects, partly from direct toxic action and partly from secondary toxins elaborated in the body, it is difficult to say. Alcohol is one of several drugs which are fat soluble and combine with the lipoids of the nerve cells and other visceral cells. The metabolism of the nerve cells is thereby disturbed, and the ordinary psychological patterns are likewise upset. Much research on the many questions involving alcoholism has been promoted in the last few years, and in time both therapy and prevention will be greatly benefited.

Aside from pathological intoxication and the mental disturbances of acute intoxication, the psychotic pictures, to be discussed later, occur only in chronic alcoholics. By comparison with the sum total of misery caused by chronic alcoholism, the number of mental cases is comparatively small. A great deal of minor and major crime and sexual irregularity, inasmuch as alcohol is to some extent an aphrodisiac, may be accounted for by acute or chronic drinking.

The other exogenous poisons require only brief mention. At one time arsenic, especially that form of chronic poisoning colloquially called arsenic eating, seems to have been fairly important in causing neuropsychiatric disorders. Such cases are practically unknown in this country today. Lead poisoning, with a variety of signs of neurological disorder and mental deterioration, does still occur occasionally, usually as an occupational disease. In babies and young children it is due to chewing the paint off toys, cribs, and other articles. Improved industrial methods and changes in paint formulas have greatly reduced these risks. Many other toxic substances are used in industrial processes and may produce neuropsychiatric disorders unless adequate precautions are taken to protect the workers.

Endogenous Toxins

Here we are primarily concerned with infectious diseases focalized in other parts of the body, but affecting the nervous system through toxins elaborated in the body's fight against the disease. Also, the effects of fever (hyperpyrexia) and some direct, though secondary, infections of the nervous system must be considered.

Any acute infection may produce disturbances in psychic functioning, either because of the fever or the circulating toxins. Diphtheria, scarlet fever, measles, influenza, pneumonia, typhoid fever, osteomyelitis, and tuberculosis are examples of common infectious diseases which may produce such effects. Typically the patient is afflicted by delirium, which may be followed by coma and occasionally by convulsions. In cases which recover, the delirium clears up, followed by complete or partial amnesia.

In addition to the toxemia, there is sometimes direct infection of the meninges, meningitis, or the brain, encephalitis. Any infectious disease, including tuberculosis and gonorrhoea, may give rise to a meningitis or a meningoencephalitis. These cases are likely to be more serious in symptomatology and outlook, and general recovery may leave some permanent defects in neurological or psychological functioning, or both. The disturbances in psychic functioning are most commonly in the intellectual field; at least the signs of disturbance are most obvious in these functions.

In severe cases of measles and scarlet fever there is also a meningeal eruption, which in turn may leave permanent scarring. Rare cases are seen in which a carefully taken history reveals a stoppage of mental development following an experience with these diseases. In some infections of the uterus following childbirth, a secondary focus of widespread infection of the brain, with death or subsequent mental crippling, may result.

While the problems here are medical, it is clear that the severity of a past disease process and evidence of invasion of the nervous system are important in assessing the present status of those who survive the illness. It is always necessary to ascertain whether there was delirium or coma, the individual's usual reaction to fever, and whether changes in personality were noted after recovery. The effects of fever may even be seen in some people with very mild infections, such as the common cold.

Mild to severe depressions may occur with fever or in the course of an acute infection. More difficult are the depression and lassitude which follow disorders such as influenza, often persisting for several weeks. Such reactions have been observed in people who otherwise showed no indications of a depressive or cyclothymic temperament. Presumably such states are related to the length of time required to bring the nerve cells back to full functioning after relatively severe disturbances.

This brings up the point that pathological processes in the nervous system, of any origin, such as toxic, infectious, circulatory, or mechanical, may be classified as reversible or irreversible. Whether a given process is reversible depends upon such factors as severity, length of time of action, degree of oxygen deprivation, (anoxia) extent of interference with cellular metabolism, and degree of toxicity for the nerve cells. For example, some poisons have a selective affinity for nerve cells and are quickly absorbed and fixed in the cell, causing quick cell death by an irreversible process. Nerve-cell death in turn may bring about death of the whole organism because of the cessation of bodily functions controlled by the affected nerve cells. Other poisons and toxins have a lesser affinity for nerve cells and are not fixated, but pass through the nerve cell, impairing cellular metabolism and function during this passage.

If the toxic action is not too prolonged or destructive effects on the nerve cells are not too great, the damage may be only temporary and the cells eventually return to full function. This, however, is a slow process in many cases. It has been shown that in some diseases producing reversible degenerative changes it requires at least three months for restoration of cells to normal functioning and normal microscopic appearance.

Congestion, edema, and other pressure-producing changes occur in many infectious and toxic disorders of the nervous system. They produce an excess of symptoms, that is, even in many nonreversible processes leading to cell death and permanent impairment of function there are acute and reversible effects which subside as the congestion and edema recede. Accordingly, many symptoms disappear as recovery, even if only partial, takes place.

The nervous system has a rather large margin of safety between the first effects of agents producing organic change and the final stage of cell destruction. This safety margin or factor is of great importance with reference to reversibility. Its significance is emphasized by the fact that once a nerve cell is dead it is not replaced, which is not true of all body organs. There is evidence that functions of one brain area may be taken over to some extent by another, but this is not universal. Furthermore, the nervous system has considerable biological resistance to disease and starvation. These points are of importance in determining the effects upon the nervous system and psychic functioning of past and present physical illnesses.

Metabolic Disturbances

Such metabolic disturbances as diabetes, chronic nephritis, malnutrition, and starvation produce changes in the nervous system and in psychic functioning. The characteristic clinical pictures are delirium and coma. The physiological mechanisms vary. In diabetes the effects are due to acidosis. With insulin treatment serious states of acidosis are much less frequent than they formerly were. In chronic nephritis the effects are due to the retention of products of protein metabolism, complicated by the accompanying elevation in blood pressure. Malnutrition and starvation produce their effects through lowered nutrition, and in all probability secondary toxins are elaborated because of the altered metabolism. These effects are reversible, unless, of course, the malnutrition is severe enough to cause death.

Mild malnutrition in childhood may possibly produce some

permanent effects in mental functioning, but this has not as yet been proved. Adults who fast over a long period report states of ecstasy, visions, vivid dreams, and often a sense of separation of soul and body. If carried far enough, an exhaustion psychosis may occur. With prompt treatment these cases are usually recoverable, though many end in death.

Endocrine Disorders

Thyroid disorders have definite effects on mental functioning. The chief clinical pictures are the excitability and instability associated with hyperthyroidism, the sluggishness and depression of myxedema, due to hypothyroidism in adults, and the physical and mental stunting produced by hypothyroidism in children, the condition called cretinism. As already noted, if cretins are recognized early and appropriately treated, they may recover approximately normal status; otherwise they are usually to be found in training schools for mental defectives. Myxedema cases must frequently be committed as psychotic, but hyperthyroid cases only rarely develop psychoses.

Hypothyroid conditions have become less frequent in mental hospitals during recent years. This is due to greater precision in diagnosis of the level of thyroid functioning and the increased availability of effective thyroid preparations. Determination of the basal metabolic rate gives accurate evidence of dysfunction and permits replacement therapy in the hypothyroid states at an early stage. Treatment can then be controlled in accordance with the metabolic rate.

Pituitary dysfunction results chiefly in physical symptoms and, as a rule, psychological effects are secondary. Overactivity of the anterior lobe of the pituitary before puberty produces gigantism, sometimes associated with sterility due to hypogonadism. Overactivity of the same lobe occurring in adult life produces acromegaly. If the pituitary becomes much enlarged, symptoms of brain tumor may appear. Lethargy, apathy, and childlike moods have been described as characteristic personality traits in hyperpituitary cases. A fairly frequent association of both hyper- and hypopituitarism with feeblemindedness has also been described. However, the precise nature of the relationship involved here is unclear, since there is no universal syndrome. By far the largest group of dyspituitary cases are not feebleminded, and, contrariwise, the majority of the feebleminded do not show pituitary dysfunction clinically or anatomical pituitary pathology at autopsy.

Hypopituitarism may be manifested in dwarfism or in adiposogenital dystrophy. The appetite is usually enormous, and sugar tolerance is high. Such cases are usually described as being indolent and submissive. It should be noted, however, that many children presenting fairly characteristic physical signs of this type of pituitary deficiency are distinctly aggressive in behavior, usually as a compensation for their feelings of difference and for frustrating experiences.

Occasionally psychotic features appear in individuals suffering from pituitary disorder. Aside from those symptoms which may be ascribed to pressure from tumor formation, I know of no psychotic picture which may be regarded as typical of pituitary dysfunction. Paranoid states occur, but present no specific features attributable to the pituitary disturbance.

Disorders of the gonads produce varied physical and mental symptoms. It is perhaps only necessary to mention hermaphroditism, eunuchoid states, and the reversal of secondary sexual characteristics to show the implications.

It must be remembered that, biologically speaking, the human being is bisexual. Despite marked differences in the two sexes, the reproductive system of both male and female are developed from an embryonic tissue mass which in the beginning reveals no indications of the direction which sexual differentiation will take. In the fully developed male and female there are vestiges of the organs of the opposite sex. Furthermore, the internal secretion of the gonads contains both male and female hormones. Obviously the amount of hormone belonging to the opposite sex is very small, if normal sexual functioning is to occur. With respect to both development and function, the pituitary, adrenal, pineal, and to some extent the thymus glands, play roles which are not as yet completely understood. These roles, especially those of the several types of pituitary secretion, are apparently particularly marked in the female with reference to the functions of menstruation, pregnancy, and lactation.

In pubertas praecox an adult libido may be found at very early ages, when judgment and emotional control are still infantile. Such children are aggressively and extensively interested in sex, and usually have large and freely utilized sexual and profane vocabularies. In the very early cases, pathology of the pineal or adrenal glands is most likely to be the causative factor. In the female, the ovary is sometimes the primary source.

Medical literature is sprinkled with cases of precocious puberty. As might be expected, the number of instances increases as the age is approached at which puberty is normally to be expected. In this country, ages are approximately thirteen to fifteen for girls and fourteen to sixteen for boys. As the more normal or average time is neared, there is less disturbance in social relations and the child becomes better equipped emotionally to deal with the changes.

Cases of pubertas praecox demand careful attention from endocrinologists, psychiatrists, educators, and social workers, particularly those children who are two or more years precocious. Their social grouping, social supervision, resolution of conflict about difference, and correction of pathological states (if any) in the endocrine system are very important. Fortunately, acceleration tends to occur in all directions, though not to an equal degree in all.

At the other side of the picture is hypogonadism, frequently secondary to hypopituitarism. In these conditions puberty is delayed beyond the usual upper limit. In boys the testicles may be undescended and the penis small. Girls may show some signs of developing secondary sexual characteristics, yet the menses may be considerably delayed. In many such cases the usual prepubertal spurt in growth is also late in developing. Such delays of a year or two beyond the upper age when puberty usually occurs may have great emotional significance for the youngster and cause serious dislocations in the social situation and relationships, yet the delay may have no great physical significance or serious physical consequences.

Many studies have shown variations in the age of onset of menstruation (the most clearly defined evidence of puberty in girls) according to geographical distribution. The relationship between climate and the appearance of menstruation is by no means clear. Some observations indicate that succeeding generations born and reared in the United States acquire the pattern of menstrual onset characteristic of its population rather than maintaining that of the climatic area from which the forebears came. It has also been noted that even the first generation offspring of immigrants from a number of European areas are distinctly larger and sturdier than their parents, and this may indicate differences in functioning which may also involve gonadal maturation. It is also true that children of the present generation tend to be larger and healthier than their parents, even though many generations of ancestors may have lived in this country.

Deficiency Diseases (Avitaminoses)

In relationship to psychiatric problems these disorders have been the subject of increasing study as more vitamins have been isolated and their functions in normal and abnormal processes have become more clearly understood. The first conditions clearly recognized as having to do with the diet, either some unknown deficiency or some unknown toxic agent * (the concept of vitamins came much later) were: scurvy, relieved and prevented by using citrus fruits and juices; beri-beri, a form of polyneuritis found by experiment to be due to the extensive use of polished rice in the diet, relieved

* Osler, in 1913, classed pellagra and beri-beri with the intoxications; scurvy and rickets with disorders of metabolism. In each case, however, he indicated the possibility of "defect of certain unknown elements of food" and quoted extensively from the studies showing the influence of polished rice in producing beri-beri.

or prevented by using whole grain rice; rickets, now known to be due to vitamin deficiency, though originally ascribed to many other causes; and pellagra, which formerly occurred fairly frequently in mental hospitals, now shown to be related to deficiencies in the B complex. For several types of neuroses and occasionally for the psychoses it is now common practice to use vitamins, especially the B complex, in large quantities. They are often used in association with endocrine therapy. While this is often done on a purely empirical basis, it is known that the vitamin deficiencies do play a part in the production of various disorders of the nervous system, in intensifying the effects of alcoholism, and in other ways. Correction of deficiencies, therefore, may be important in laying a foundation for other therapy. Vitamin A has been shown to play a special role with respect to vision, especially the reinforcement of night vision.

Acute and Chronic Organic Nervous Affections

There are a number of acute and chronic diseases of the nervous system which play an important part in the production of personality deviations, including the psychoses. Two of these, poliomyelitis and epidemic or lethargic encephalitis, are infectious diseases, though the specific organisms have not been isolated.

Poliomyelitis, as the name implies, is chiefly an affection of the gray matter of the spinal cord. It involves primarily the region (anterior horns) where the motor cells are, and its paralytic effects are due to destruction of these cells. The early paralysis is always greater than the residual, which may be very slight or nonexistent. If parts of the brain are involved, the condition is usually called polioencephalitis, and the result may be death from paralysis of respiration, or if the patient survives, there may be cessation of intellectual growth and a retention of childish impulses and emotional reactions. Many patients show marked feelings of difference and compensatory behavior in reaction to the peripheral crippling.

Epidemic encephalitis is, again, what the name implies—an inflammation of the gray matter of the brain occurring chiefly in epidemics. As such, the disease was first clearly recognized and described when it appeared in epidemic proportions, originally in Europe and then in this country, following the great pandemic of influenza in 1917–1918. A number of smaller epidemics and many sporadic cases have occurred since then. Two major types of psychological reaction have been described. These may or may not be associated with the characteristic tremors and other signs of paralysis agitans, an organic neurological disorder and a frequent sequel to encephalitis of this type.

The first type of reaction is particularly common in children. There is evidence of a cessation of mental growth and considerable disturbance in behavior occurs. Responses are to the highest degree impulsive and uncontrolled. They tend to be total and not in any way graded according to the strength of stimulus. Violent temper outbursts occur. Delinquency is frequent. Treatment, except in a closed psychiatrically oriented environment, is usually unsuccessful. Several states have established special wards in one or more state hospitals for the treatment of such patients.

Psychotic reactions, usually depressions or paranoid states, occur in adults, but not regularly, and it cannot be said that there is a particular psychotic reaction type. Paralysis agitans as a neurological disorder not known to be related to epidemic encephalitis, has been recognized for many years. Some intellectual deterioration has been noted in advanced cases of long duration, but there is no special psychosis.

Brain tumors occur only in a very small percentage of cases in mental hospitals. The mental picture depends upon the localization of the tumor. Frontal lobe tumors especially affect the intellectual functions. Tumors may be associated with focal epilepsy and with several types of affective disturbance.

Head trauma also is not a frequent cause of psychotic reactions leading to admission to mental hospitals. Skull fracture, cortical laceration, hemorrhages, and scarring in cerebral tissue can and do produce changes in psychological functioning. In one type there are fairly specific personality changes, called post-traumatic constitution. Deterioration sometimes follows trauma, and in some cases an epileptic reaction ensues. There may, of course, be many focal signs, depending on the particular areas involved.

Degenerative disorders include a number of diseases of the nervous system of unknown etiology, and when the brain is involved, psychotic symptoms appear. As types, paralysis agitans and Huntington's chorea may be mentioned. The latter is also a familial disease and involves the appearance of both marked choreiform movements and mental deterioration at ages thirty-five to forty-five.

Arteriosclerosis, involving the arteries of the brain, has become one of the commoner causes of psychoses and of admissions to mental hospitals. Temporary and permanent closure of large or small arteries, occurrence of large and small hemorrhages, reduction of oxygen supply brought about by lessening of the arterial bed and thickening of vessel walls, all operate to produce symptoms. Massive hemorrhage usually results quickly in death. The initial symptoms, involving both intellect and emotions, are usually episodic, occurring as periods of confusion and disorientation, unconsciousness, overactivity, or depression. There may be good recovery from several such episodes, but sooner or later grave deterioration or death results. In many cases a paralytic stroke is physically incapacitating, but the mental faculties may remain relatively clear and unimpaired. Such paralytic strokes are not necessarily due to cerebral arteriosclerosis. Especially is this true in younger people in whom such accidents result from emboli (i.e., pieces of blood clot broken off from some other area, such as a heart valve, or following a surgical operation) lodging in a small vessel in the brain. Or the embolus may be of air or fat, especially in the case of severe accidents.

Senile changes are general, consisting of atrophy and, in the case of bones, rarefaction. Such atrophy is not uniform, and in cases in which the atrophy is especially marked in the brain, senile deterioration results. In typical cases there is no vascular disorder. In fact, there is no clear evidence of the cause of the atrophy aside from the changes of old age. It must be remembered, however, that old people may have psychoses other than senile dementia. Some people live to extreme old age without showing such deterioration; in other cases, fairly characteristic senile symptoms occur considerably earlier than the age at which they might be expected.

Aside from the pathological etiological factors mentioned above, the psychiatrist is confronted with numerous cases in which no etiology of a physical or physico-chemical nature has been demonstrated, despite a great deal of research. Personality disorders, the neuroses, schizophrenia, and the manic depressive psychoses are all disorders of unknown etiology in this sense. The neuroses most clearly demonstrate a psychic, or better stated, a psycho-social genesis. Such an origin is least clear in the schizophrenias, which may be due to the relative inaccessibility of these cases. Involution melancholia is an example of a type of disorder in which both physiological and psychological factors interplay so that in cases superficially similar, now one treatment and now the other is efficacious. In state hospitals the cause of the afflictions of nearly half of all admissions are unknown. In time it will be possible to delimit etiology in these "functional" cases in accordance with their psychopathology and psychogenesis, or perhaps in terms of organic factors which have not yet been discovered.

CHAPTER IV

CLINICAL COMBINATIONS OF SYMPTOMS

IN THE ATTEMPT to arrive at a clear understanding of patients and their difficulties, I have found it useful to think in terms of certain combinations of symptoms. These clusters of symptoms are not equivalent in value to the symptom complexes or syndromes which are characteristic of particular disorders. They are, however, suggestive of the general type of disease process, organic or functional, from which the patient suffers. Because of their indicator value, these combinations also point to further laboratory and clinical studies which are necessary for purposes of differential diagnosis.

There has been a recent tendency to decry the need for complete study and accurate diagnosis in dealing with problems of personal adjustment. There has also been a tendency to minimize the essentially psychiatric nature of many problems of maladjustment, and attempted treatment has been ineffective as a result. Organic and constitutional factors are often ignored, with resulting unjustified optimism as to treatment possibilities. These attitudes have been stimulated, at least in part, by the great flood of popular and semi-popular literature in the psychological and psychiatric fields. There has been a marked increase in the utilization of psychotherapy by both the trained and untrained. I shall have more to say of this later, but here it may be emphasized that psychotherapy of any type, and the types appear to be legion, is a most dangerous tool in the hands of poorly trained, unsupervised workers, no matter what the *theoretical* background of professional training may be.

It is essential for the social worker to be aware of the indicator symptoms of mental disorders and their variations. If the worker's efforts are to produce results and the area of professional functioning is to be delimited from that of the psychiatrist, there must be a clear idea of treatment possibilities. This is true even when it is recognized that there are many conditions which *either* social worker or psychiatrist may treat with entire adequacy. However, the ability to recognize conditions which are clearly psychiatric will assist the social worker to avoid wasting effort on cases which are either untreatable or present problems which are outside the province of case work treatment.

It must always be remembered that about one half of the cases whose condition requires hospitalization present some type of definite physical pathology as the essential causative factor in the mental breakdown. Among the groups which do not present any known physical pathology, patients in the largest group (schizophrenia) are not ordinarily susceptible to psychotherapy.

Adequate study and diagnosis are of first rate importance in determining the types of treatment to be used. Various measures are employed, including medical and surgical treatment, hydrotherapy, occupational therapy, group therapy, and shock therapy, as well as psychotherapy in selected and suitable cases. The organization of the hospital and the interrelationships of patients are also important factors in treatment.

To revert to the combination of symptoms, perhaps the most important distinction to be made is between states presenting as central or outstanding symptoms disturbances of consciousness and memory and those which do not. However, there are states in which disturbances in the field of emotion or motor activity are the predominant or primary symptoms. Discussion of these several groups will clarify statements made above.

Symptomatology Primarily Centering in the Intellect

Intellectual disturbances may be classified into two broad groups in accordance with the presence or absence of clouding of consciousness. As related to this broad principle of classification, there are differences in causation, in treatment, and in outcome.

With clouding of consciousness.—This phrase implies that there is disturbance in the field of awareness, i.e., the perception and fixation of external facts or events and the accurate knowledge of one's own mental operations, sensations, and whereabouts. One of the cardinal signs of clouding of consciousness is the symptom known as "disorientation." This occurs with respect to time, place, and persons. Disorientation for time is considered to exist when the patient is more than three days out of the way on the day of the week, or the date. The disoriented patient may miscall the season of the year, the month, the year, the period of the day— morning, afternoon, night. Disorientation for place may involve the immediate surroundings, the city, state, or even the country. Disorientation for persons may include failure to recognize those in the immediate vicinity, friends, or members of the family. The last bit of orientation to be lost is, as a rule, the knowledge of personal identity.

It is true that disorientation occurs in functional disorders and that awareness of what is going on in the immediate environment may be, or at least seem to be, quite unimpaired. But disorientation is most frequent of all in the toxic-infectious and organic cases; especially in the former it may be associated with delirium. In organic cases there are usually associated disturbances of memory, judgment and reasoning—in other words, a generalized intellectual impairment or deterioration.

Loss of memory, or amnesia, has certain characteristics which vary in accordance with the underlying causative factors. It may be circumscribed and refer only to a particular period of the patient's life, while retention of memory for previous and subsequent events remains. Such circumscribed amnesias occur as a result of many acute febrile disorders; covering the period of an epileptic attack or its equivalent; in attacks of arteriosclerotic confusion; after too much alcohol; as a result of head trauma; after acute psychoses, with great excitement or confusion; and in cases of hysteria.

A limited amnesia of this type may be the only sign of mental disturbance. Thus, in cases of head trauma with loss of consciousness the patient may or may not later show signs of a continuing mild to severe personality disturbance. There will, however, be a period of amnesia, and in typical cases with severe trauma there will be loss of memory not only for the period of unconsciousness but also for the accident itself and for a variable length of time before the accident. Sometimes this will be only a few hours, but it may extend for weeks or months. One of my patients suffered a fractured skull in an automobile accident and was unconscious for seventy-two hours. He made an uneventful recovery, but careful testing a year later revealed a complete amnesia for all events during approximately three weeks before the accident. Aside from this circumscribed amnesia, the only signs of altered personality were diminished ambition and a tendency to be too casual about matters which he had formerly considered important.

By contrast, the amnesias of functional or neurotic origin are usually characterized by clear-cut limits, both at the onset and at the end. For example, one man after having a severe quarrel with his wife, the culmination of a long period of domestic difficulties, left home for his office. He put his keys in his desk, and remembered nothing more until three weeks later, when he "came to himself" walking in the streets of a city some two thousand miles from his home. His only memory for the intervening period was that the soles of his shoes were pounded while he was apparently sleeping on a bench in a railroad station. Where this was, how he made the trip, where he ate or lodged, or any other experiences he could not recall.

This brings out another point regarding attacks of amnesia. A patient may automatically act in a manner which seems, at least to casual observers, to be normal. Or, as in many cases of amnesia reported in the newspapers, the patient may be aware of the loss of knowledge of personal identity and may appeal for help on that basis. Such individuals retain their language usage and ability to travel, but cannot remember who they are or where they came from.

There are many variations of these "twilight" states. Personal identity may not be lost, but loss of memory for past experiences or loss of language usage may occur. Activity may be carried on which has a high symbolic value, but it is divorced from reality, sometimes delinquent, and for it the patient has or develops a complete amnesia.

Such automatic activity, with or without evidence of confusion, also occurs in cases of epilepsy, as one type of so-called epileptic equivalent. Various states of activity also occur, often in the nature of a furore; blind assaults may occur, resulting in serious injury or even death to the person assaulted.

In some cases alcohol in even small quantities produces a state of automatic activity, with apparently clear faculties and good co-ordination, but with complete amnesia later. The behavior may be quite ordinary, or it may have unusual or even bizarre features. States of extreme rage may also be succeeded by amnesia, which, however, is not complete.

Certain aspects of amnesia are regarded as normal because they are so frequently encountered. A conspicuous instance is the amnesia for the events of early life. Thus, the average adult can spontaneously recall few or no events of his first four or five years.

A few people will place the earliest memories in the third year; others are unable to recall anything before the age of ten or even twelve. In addition to this inability to recall early experiences, some people have very imperfect memories for certain types of experiences, particular categories of knowledge, classes of objects, or categories of words. On the other hand, in the feeble-minded and in the deteriorated diffuse defects of memory are common.

There is a selective process in memory, dependent in large part upon the degree of impressibility for an individual experience. A group of people undergoing a similar experience who compare notes some time later will remember different details; sometimes there is no common core of facts remembered by all or most of the group. This brings out the point that impressibility is conditioned by the emotional values of an experience, as well as by the intensity of the experience as a stimulus and by the degree of attention at the time.

In the deterioration which accompanies senility, it is the memory for recent events which suffers first. As the deterioration becomes marked, more and more of the recent past is blotted out, the amnesia progressively extends backward, and daily experiences seem not to be recorded at all. A senile completely disoriented for time, place, and the persons around him may, however, give a detailed and reasonably accurate account of his past life up to the age he claims to be.

The amnesia in other organic disorders, such as general paresis, meningovascular syphilis, and arteriosclerotic cerebral disease is likely to be patchy. The material forgotten by the patient may vary from time to time, so that at some times certain things are remembered which are forgotten at other times. Orientation is also variable.

Confused patients are disoriented, irrelevant, and incoherent in speech, often poorly co-ordinated in motor activity, and not in contact with their surroundings. They do not enter into a definite conversation, since their attention is gained only with difficulty and cannot be held. There may also be hyperactivity of a rather aimless type. Such conditions are usually organic, less often toxic, in origin.

Delirium is characterized not only by confusion and often overactivity but also particularly by hallucinations. Delirium is usually of toxic or infectious origin, and the hallucinations are predominantly visual, though any of the senses may be involved. Often they are scenic or panoramic in type. Since the hallucinations are likely to be vivid, they may be remembered when all other events of the delirious period are forgotten. People of all ages, including those in the senile period, may become delirious. It is especially important to remember this concerning the aged and women after childbirth. One old lady was twice sent to a mental hospital with a diagnosis of senile dementia. Incision of an acute purulent infected parotid gland, first on one side, then on the other, promptly relieved her delirium during both admissions. Each time the delirium cleared up, she appeared to be a normal elderly woman.

Associated with delirium are the usual physical signs of toxemia, varying somewhat according to the cause. Temperature elevation, rapid pulse, and other signs are to be expected if the disorder is due to infection. The classical picture of alcoholic delirium tremens does not show elevation of temperature, but there are physical signs which, together with the history, make diagnosis possible.

One interesting variant of this picture, originally described by Korsakow and called by his name, is a confabulating delirium usually associated with polyneuritis. Hallucinations are not as prominent in this condition as in true delirium. Such patients seem alert to what is going on, but actually remember nothing. They are disoriented for time and usually for place. Being highly suggestible, they will elaborate on any experience, real or only suggested. While Korsakow's syndrome is most commonly due to alcohol, it does occur as the result of other toxic and infectious disorders.

Coma is the end result of many disease processes. It is to be distinguished from stupor by the state of unconsciousness which, as such, is not an integral part of stupor. In and of itself, coma is a grave sign, and it is usually followed by death. Today, when diabetics administer insulin to themselves, comatose states sometimes occur unexpectedly because of the fall in sugar level. Any form of sugar given while the patient can still swallow, or sugar given intravenously, will clear up the coma immediately.

Finally, there is the loss of consciousness occurring in cases with convulsive disorders. These are discussed in detail in another section, and it is only necessary here to state that loss of consciousness may occur with or without an actual convulsion. It has already been mentioned that circumscribed amnesia results. It is the ultimate fate of many epileptics to become psychotic or to deteriorate.

There is some reason to believe that the beneficial effects of shock therapy, so widely employed today, may be due to a minor degree of intellectual loss, affecting recently formed constellations of ideas.

With clear consciousness.—It has been mentioned that few people are able to recall their early years with any great clarity or accuracy. Individuals have been encountered who claimed ability to recall particular isolated events at as early an age as one year. But these cases are rare; in fact, it is uncommon to find a person who can recall many events before the age of three or four. As a general rule, people recall events of the recent past more clearly and in greater detail than they do more remote events. However, it falls within the domain of the abnormal for an individual to be unable to recall events occurring before the age of ten or twelve. If the person is of average or superior intelligence, such a memory defect must be ascribed to a psychic trauma or to a series of them. Such traumata, being repressed, carry with them a great many nonrelated ideas, experiences, and emotions.

The mentally deficient, on the other hand, never develop good memories, but the memory defects are usually generalized. At the same time, the idiot-savant type may have a remarkable memory for a particular type of detail. It appears to require a mental age of at least eight to be able to give correctly the birth date and year, as well as age. The mentally deficient are defective in all the three elements requisite for good memory—impressibility, associations, and recall.

The feebleminded and those with intellectual deterioration also show defective reasoning and judgment. They cannot reason from cause to effect, or vice versa; the ability to make simple arithmetical calculations is absent; logical synthesis is impossible.

Delusions are classified as disorders of judgment, since they are false beliefs. They occur in cases with clouding of consciousness, with mild to severe intellectual deterioration, but even more commonly in cases with clear consciousness, good orientation, and without particular signs of intellectual dilapidation. Delusions may be classified into several types according to the content of the delusions, or according to whether they are directed toward the self, the somatic and grandiose delusions, or toward the external world in the form of delusions of persecution.

Delusions may be very convincingly presented and are almost invariably supported by masses of evidence. Somewhere, however, in the content of the ideas or in the evidence adduced in their support, there will appear inconsistencies, contradictions, and impossibilities which reveal the delusional nature of the ideas. At the same time, it is imperative in many cases to make rather extensive investigation of alleged false ideas before the delusional nature of the beliefs can be demonstrated. This is particularly true in situations of marital disharmony when one partner suspects the other of infidelity and in some cases in which assault, attempts at rape, or even murder may be claimed.

The most common delusion is that of persecution, the essential or basic delusion of all the many types of paranoid psychosis. People actually are persecuted as individuals or in groups, so that here again not all ideas of persecution are *ipso facto* delusions. Common to all people, also, are ideas of reference—that a particular remark, event, or action has specific reference to them—which may not be at all true. Probably everyone has had the experience of suspecting that he was the subject of a conversation which stopped abruptly when he joined the conversers. Such ideas only become important as indicators of mental disturbance when they occur so frequently and in such a wide variety of settings that in some instances they cannot possibly be true. These ideas of reference, associated with increasing tenseness and suspicion, frequently exist for some time before actual delusions emerge in recognizable form. Delusions of persecution have been given an interesting interpretation by Freud, at least for the so-called paranoid states. But delusions of persecution occur in every type of psychosis; the organic, toxic, and infectious types, as well as in the schizophrenic, cyclothymic, and other functional disorders. In cases regarded as paranoid personalities, but not psychotic, the mechanism which is most obvious and most used is that of projection. That is, the individual accepts no personal responsibility for anything that happens to or about him, even though it is his own behavior which provokes the reactions of others. Mingled with this attitude are ideas of being different, usually in a superior way, of being inadequately appreciated, of being misunderstood or even persecuted in an organized manner.

Freud's interpretation of delusions of persecution is based on the idea that there is an underlying homosexual trend which is repressed, but unsuccessfully so. The trend is unacceptable to the superego; the formula "I love him" (in the male) is insupportable and becomes "I hate him." This, too, is untenable, and so it becomes "He hates me," and the idea of persecution is fully formed. The formula is adequate, even if a homosexual trend cannot be demonstrated.

Delusions of grandeur are particularly common in general paresis. They occur in the paranoid conditions, apparently as rationalizations for the persecutions being suffered. In the manic phase of cyclothymia they are also common and are usually characterized by their essential plausibility.

In the paranoid, the ideas of grandeur may be quite bizarre. It is among these cases that identifications with great people of the past are developed, such as ideas that the patient is Napoleon, Christ, or Queen of the World. Delusions of being God are extremely rare; I have seen this in only one case that was not delirious. Many patients communicate with God, have been given special missions by Him, and are His agents on earth. Delusions of being the second Christ, and among women delusions of being pregnant by immaculate conception, are quite common.

Delusions of self-depreciation occur in depressions. Such ideas as having committed the unpardonable sin, of being condemned to eternal torture, and of having no future are representative. Hypochondriacal or somatic delusions are also common in depressions, especially in the agitated depressions so characteristic of the involution period. That the bowels are obstructed, there is no heartbeat or circulation, or the stomach is gone, are representative ideas.

Of course, many people have hypochondriacal ideas without a psychosis. These are the chronic neurotic invalids whose neurosis finds expression in subjective physical symptoms and unusual ideas about their personal anatomy and physiology. These are not to be confused with the psychosomatic cases.

Basic to intellectual operations are perceptions; these derive from the general and special senses. Some of these are internal, such as the visceral sensations and the kinesthetic impulses from muscles, bones, and joints, which provide the basic information regarding the position of the various parts of the body. Other sensations are derived from the skin, through contact. Temperature, pain, and discrimination of the size of touching structures and their locations are all functions of skin sensibility. The sense of taste is also one of contact. But the senses of hearing, vision, and smelling operate from a distance and represent the perceptions by which one is, for the most part, in contact with the more remote environment.

False sensory impressions may be of the nature of illusions or of hallucinations. Illusions are fairly common; they represent misinterpretations of things actually seen, heard, felt, or smelled. A fluttering curtain may be incorrectly interpreted as a moving person, or sounds may be given quite wrong values. In these instances the misinterpretation is usually seen in terms of a threat, and the emotional reaction would very likely be fear.

Hallucinations, on the other hand, are endopsychic in origin and represent sensory impressions without objective stimulus. Voices are heard when no one is around; visions appear which no one else sees; odors of gas and the taste of poison are seemingly detected; various tactile sensations, such as bugs crawling under the skin or the tactile and inner sensation of electrical currents being passed through the body, occur. All these appear in the absence of any visible or palpable sources of stimuli. Hallucinations and delusions usually occur together, and they usually have the same general type of content. However, either may occur without the other, and they may not have the same affective values.

Visual hallucinations are most common in the toxic-infectious, exhaustive types of disturbance. Auditory hallucinations are most frequent in schizophrenia and in the paranoid conditions. They also occur in one type of alcoholic psychosis, the nondelirious state of acute alcoholic hallucinosis. Hallucinations in the other sensory fields are less common and, while they do occur from many causes, are most frequently found in schizophrenics. Hallucinations of smell occur in organic brain disease, especially in brain tumor. "Hypnagogic hallucinations" is the term applied to exceptionally vivid sensory images occurring in the twilight state between sleeping and waking, but recognized for what they are on awakening.

Symptomatology Primarily Centered in the Emotions

In general, we speak so much at present of emotional disturbances, complexes, and conflicts that there is a tendency to forget the more serious psychotic symptom pictures in which alterations of mood are in the forefront. In the typical picture there are also disturbances of activity, which in certain psychoses are harmonious with the mood. In other psychoses the activity or the emotional reactions, or both, are paradoxical; that is, they are not in agreement. There are three principal types of pathological emotional states, chiefly psychotic in nature.

Depression.—In this state the patient feels, appears, and acts sad. Nor is the gloom lightened by events which would make a normal individual happy or cause laughter. Obviously this mood far exceeds anything that could be called normal unhappiness in the face of untoward events. Furthermore, such states extend over long periods. In many, perhaps most, instances the patient or the family attributes the depression to some external event or series of events. In many cases depressing events really have occurred and have acted as precipitating factors, but the ensuing reaction is both excessive for the stimulus and prolonged far past the time when under ordinary circumstances it would disappear or at least lighten.

The patient describes his mood as an intense and truly painful dejection. This is combined with slowness of thinking and paucity of ideas, which the patient also recognizes. Everything is seen through dark glasses and viewed with alarm; pessimism and worry dominate thoughts of the future. In more advanced stages the future is utterly black, and the patient feels doomed both in life and after death. Feeling utterly hopeless, patients develop suicidal ideas and attempt self-destruction. As depression deepens, such ideas are not given up, but inhibition of thought and especially action are so great that suicidal attempts are not made. As depression and inhibition lighten, the suicidal impulse is still present, and many cases of suicide occur in this recovering period. In fact, this is the most dangerous period in depressions; since the patient seems much improved, vigilance is relaxed. Many reports of suicide read that the person "was recovering" or "had recovered" from a "long illness." Though usually it is not stated that the illness was a depression, evidence in the stories often proves that this was so.

Minor depressive reactions occur to everyone under appropriate conditions. Major depressions occur in many psychoses, but the typical psychotic depression is that of cyclothymia, which in the past has customarily been designated as melancholia, usually divided into several types. Thus, "acute," "chronic," and "recurrent" melancholia are terms frequently found in the older literature.

The depressed patient's delusions are directed against himself; they are self-accusatory and self-deprecatory. Patients are sure they have committed the unpardonable sin, which usually turns out to be some very minor delinquency, often in childhood. Somatic or hypochondriacal delusions are common and often nihilistic. In rare cases the ideas are projected in paranoid style, and the patient blames others for his troubles.

Depressive reactions may also be secondary to hallucinations of a threatening nature. Fearful reactions are likely to occur along with these reactions, though they are not especially common in the cyclothymic depressions.

In true depressions weeping is uncommon except in the earliest stages. If it continues to be marked, the chances are that the depression is secondary rather than primary and that the weeping does not so much indicate depression as it does self-pity, fear, anxiety, or even hostility.

Elation or excitement.—Excitement is even more common among psychotic patients than is depression. Here, again, elation is a normal experience for all at some time or other, but pathological states of elation are excessive and prolonged in relation to the stimulus or, more commonly, appear without specific stimulus. Along with the elation is likely to be euphoria, which is essentially a feeling of great well-being. These excited states occur in practically all types of psychosis, though in many they are short-lived. The paradigm of such states is the manic phase of cyclothymia. Such patients say that they are happy, feel very healthy and strong; nothing can possibly be wrong with them, they insist, because they feel so well. Delusions are self-maximating or grandiose, though occasionally they will have a paranoid coloring. Manics are usually irritable, but are also easily distracted from the cause of irritability.

Hyperkinesis, or excessive motor activity, is, perhaps, the most obvious outward sign in states of elation. Such patients are very talkative and very busy. Characteristic of the stream of speech is the fact that it wanders widely and the goal is rarely, if ever, reached. Furthermore, the patient is easily distracted from his train of thought by sounds, comments, and sights. General activity tends to follow chance stimuli or vagrant thoughts. Left to themselves, such patients can squander unbelievable amounts of money, travel great distances for no special purpose, or become involved in divers inappropriate situations. One patient spent more than twelve hours in driving to a town forty miles distant, because he could not resist turning into each side-road he saw. The real mystery is how he ever reached his destination, but he did have a joyful time.

Elation may become extremely painful to the patient because of the intensity of the long-continued process, or it may give way to great irritability. Exhaustion, coma, and death may supervene as the excitement increases. Usually patients lose weight during these manic phases, and one of the early signs of improvement is likely to be an increase in weight.

Apathy, indifference, and paradoxical emotional responses.— These are important and ominous signs when they apparently dominate the mood. At the very least, they are evidences of a schizoid personality, and when well developed these types of emotional response are among the cardinal and most important signs of schizophrenia itself. Apathy and indifference are frequently found in organic types of dementia or with lesions in certain areas of the brain without obvious intellectual deterioration. The paradoxical emotional responses of the schizophrenic are not necessarily or usually expressed by laughter or weeping. Instead, satisfaction at some experience which should be depressing, or a gloomy response to what should be cheerful news, may be verbally expressed or shown in behavior.

The schizophrenic is absorbed in his own inner world, and it must be emphasized that the apathy and paradoxical responses apply only to external events. If the schizophrenic's world can be penetrated, lively emotional reactions to the inner ideas will be found. It is the relative inaccessibility which makes the apathy stand out so sharply by comparison with impassivity in the normal and the obtuseness of the organic dementias. The latter cases are accessible: the one will explain that subjectively he does not seem to feel as intensely as other people do; the other will show general evidences of dilapidation, the impoverishment of affect being only one part of the total picture.

Symptomatology Primarily Centered in Activity, or Kinesis

It is the state of activity, including speech, which ordinarily calls attention to the psychotic individual. States of hyperkinesis occur in many types of psychoses and are among the most troublesome of all in treatment. The degree of hyperkinesis varies greatly, from that of the mildly stimulated hypomanic to that of mania furiosa. Other symptoms, of course, enter in to make differential diagnosis possible. For example, sometimes overactivity is based on fear aroused by threatening hallucinations and delusions, or the hyperkinesis may be accompanied by delusions of grandeur, a general state of euphoria, and the deterioration of general paresis.

A popular idea about the psychotic person is that he is continuously overactive, extremely talkative, and more or less incoherent in speech. One thing which always impresses the visitor to a mental hospital is what a contrast this is to the truth.

No satisfactory explanation has been advanced for the fact that states of excitement are more common among psychotic women than among psychotic men. It is hardly to be explained by the statistically significant differences in the types of psychoses affecting the two sexes, since excitement also characterizes the psychoses which are more predominant among males.

States of underactivity, or hypokinesis, are also common to many psychoses. There is, again, a considerable range of variation, from slight degrees of retardation and underactivity to states of stupor in which voluntary activity is completely suspended, or nearly so. However, the patient remains conscious, as is shown in various ways, and this is the feature which distinguishes stupor from coma. As already stated, coma occurs in many organic and toxic conditions, and the prognosis is always grave. Stupor, by contrast, occurs chiefly in the so-called functional disorders, especially in schizophrenia as catatonic stupor, and in the depressed phase of cyclothymia. There are also trance states in hysteria, but in these there is usually also apparent suppression of consciousness or, perhaps, an alternate personality in charge.

Paradoxical or parakinetic responses, in which the actions are beside the point, that is, do not fit the stimulus, are found almost exclusively in schizophrenia. Most prominent in schizophrenia are the negativistic responses, especially marked in the catatonic type. Here the tendency is to do the exact opposite of what is requested or ordered. Asked to open the eyes, the patient shuts them tightly; asked to come forward, he backs away. Other types of activity which seem unmotivated to the observer are stereotyped modes of action and repetitive speech. Mannerisms occur in all people to some extent and under some circumstances, but the stereotypies of the schizophrenic are both peculiar and most difficult to understand.

Posturing is one type of paradoxical activity which appears strange and unmotivated. Catatonic patients, especially, assume difficult postures and hold them for long periods. The crucifixion position, the position of prayer, and standing with the back pressed closely to the wall are typical examples.

All these variations in degree and type of activity are also found in well people, but not in the extreme degree which characterizes the psychotic or the neurotic. When working with so-called problem children, it is usually possible to ascertain environmental factors which determine deviation in the type and degree of response. If such causes cannot be demonstrated, we must turn to constitutional factors, pathological or otherwise, to explain the situation. For example, chronic fatigue often produces a state of hyperkinesis with loss of appetite, irritability, and insomnia. The fatigue, in turn, may be due to physical or mental causes or to a combination of both. Particularly common in children, this syndrome is also frequently overlooked. As an important emotional cause, the feeling of being rejected is outstanding in children. On the other hand, in many cases of emotional and kinetic disturbance no specific factor, such as fatigue, some nervous disorder, rejection, or an endocrine disturbance, may be found. Under such circumstances it is necessary to fall back upon relatively unsatisfactory concepts of an abnormal personality of uncertain origin. Especially in children, however, disorders of activity will usually be found to be compensatory for some sort of disturbed emotional relationships, centering primarily in the family.

Summary

It is clear from this résumé of the clinical combinations of symptoms that not all mental disorders are due to emotional conflicts or complexes or to disturbed interpersonal relationships in childhood. In recent years there has been a pronounced tendency to view all types of social maladaptation as related solely to emotional conflicts. It is often forgotten that even emotional and environmental causes may become so thoroughly internalized that a fixed, crystallized deviation in personality results and may be extremely intractable to treatment. Furthermore, there are conflicting drives within the individual which can and do result in disturbed mental states without either organic or environmental pathology. This statement holds particularly true for schizophrenia and cylothymia, neither of which has revealed any consistent personal or interpersonal pathology or psychopathology.

CLINICAL GROUPINGS, ESPECIALLY OF THE PSYCHOSES

Many classifications of mental disorders have been proposed and used for longer or shorter periods of time. In retrospect, some of them are amusing because of the evidence they reveal of the poor understanding of the natural history of mental disorders. Many disorders were "isolated" on the basis of particular symptoms; there was no "seeing through" the total clinical picture to causative factors, the basic process in true diagnosis. The fact that over a long period of time medicine in general was dominated by the doctrine of mono-causation in disease contributed to the confusion. Another point is that psychology only slowly emerged as a science, and then for a considerable period was concerned chiefly with learning processes and choice of activity; little was done in the field of emotions. The development of experimental psychology, of mental tests, and finally of psychoanalysis, with its emphasis on the unconscious mechanisms, brought psychology into psychiatry as a dynamic force.

As has already been pointed out, the development and use of several laboratory tests, the latest being the electroencephalogram, gave psychiatry its first precise diagnostic tools. However, in most psychiatric cases, as will shortly become clear, there are no exact clinical differentiating signs or symptoms; psychiatric diagnosis is still an art requiring careful history taking, close observation, and meticulous examination; in other words, thorough and adequate clinical study. Diagnostic data must be complete and then carefully interpreted against a background of experience with all sorts of abnormal mental conditions, plus a knowledge of normal or usual reactions in varied life situations. All opinions to the contrary notwithstanding, accurate diagnosis is of first-rank importance in psychiatry because of its indispensable relationship to the choice of treatment approach. Diagnosis is not an end in itself and is most useful in psychiatric cases when it is not categorical, but results in a dynamic synthesis.

In order to choose the proper treatment methods, it is important to divide psychiatric cases into those who have insight into their condition, and those who do not. What is it that brings the person with a psychiatric problem to the psychiatrist, the psychiatric clinic, the child guidance clinic, the psychoeducational clinic, the social agency, or the social worker? There are three possibilities to be borne in mind.

1. The patient recognizes that he has a personal problem, that he is ill or is not adjusting well in one or more of his general relationships, that there is something wrong with him, due to "nerves" or "emotions," which can be treated and either cured or ameliorated. The patient who voluntarily comes for treatment has insight and is a suitable subject for psychotherapy or any other type of therapy indicated by the physical and mental findings. The insight is not complete, since if it were he would presumably be well and in no need of treatment. In this group will be found the psychoneurotics, cases of epilepsy, and many incipient and some recovered psychotics. The latter recognize a vulnerability in themselves, wish to avoid further difficulties, and therefore apply for treatment.

2. A disturbance in functioning is recognized, but not by the patient. There is usually a change for the worse in behavior and social relationships, or a failure to change the behavior in a manner consonant with the growth and development of the individual. Such patients, whether adults or children, are without insight and are brought for treatment by another person. If such a patient sees any problem, it is usually a different one, and even that is cus-

tomarily not seen as it actually is. In this group of patients will be found the psychotics, the deteriorated epileptics, many mental defectives, and most psychopaths.

3. Acute or chronic breakdowns of social adaptation include such commonplace behavior patterns as inability to make normal progress in school, to hold a job, to behave in reasonable accordance with accepted standards, or to establish and maintain effective personal relationships. Frequently these breakdowns or failures are the sources of concern to someone other than the patient. The latter may, however, be distressed by his situation, even though true insight is only partial or absent. A patient with delusions of persecution may be irritated or upset by the imagined persecutory activities, but have no insight into the endopsychic origin of the delusions. In fact, such patients reject any suggestions that they may have delusions and react to such ideas with hostility and suspicion directed at the one who offers an explanation.

Conventionally, the mental disorders are grouped in six categories: (1) psychoses, (2) mental deficiency, (3) epilepsy, (4) psychoneuroses or neuroses, (5) psychopathic personality, and (6) primary (or reactive) behavior disorders. Discussion of the use of some of these terms seems appropriate here, though more precise definitions are given in connection with the description of the individual conditions.

Psychosis is literally defined in the dictionary as "a disease of the mind, especially one without demonstrable organic lesions. Any morbid mental state." The ending "osis" means "condition of" or "state caused by." Hence the term psychosis should logically be applied to psychogenic diseases. In actual practice the term is used to cover all the frank mental diseases, both those with known organic pathology and those without. These mental diseases are, except in some cases in the incipient stage or after complete recovery, characterized by complete absence of insight into the fact of illness or the presence of a mental disorder. These patients require treatment against their will, and as a result legal methods of commitment are provided.

Most states have provisions for voluntary admission to mental hospitals, even for psychotics, and also provision for temporary care through police action or on a physician's certificate. It is usually necessary to commit the psychotic patient. In many states this requires on a prescribed form a report of an examination by two physicians and a hearing before a judge of a probate or other court of record. The patient may have the right to a trial by jury on appeal. In some states commitment is by a jury trial, while in others there are insanity commissions, often made up of a doctor, a lawyer, and the county clerk.

In practice, therefore, the medical term "psychosis" is synonymous with the legal term "insanity," though it must be remembered that some psychotic people are not committable; at least a judge or jury may so decide. The term "insanity" (earlier, "lunacy") was formerly a respectable medical term. Because of narrow legal definitions, plus the increasing recognition of the fact that there are medically many kinds of "insanities," whereas there is only one legal variety since one is either sane or insane before the law, the medical profession adopted other terms—"mental diseases" and "psychoses." "Lunacy" and "lunatic" were dropped from the nomenclature when the notion was dispelled that mental disorders were caused by the moon's phases. The term "psychiatry" has largely replaced the term "mental diseases"; "psychiatrist" has replaced "alienist"; "neuropsychiatry" and "neuropsychiatrist" are terms which have considerable vogue, especially among those who practice both neurology and psychiatry. Psychoanalysts are, or should be, well-trained psychiatrists who have made a special study of psychoanalysis and tend to or do select for treatment only cases suitable for that particular type of psychotherapy.

Neurosis is defined as "any morbid nervous state. A functional disease of the nervous system—a disturbance of the nerve centers or peripheral nerves not due to any demonstrable structural change." Presumably such changes might be due to physicochemical alterations not demonstrable by the techniques at our command. Psychoneurosis is defined as "mental disease independent of organic lesion," practically equivalent to the definition of psychosis. It will be seen that the definition is quite different from that of neurosis, yet these two terms are used interchangeably in psychiatric literature. "Neurasthenia" and "psychasthenia" are two of the classical psychoneuroses. Neurasthenia is defined as "a group of symptoms resulting from debility or exhaustion of the nerve-centers"; psychasthenia, as "mental fatigue." Finally, "neuropsychosis" is a "combined nervous and mental disease."

Accordingly, if our usage of words were more literal and logical, we should have the following groupings: (1) neuropsychoses, including about half the psychotic patients; (2) psychoses, including the other half of the psychotic patients and all the psychoneurotics. It is unlikely that any such change will occur; present usage has too much tradition back of it. We shall therefore use the terms psychosis and neurosis, or psychoneurosis, in the sense of their acquired and general usage. It has been proposed that the psychoneuroses be defined and classed as minor psychoses, but the suggestion has never been officially adopted.

As a rule, neurotic people recognize that there is something wrong with them and sooner or later seek treatment. They may seek treatment for somatic symptoms, for nerves or nervousness or nervous breakdown, and may be reluctant to admit that disturbances in mental functioning, especially in the emotional field, are the real causes of their symptoms. Psychotic people, as already stated, ordinarily are without insight and do not voluntarily seek treatment.

This discussion of the usage of terms has been presented in such detail only because the points made emphasize the confusion which has always existed, and still does exist, regarding the relationships between body, including the nervous system, and mind. If "nerve," "nervous," and "neuro" refer to that structural system in the body called the nervous system, then there should be evidence of structural change if we are to speak of "nervous breakdown," "nervousness," or "neurosis." The statement that no physical changes are demonstrable is usually met by the assertion that our methods of anatomical and chemical analysis are not sufficiently refined to bring out the delicate changes which must underlie the functional disorders; that is, in the neuroses and several of the psychoses. Such a view tends to deny the reality of mind as a biological function of the organism. The brain is the anatomical substrate for the mind, and without a well-developed brain no symbolic, creative, non-material activity is possible.

The mind functions as an organ in social relationships. With no intention of arguing about monistic or dualistic philosophies, the point that the mind is the social organ of the individual must be emphasized. Mind is complex, and it has been subjected to several sorts of analysis. There is the old "faculty" analysis, including sensation, perception, apperception, association, memory, emotion, instinct, will, and action. With some modification, these categories are still important in understanding mental operations. In more modern terms, there are unconscious and conscious aspects of mental operations. Furthermore, the mind is compounded of the id, the ego, and the super-ego, and the way in which these function consciously and unconsciously has important effects on behavior and adaptation.

With the exception of the so-called primary behavior disorders, the several groupings other than the psychotic are sufficiently defined in their respective sections. Primary, idiopathic, or essential means, in general medical literature, that the cause or causes for a disorder are unknown. Primary behavior disorders are, accordingly, behavior difficulties not due to the presence of psychosis, mental defect, epilepsy, neurosis, or psychopathic personality; that is, the diagnosis is made by negative exclusion.

The disorders of behavior which interest us are the outward manifestation of inner reactions of the individual to stresses and strains within himself or in the outer world of reality. Most commonly, they result from difficulties in interpersonal relationships. For these reasons I prefer the term reactive behavior disorders, and have so designated them throughout.

In the immediately succeeding sections the psychoses are discussed. They have been divided into two major categories: (1) the psychoses of known organic pathology or etiology or both; and (2) the psychoses without known pathology or etiology or both.

The psychoses in group one are: neurosyphilis, organic brain diseases, senility, the toxic-infectious, endocrine and metabolic disorders, and those which are caused by exogenous poisons. The presenile or involutional disorders are between groups one and two. The second group comprises schizophrenia or dementia praecox, cyclothymia or the manic depressive reactions, paranoia and paranoid conditions. The psychoses which occur in mental defectives, in those with convulsive disorders, and in psychopaths are taken up in the sections dealing with the basic disorders. That the psychoses are discussed first, and in the particular order in which they are presented, is a matter of deliberate choice. This procedure has value in terms of orderly exclusion and has a further virtue in focusing attention on the conditions which may more easily be forgotten in working with the average client. Furthermore, knowledge of the psychoses gives the necessary broad base for the study of the psychopathology of other conditions.

For each psychosis and other clinical entity there is discussion of presenting problems, data from the several examinations, pathology and etiology, psychopathology, prognosis, and treatment. Special stress is laid on the social worker's possible participation in treatment.

CHAPTER V

PSYCHOSES OF ORGANIC ORIGIN

SYPHILIS OF THE NERVOUS SYSTEM

SYPHILIS invades the nervous system, with resulting pathological changes in structure and disturbances in function. One type of pathology is similar to that found in other organs, characteristically an inflammatory reaction around blood vessels, giving rise to disturbances in circulation and so in the functioning of the nerve cells. This type is frequently complicated by meningitis, and the varied clinical pictures are ascribed to the meningo-vascular changes.

In a second type, occurring especially in the spinal cord and in the optic nerve, there is degeneration of fiber tracts, with resulting irremediable loss of function. This is the case with tabes dorsalis, an anatomical term for a disorder also known by a clinical descriptive term, locomotor ataxia. Sometimes there is a combination of this and the third type of change, when the condition is called taboparesis.

In the third type the changes occur in the gray matter of the brain, the cortex or parenchyma, and consist of inflammatory changes around the blood vessels, a mild degree of chronic meningitis, nerve cell destruction, and scarring due to gliosis. This meningoencephalitis represents the pathology of the clinical disorder, general paresis.

The meningo-vascular disorders occur in the first, second, and third stages of syphilis. In the third stage, gummata sometimes occur in the brain or the meninges, giving rise to symptoms which are clinically more or less identical with those of brain tumor.

General paresis and locomotor ataxia, on the other hand, occur late in the history of syphilis, usually long after the subsidence of all signs and symptoms of general or systemic syphilis. As already noted, in many of these cases it appears that the early signs of syphilis were either so mild or so transitory that they were not noticed or were thought to be some milder disorder not fraught with such grave future possibilities. This point explains in part the fact that it was nearly a century after "general progressive paralysis of the insane" was first described and established as a clinical entity before it was conclusively proved that all such cases were due to syphilis and only to syphilis. Alcohol, exposure, certain heavy labor occupations, and other factors had for many years been regarded as causes. Final proof that syphilis is always the cause came with the development of laboratory tests, the Wassermann reaction in blood and spinal fluid, other tests of the spinal fluid, and finally, a most difficult and brilliant demonstration of the causative organism, the spirochaeta pallida or treponema pallidum, in the brain in cases of general paresis.

The story of the development of our knowledge of general paresis presents a classical picture of the way in which medical knowledge develops and the various stages through which it must pass before it is complete, which is true for a comparatively limited number of diseases.

According to several historical accounts, general paralysis of the insane, or dementia paralytica, was established as a definite entity by its description in 1826. However, one reliable historian dates the first description in which one could definitely recognize general paresis as being written in 1672. Accurate descriptions are also recorded in 1798 in England and in 1822 in France. In the first American work on diseases of the mind, by Benjamin Rush in 1812, there is nothing to indicate recognition of the disorder in this country.

The early descriptions are, in general, adequate so far as clinical symptomatology is concerned. The gross pathology of the disease, especially of the cranium, meninges, and nervous system, was well established in the 1870's and 1880's, followed by refinements in the knowledge of gross pathology and of microscopic changes through the development of better technical methods.

Great debates raged over causation. It was not until the 1850's that syphilis began to be seriously considered as, perhaps, the chief cause. Clouston, a leading English psychiatrist, wrote in 1884 that the causes were "over and promiscuous sexual indulgence combined with hard muscular labor, a stimulating diet of highly fed flesh meat, the brain being all the while excited and poisoned by alcohol and syphilis, all these things being begun early in life and kept up steadily. Hard study, or severe mental shocks, or traumatic injuries, or continuous anxiety, will also produce the disease. I do not think there is any proof that it is syphilitic in origin." Clouston regarded general paralysis as "not only a variety of insanity, but a true cerebral disease." He said that "its study has somatized and definitized the study of all mental diseases, and has added . . . to our knowledge of the connection of mind with body." He noted that it was a disease of the cortex characterized by progression and stressed the factors of mental enfeeblement and mental facility on the one side, and motor deficiencies of speech, stages of convulsions, inco-ordination, paresis, and paralysis on the other. Clouston regarded it as a premature, pathological, quick, senile condition, the "trophic energy" being exhausted by overstimulation. He mentioned pupillary changes, but did not, apparently, lay great stress on them.

Clouston was writing toward the end of a period when medical thought in general was much confused about the origin of disease. He had been professionally trained in a school in which "moral causes" were considered to be predominant in the production of mental disorders, just as the trend now is to ascribe them to psychogenic causes. It was during his time, the period from about 1860 to about 1890, that the first definite proofs of the localization of cerebral function were discovered, and the relationships of bacteria to the production of disease began to be proven. In none of the writings of psychiatrists and neurologists during this period have I encountered anything to indicate that they had any special idea of the cause of syphilis beyond the idea that it was contagious and transmitted by some kind of "virus."

Refinements in neurological examination steadily built up a picture of degenerative processes in the nervous system in general paresis. Chief among these were: pupillary alterations, especially of the type, the Argyll-Robertson pupil, now known to be practically pathognomonic for the parenchymatous types of neurosyphilis (general paresis, juvenile paresis, tabes dorsalis), reflex changes, speech defects, and memory and reasoning defects. Eminent men argued for syphilis as a cause, pointing to various statistical and inferential data, but they were opposed by others equally eminent, who relied on other statistical and inferential data.

The point was, as previously mentioned, that histories given by paretics are sometimes highly unreliable with respect to syphilis and, in the absence of reliable or infallible objective tests for syphilis in the individual case, only indirect statistics and inferences based upon inadequate premises were available. To be sure, as early as 1886 it was noted that paresis occurred sixteen to seventeen times as frequently in syphilitics as it did in "healthy" persons, but even that conclusion was obviously based on inadequate data. In 1897 it was reported by a thoroughly reliable observer that inoculation of nine paretics with syphilitic virus had failed to produce syphilitic symptoms, regarded as a sure sign of previous syphilitic infection. However, other equally competent observers reported infections in cases of paresis similarly inoculated with syphilitic virus.

Perhaps this is as good an example as can be adduced to demonstrate the difficulties which beset the determination of etiological factors in situations in which all the data are not available, perhaps because of inadequate observation or, as in this instance, because technical methods were inadequate. A complication here was the fact that paresis and tabes were not amenable to the usual antisyphilitic remedies. This led to their being called "metasyphilis" or "parasyphilis," whereas general evidence made it more and more clear that syphilis was an extremely important, if not the only, factor in the production of these disorders. Furthermore, these affections occurred late in the natural history of syphilis, from five to twenty years after infection, the largest group occurring ten to fifteen years later. Those affected were chiefly men, usually vigorous, active, aggressive, and often rather successful individuals. Many were married and had healthy wives and children. In other cases there was a typical history of infection in the wife, with miscarriages and eventually the birth of congenitally syphilitic children.

In the case of paresis, however, advances in the study and treatment of syphilis in general eventually provided technical methods which proved the syphilitic origin of paresis and forged the last links in the chain of cause and effect. One of the first was the technique of lumbar puncture, developed by Quincke in 1895 in the treatment of acute cerebrospinal meningitis. Applied to the study of the spinal fluid in mental diseases, its full value was not realized until some two decades later, when technical methods of examination of the fluid permitted a considerable measure of differential diagnosis.

The demonstration of the treponema pallidum as the causative organism of syphilis by Schaudinn, in 1905, was followed in 1913 by Moore's and Noguchi's demonstration of the organism in the brains of paretics. From a practical standpoint, the development of Wassermann's reaction, in 1906, was of the highest importance. For here is a test which is applicable to both blood and spinal fluid and is accurate in an extraordinarily high percentage of cases. The use of the Wassermann test on the blood of all admissions was made a routine in several mental hospitals in 1912. In the same year several hospitals developed the use of spinal fluid examinations in all cases with positive blood Wassermann and in those with clinical signs indicating the possibility of positive tests in the spinal fluid, even though the blood Wassermann was negative.

For the first time psychiatry was equipped with definite, objective, reliable tests to determine the presence of syphilis of the nervous system, and in the case of the spinal fluid tests other than the Wassermann, of aid in the diagnosis of certain other organic processes. It should be remembered, however, that these laboratory tests do not give a diagnosis of the clinical state or condition of the patient, although they do differentiate pretty well the type of pathological process. Thus, the spinal fluid may give a typical test picture of paresis although the patient is free from clinical signs and symptoms.

Treatment of paresis has undergone several changes. Ehrlich's patient experimentation which resulted in the production of salvarsan in 1907 led to several chemotherapeutic attacks on the problem of paresis, such as intraspinous and intraventricular injections of salvarsanized and mercurialized serum, and intensive intravenous treatment with salvarsan and its successors. Treatment by induced malarial and electrical fever, often with penicillin, is the latest and apparently the most successful method. While these treatment methods have greatly improved the prognosis in general paresis, it is still not universally good, and most of the victims still die within five years after the onset of clinical symptoms.

This brings up two important and still unsolved questions: Why do about two percent of syphilitics develop paresis? Why are there about four times as many male as female paretics? The only answers at present are in terms of other questions. Is there a special strain of spirochaete, with a selective affinity for the nervous system? Or do some individuals have a specially receptive nervous system, where, perhaps, immunity in other parts and systems of their bodies is so great that the organisms find a host only in the nervous system? The data are too confused to give an answer at present.

But there is the history, from the stage of early recognition of a pattern of symptoms, through confusion of recognition, then delimitation of pathology, to etiology and attempts at specific therapy. As with many another disease, prevention rather than treatment still holds the greatest promise, for without being infected by syphilis, no one can develop any of the neurosyphilitides.

As already indicated, general paresis appears predominantly in males (75% of 6,000 first admissions were males). Nearly one half the paretic first admissions occurred in the age range thirty-five to forty-nine. However, there were cases in all age groupings; approximately 3 percent were under twenty-five years of age, and 4.3 percent were sixty-five years and over. It occurs in practically all races, at least cases have been so diagnosed in twenty-six of the thirty-three races listed in the New York Department of Mental Hygiene Report for 1938. It appears with greatest frequency in residents of large cities. Thus, 63 percent of first admissions in New York State in 1937–1938 were from New York City alone, while only 9 percent were from rural areas, and 28.7 percent were from communities of 2,500 and up. It occurs in people of all degrees of education, from the illiterate through college graduates, and in about the same percentage in the several educational groups as for the whole number of first admissions. Similarly, it occurs in all economic groupings, and again in about the same percentages as for the whole number. To sum it up, general paresis, like syphilis, is no respecter of persons, age, sex, education, vocation, or economic status.

Since about one fourth of the patients are of "dependent" economic status and another two thirds are of "marginal" level, the problems presented to the social worker may be phrased by patient or family in terms of economic need rather than in terms of disease. The usual picture, however, is that of a man from thirty-five to forty-five years of age who has undergone a relatively rapid alteration in personality characteristics, without visible external cause or any manifestations of an acute or chronic physical disease.

The earliest clinical symptoms are likely to be in terms of sharp changes in personal habits and in social relationships. Thus, the behavior of the individual may become extravagant in many ways; there is an expansive feeling of well-being called euphoria and he has ideas of grandeur which lead to wild claims of power and wealth. Though there is great motor activity, he accomplishes little. A person of previous reasonably frugal habits may become a spendthrift and very quickly dissipate the savings of a lifetime on trivial inconsequentials or in inane speculation. Changes in habits and language occur, showing both dilapidation and coarsening. Sexual activity, especially promiscuity, may greatly increase; arrant alcoholism may develop. Physical signs, such as tremor, especially of the facial muscles, speech defect, or handwriting defect, may precede or follow the outbreak of socially disturbing behavior. These symptoms are ordinarily overlooked, unless a physician is consulted, and the patient may feel so well that he is not aware of any occasion to call on a physician.

Disturbance in the ability to calculate may be an early sign of the disease, as it is certain to be later. One of my patients first sought help because he found it impossible to strike a correct trial balance. The gravity of his condition was not, however, appreciated by his physician or by his family until he had dissipated his small fortune of some $60,000 in wild stock market speculations and foolish and unnecessary purchases. Later, while receiving intensive salvarsan therapy, he became hallucinated, talked with God, and developed the delusion that he was Christ. He was one of very few otherwise typical paretics in whom I have ever seen such developments.

This, briefly illustrated, is one type of paretic, the grandiose, or expansive. Such an individual is happy, though irritable; he is full of delusions of grandeur, many of which are bizarre; he is overactive and talkative. He may decide he is some noted person, a king or all-powerful, while still good-naturedly doing menial work on the ward. One patient claimed to have a miraculous telescope with which he could see for twenty miles, and a rifle which would hit any chosen target regardless of the direction in which it was aimed. He offered the physician a solid gold suit of clothes and a million dollars for release from the hospital, but he good-naturedly accepted the doctor's refusal to release him until he was able to make the fantastic payment. Logically enough, the patient said he could not make the payment until he was out, but at the same time made no effort to use his miraculous rifle to attain his ends and cheerfully accepted his incarceration.

Episodes of excitement and violence occur and may be very

difficult to deal with. In fact, in a small group of cases, often with sudden onset, extreme excitement develops, and the course from onset of recognizable symptoms to death is short.

This expansive type was long regarded as the classical syndrome of general paresis, probably because it is the most spectacular. But states of depression or anxiety, with hypochondriacal or self-accusatory delusions, also occur. In the early stage these patients give the impression of being more deteriorated than do the grandiose patients at a similar stage of progression, probably because of their slowness, their paucity of speech, and the narrow range of activity. Suicidal attempts may occur, and there may be intercurrent episodes of excitement and violence. Hallucinations, while not common, may appear. When a depressed state is marked from the beginning of symptoms, the course is believed to be shorter than usual.

Actually, the most common clinical picture is that of a progressive dementia. In fact, whatever the state of activity and whatever the mood, the only definitely characteristic mental symptoms in general paresis are those of intellectual deterioration. Forgetfulness, loss of recent and remote memory, defective judgment and reasoning, and loss of ability to calculate are present early in the clinical picture. These become increasingly marked as the disease progresses, until the patient becomes disoriented for time and place and even unable to respond. Characteristic also is the patient's indifference to the effects of his behavior upon other people. As previously noted, this behavior may be greatly coarsened and flagrantly delinquent or even criminal. To the layman this deterioration in morals is often the most conspicuous sign. It may lead to condemnation on moral, ethical, or legal grounds rather than to recognition that a state of disease is present and responsible for the altered conduct and standards of social relationships.

General paresis, then, is a disease in which the diagnosis rests ultimately upon the results of laboratory tests; but there are such characteristic physical signs attendant that the diagnosis cannot be missed when they are present in typical combinations. The mental symptoms are the least clear-cut of all. Indeed, most of them occur in disorders having other causation, though not in the same constellations. Progressive deterioration in the intellectual faculties constitutes the central core of the mental changes in paresis. In the brain, the frontal lobes (regarded as the areas primarily concerned with intelligence, association, memory, and judgment) show the greatest atrophy and hardening (as a result of gliosis). This is an interesting point, since one of the common lay names for general paresis in the past was "softening of the brain." It is of interest in passing to note that not all apparently expansive ideas of the paretic are *ipso facto* delusions. For example, patients may assert that they are the best persons at their particular work or have the highest of reputations. This may turn out to be true, but only for their past performances.

The course of general paresis, if untreated, is generally quite rapid, and death usually ensues within two to five years of the outbreak of clinical symptoms. While death may be due to some intercurrent disease, such as pneumonia or other infections, trauma, or other processes, it is actually due to general exhaustion from the paretic process in about 75 percent of the cases. During the course of the disease the patient may pass through one or several cycles of increase in weight, followed by loss of weight and increasing weakness and inco-ordination. Such severe generalized tremor may develop that the patient becomes bed-ridden, incoherent, has difficulty in swallowing, is incontinent or retentive of urine and feces. In such a stage he may die, or a remission may develop even when death seems imminent. He may then gain weight and show reduction in tremor and speech defect, be out of bed and able to feed himself. If convulsions occur in the stage of rapid decline, death usually results.

More remarkable, however, is the fact that in about 10 percent of untreated cases a fairly complete to a remarkably complete remission of symptoms occurs, and the patient may for a longer or shorter time be able to resume life adequately outside an institution. It was observed that paretics who had erysipelas, formerly one of the scourges of mental hospitals, and recovered from it were more likely to have such remissions. It was this which led Warner von Jauregg to seek a fever-producing organism that could be controlled. Various types of infective agents were tried but were too dangerous. Malaria was finally chosen, and the results were definitely encouraging. The discovery that the induced high temperatures were the essential elements in therapy led to the development of methods for electrically inducing high fever which could be controlled at will and did not involve the introduction of another disease. Fever therapy, often supplemented by therapy with arsenicals, mercurials, bismuth, or penicillin, has resulted in a several-fold increase in the rate of remissions. Whether the remission is spontaneous or induced by treatment, there is always the possibility of relapse. Treatment should be undertaken at the earliest possible moment in the course of the disease, when many symptoms are dependent on reversible changes in the nervous tissues.

The social worker serving the family of a paretic must never forget, as an important item of responsibility, that the family of a paretic is the family of a syphilitic. Hence the spouse and all the children should be examined and have at least blood Wassermann tests. The wife and all the children may be syphilitic, or none may be. The children of paretic women will show signs of congenital syphilis in the majority of cases, though the husband may escape infection. Rare cases of conjugal paresis have been described. One woman, who later developed nonparetic neurosyphilis, bore twin boys who were regarded as identical twins. From the early photographs they certainly appeared to be identical, but a few years later developed a marked divergence in appearance. One boy showed the typical facial appearance of the congenital syphilitic; the other did not. At age sixteen the latter boy developed an unusual type of episodic psychosis, never precisely diagnosed, but there was no clinical or laboratory evidence of neurosyphilis. Provocative doses of salvarsan left both blood and spinal fluid examinations still quite normal. Such an unusual situation merely emphasizes the need for careful examination of all members of the family of all syphilitics, including those of paretics.

In tabes dorsalis, as already mentioned, there is degeneration of the posterior columns of the spinal cord. These tracts contain the nerve fibers which carry the sensory impulses derived especially from the muscles, bones, and joints. Degeneration of these fibers leads to a loss of deep sensibility, atrophy, loss of tone of muscles, and a characteristic disorder of gait. These patients need to look at the ground when walking, and in later stages may be unable to walk at all. The gait is characterized by a wide base, with a peculiar slapping forward and down of the feet.

In some cases there are symptoms of general paresis, occurring at any time from the onset of tabetic symptoms to late in the course of the ataxia. Hallucinations, especially in the visual field, are likely to occur, since the optic nerve is usually involved in a primary atrophic process; blindness usually supervenes. Where both the tabetic and the paretic processes are present, the condition is called tabo-paresis.

Juvenile Paresis

This is a disorder of the young child, up to adolescence, and is nearly always the result of congenital syphilis. Sometimes development is inhibited, and if convulsions are present the diagnosis may be obscure. However, there may be a history of normal development during several years, and then the appearance of deterioration, excitement, and perhaps delusions will mark the onset of paresis. Neurological and serological study will show the true nature of the disturbance in functions. Trophic changes are common and may be extreme. One case of congenital syphilis known to me assumed first the clinical picture of tabes, with all the relaxation of muscles and joints which that disease of the spinal cord brings about. The boy was trained as a contortionist for his family's small street carnival. At about the age of twelve his knee joints began to swell, and the ends of the bones enlarged, the typical Charcot joints. He became progressively weaker and more ataxic and developed a psychosis characterized by hallucinations and a type of fabricating pseudodelirium more commonly seen in toxic psychoses.

Cerebral Syphilis: Meningo-Vascular Neurosyphilis

A major clinical contrast between cerebral syphilis and general paresis is the focal and episodic nature of symptoms in the former. Thus, paralysis involving individual nerves, for example, those supplying the eye muscles, are common in cerebral syphilis. So are transitory periods of dizziness, confusion and disorientation, amnesia, delirium, and even coma. Brain hemorrhage occurs, with resulting spastic paralysis, perhaps hemiplegia, which is a stiff paralysis of one side of the body. The clinical signs and symptoms may change with considerable rapidity, or, depending on the nature of the lesion, they may be fixed. Headaches and blurring of vision are related to increased intracranial pressure. With single or multiple gummata, the classical signs of brain tumor—headache, blurring of vision due to optic neuritis, and projectile vomiting—may be present.

As already noted, meningo-vascular neurosyphilis tends to develop rather early in the course of general syphilis. This type of neurosyphilis yields fairly easily to intensive chemotherapy, especially tryparsamide and to penicillin, but fever therapy is not generally as effective as it is in paresis. However, in any case of syphilis which does not yield readily to other therapy there is a tendency to use fever treatment.

The differentiation of general paresis and cerebral syphilis is not always easy, either clinically or serologically. States of excitement occur in both, and even with well-marked disease of the blood vessels the symptoms may be of general cerebral disturbance, rather than focal. Apparently only the most marked meningo-vascular cases, or perhaps only those most resistive to treatment, reach the mental hospitals. In any case, the admission and discharge rates for all forms of cerebral syphilis are only about one fifth as great as those for paresis. Furthermore, 23.5 percent of cerebral syphilis cases were discharged as recovered, and another 71.5 percent as much improved and improved, leaving 4.7 percent as unimproved. The corresponding figures for 426 cases of paresis were 18 percent, 74.9 percent, and 7.2 percent, respectively.

Paranoid State

One of the interesting and complex pictures occasionally found in neurosyphilis is a typical paranoid psychosis, which may be mistaken for a schizophrenic or other etiological type of paranoid condition. From the clinical standpoint the neurosyphilitic paranoid state tends to be characterized by numerous and vivid auditory hallucinations, often accusing the patient of delinquency and immorality, and by a marked emotional response which fits the character of the hallucinations and delusions. The latter are profuse and are most likely to be depressive, fear-producing, and persecutory in content, again in line with the threatening and accusing hallucinations.

Focal or other signs of the organic process in the central nervous system may be very slow in appearing, though these patients may have had occasional convulsions for a number of years prior to the development of focal signs. Occasionally cases are seen in which the disease runs a very rapid course, and death occurs in a few weeks or months in spite of treatment. Such cases usually show at autopsy a very marked meningitis, often with thromboses in the meningeal veins.

Unless these cases are studied serologically, the presence of neurosyphilis may not be suspected from the history or the physical signs. Psychiatric symptoms of intellectual deterioration, so characteristic in neurosyphilis, may not be present for a long period, or at least not obvious. Under such circumstances the case is likely to be classed as schizophrenia. Serological examination of blood and spinal fluid will usually clear up the diagnosis. These cases, in my experience, are quite refractory to chemotherapy. The course tends to be long, and characteristic focal symptoms of cerebral syphilis appear late. Thus, tabes, blindness, aphasia, intellectual deterioration, hemiplegia, paraplegia, and other signs may only appear after the paranoid state has endured for some years.

Comment

General systemic syphilis may occur in persons suffering from mental disturbances not due to syphilis. The further course of infection, with special reference to the development of neurosyphilis, is probably more related to the extent and effectiveness of treatment than to the existence of a mental disorder.

Congenital syphilis with involvement of the nervous system is found to be a causative factor in a small percentage of the feebleminded. General syphilis, as shown by positive Wassermann or other tests of the blood, occurs with somewhat greater frequency, but the significance of such systemic infection in relation to the feeblemindedness is obscure. Syphilis in more remote ancestry has been speculatively considered as a cause of feeblemindedness through degenerative effects on the germ plasm. The same views have been expressed with respect to alcoholism, but in this case experimental work has not verified the hypothesis. There is little or no direct evidence to support such a view with regard to syphilis.

Syphilis enters into one type of neurosis, the so-called syphilophobia, since the content of the patient's fear is that he has or may acquire syphilis. Actual infection is not, of course, present, and the real problems are related to guilt and anxiety. The treatment is the same as that outlined in the section dealing with phobias.

PSYCHOSES WITH ORGANIC BRAIN DISEASE

These psychoses have a symptomatology characterized primarily by disturbances in the general field of the intellect, such as amnesia, deterioration of judgment and reasoning powers, all combining as dementia. To these may be added loss of emotional control. There are usually neurological signs indicating the organic nature of the disease process and often the affected area in the nervous system. The largest number of cases fall into the arteriosclerotic group.

In general, these disorders present problems for medical and surgical treatment. By the time they reach the psychotic stage, if indeed they do, the cases demand hospital treatment. There are, of course, many more cases of these organic types of neurological disease than ever develop psychoses. Those who do develop psychoses have a longer or shorter prodromal period during which neurological and mental symptoms develop. It is in this period that the social worker may most often be called upon and may be of the greatest service in recognizing the origin in disease of various symptoms of social maladaptation. The worker may then guide client and family to proper medical care. Assistance may be necessary in several directions, especially since organic cases tend to occur in later life and the patients frequently have responsibilities which their illness makes impossible to continue. Economic problems may then arise, or, if a dominant personality is stricken, other members of the family may not be able to assume the necessary responsibility for decisions.

A great deal of supportive activity, both personal and economic, may therefore be necessary from the social worker. A knowledge of specialized resources for particular types of organic cases, such as neurosurgery, is also of value. But one of the most important functions of the social worker when these conditions are prominent is to see that competent medical attention is secured.

Psychoses with Cerebral Arteriosclerosis

These disorders stand next to schizophrenia among causes for admission to mental hospitals and account for 16.0 percent of admissions with psychoses to all state hospitals in the country in 1945. In New York State the admission rate per 100,000 population increased from 1.8 in 1912 to 20.4 in 1945, while the percentage of arteriosclerotics among first admissions increased from 2.9 to 22.8. These were the largest relative increases reported for any group of psychoses. The death rate in these conditions is also high. Approximately 62 percent of the deaths occur within a year after admission; 22 percent within the first month.

The marked increase in incidence of the arteriosclerotic disorders correlates with the longer duration of life and consequent greater likelihood of the development of arteriosclerosis. Approximately 10 percent of the population of the country was sixty years of age and over in 1940, the preponderance of women becoming more marked in successive semidecades beginning with age sixty-five. This means that there were approximately 13,800,000 people in these age groups. The total admissions to all state hospitals in 1937 of patients age sixty and over with psychosis, some 17,255, represents less than .2 percent of those of presumed arteriosclerotic age. However, 25 percent of nearly 70,000 first admissions with psychoses to all the state hospitals were sixty years of age and over, as were 80 percent of the New York first admissions of arteriosclerotic psychoses.

The average duration of hospital life of the arteriosclerotics who died in hospital was 1.5 years, the shortest of all the groups. By comparison, the average duration òf hospital life of schizophrenics was 17.6 years. Another useful contrast is in the number of deaths per 1,000 cases of the same disorder under treatment. For schizophrenia this rate was 25.3; for the arteriosclerotics, 237.4.

It is clear that the arteriosclerotic psychoses present a serious problem to the mental hospitals. Aside from high admission and death rates, with relatively short hospital residence, another point is of great importance with reference to the care of such patients. This is the factor of physical disability, which is so great that a high proportion of these cases require bed care and an unusual amount of nursing. To a large extent this also explains the considerable increase in the number of infirmary beds and buildings which have become necessary in mental hospitals.

Arteriosclerosis is a generalized disease of the arteries, which may differentially affect the nervous system or secondarily affect it in ways to be discussed later. In the arteriosclerotic psychoses, as well

as in organic nervous disorders without psychosis due to arteriosclerosis, the outstanding feature of the clinical picture is the
episodic character of the manifestations. This is true up to fairly
advanced stages of dementia, which is characteristically in the
intellectual field.

Thus, in cerebral arteriosclerosis so-called "strokes" occur, with
one of several results: death, permanent paralysis with or without
mental symptoms, or comparatively complete recovery. Similar
episodes, but without paralysis, occur as periods of confusion, often
with aphasia, vertigo, ringing in the ears, and similar symptoms. In
early stages of the disorder such episodes usually clear up fairly
completely, often with some degree of amnesia. Death may occur
in such episodes, or dementia may supervene. As more episodes
occur, a variable amount of dementia is sure to develop. Death is
usually due to "disorders of the circulatory system," though various
infections, particularly respiratory diseases, may be the terminal
factor.

The blood pressure is not necessarily especially high in these
psychoses. In many cases there is little or no evidence of peripheral
arteriosclerosis, while both clinical and laboratory evidence of
marked cerebral arteriosclerosis may be very definite. The converse of this is also in general true; that is, there may be marked
evidence of peripheral arteriosclerosis, with little or no evidence
of sclerosis of the cerebral vessels.

The clinical picture may therefore be summed up as one in which
episodes of dizziness and confusion, patchy amnesia becoming
more and more complete, deterioration, various organic nervous
affections, such as paralysis of one side of the body, motor or
sensory aphasia, and apoplectic strokes all may occur in a variety of
combinations. Treatment is primarily medical and, in general, is not
too successful once mental symptoms appear. A moderate degree
of general sclerosis is common in later life; the number of persons
who have the disorder, with or without general symptoms, is
certainly vastly greater than the number who develop neurological
or mental symptoms. Forgetfulness, loquacity, and a tendency to

live in the past are general characteristics of old age. If there is some patchy memory defect, perhaps uncontrolled and unstimulated short outbursts of laughter and weeping, together with any other evidences of episodes of the nature described above, an arteriosclerotic brain condition may be suspected.

The chief differential diagnostic problem is to distinguish the senile psychoses. This problem is further discussed in connection with the latter group. Various clinical and laboratory examinations, together with the history of onset and development, are usually sufficient to clear up this question. Syphilitic nervous diseases must also be differentiated. For the social worker, the chief issues are to remember the episodic character of the manifestations occurring after age fifty, especially after sixty, and that fatal cerebral hemorrhages are common and may occur at almost any time in the course of arteriosclerotic disorders. The family should be prepared accordingly, once the diagnosis has been made. The patient may become very much disturbed, suddenly and at almost any time. Finally, for safety and for the best possible care patients should be hospitalized as soon as any symptoms of a psychosis appear.

Traumatic Conditions

Despite a tendency on the part of many, especially parents, to overemphasize the importance of falling on the head or other types of head injury, it is striking that psychoses due to head and therefore cerebral trauma are really very rare—only about one half of one percent of admissions to state hospitals in peacetime. In fact, the vast majority of people suffering head trauma show no sequelae. For symptoms to continue or to increase after recovery from the immediate shock, it is necessary that the head injury be severe, with lacerations and destruction of cerebral cortex, or that there be permanent pressure from a depressed fracture or an organized blood clot. In many instances some type of operative procedure, such as decompression, elevation of depressed bone, removal of splinters, or hemorrhagic clot, is necessary in the period immediately following the accident. Results may be excellent to poor, depending upon the nature, extent, and location of the traumatic lesions. This phase of diagnosis will not be discussed here.

The so-called post-traumatic mental states have usually been described under three heads: post-traumatic constitution, dementia, and confusional states. Post-traumatic states severe enough to produce recognizable changes in personality usually have one characteristic in common, viz., an amnesia for a variable period of time prior to the accident. This may be for only a few hours, or it may extend back for several weeks or even several months. The post-traumatic constitution presents many characteristics of the psychopathic personality, but in this instance the changes are related to a definite organic lesion. Forgetfulness, impaired concentration, fatigability, social irresponsibility, irritability, with violent temper outbursts, lowered moral standards, and loss of or indifference to goals are among the traits common to these cases. An outstanding characteristic is such a heightened reaction to alcohol that very small amounts produce a severe intoxication, even to the extent of automatic activity or violent outbursts with subsequent amnesia. This is similar to the reaction in pathological intoxication, to be discussed later, which has no known organic basis.

A few cases have been seen in which there are widely separated psychotic episodes, sometimes with typical symptomatology of other psychoses, such as paranoid states. The episodes may clear up in a comparatively short time, with amnesia for the psychotic period as the clinical characteristic distinguishing the traumatic origin of the condition. It should be pointed out that similar episodes, with varying symptomatology and later amnesia, occur from other causes, particularly hysteria, which is a functional disorder.

Convulsive states occasionally follow head trauma. In some of these cases, due to pressure, operative procedures may relieve the condition. In others, where the lesions are cortical or subcortical, operation is ordinarily of no avail.

More usually there are either episodes or prolonged periods of confusion and overactivity, often with hallucinations and scattered delusions. These may clear up after a time, or they may go on into the most common of the post-traumatic psychotic conditions, a dementia involving primarily the intellectual processes. According to the severity of the lesions, the deterioration may be slight to great. There may be various types of neurological impairment as well.

It is clear that the problems involved in dealing with these traumatic conditions are medical and surgical. Many victims who are not instantly killed die within a short time. In cases of partial recovery, problems of employment re-education, and social supervision do arise. These needs were tremendously magnified among returning wounded soldiers. The principles involved in dealing with such conditions are the same as those applicable to other psychotic or neurological conditions where rehabilitation is attempted. These principles are discussed in another section.

Psychoses with Brain Tumor

Psychoses associated with or due to brain tumor are extremely rare among admissions to mental hospitals; they comprise less than two tenths of one percent of all first admissions. Undoubtedly many, if not all, cases of tumor of the brain, whether primary or secondarily developed by dissemination or metastasis from tumors originally located elsewhere, develop mental symptoms of one sort or another. Mortality in brain tumor is high, and the mental symptoms may play a very minor part. Operative interference may be successful and may bring relief from mental symptoms along with other improvement.

Aside from localizing clinical signs and laboratory studies, the cardinal symptoms of brain tumor are headache, with blurring of vision, optic neuritis, and projectile vomiting. The great developments in brain surgery within this century have facilitated early diagnosis. It is not, however, especially likely that the social worker can do more than see that such obviously ill persons receive medical attention or the kind of after-care social work the doctor decides the patient can use.

Epidemic Encephalitis

The acute phase of epidemic encephalitis is dramatic in symptomatology, and in typical cases is not difficult to diagnose. The disorder has been intensively studied since its first recognition in epidemic form in this country in 1918. Commonly known as "sleeping sickness," it occurs sporadically throughout the country, but there have been no large epidemics recently. In the early phases the mortality is comparatively high.

The acute symptomatology is quite varied. Most commonly there is excessive sleeping, from which the patient may be roused for short periods. There may be marked insomnia, or the normal sleep rhythm may be reversed. Confusion, amnesia, hallucinosis, chiefly visual, and excitement may occur. It will be noted that these are, in general, signs of delirium. In securing histories of individuals in later life, it is essential to inquire for the various symptoms of encephalitis if unexplained temperatures or somnolence are reported as having occurred in the early years.

For present purposes it is the so-called postencephalitic disorders which engage attention. These are really chronic, mildly progressive developments after the acute state has subsided. In adults the most common after effects are the development of the syndrome of paralysis agitans, often with confusion and some signs of deterioration. That the incapacitation symptoms are usually physical rather than mental is shown by the very small number of patients with psychoses due to encephalitis admitted to mental hospitals.

A few hospitals in the country have provided special wards for children with behavior disorders following epidemic encephalitis. Many encephalitic children have been cared for at home, with or without the benefit of clinical or social service supervision. Many are also continued in public school, unless their behavior becomes too troublesome. Especially in the early days, many were committed to correctional schools, where the more disturbed cases presented serious problems to the authorities and to the other inmates.

It must be emphasized that in general the pathological process in the nervous system is a chronic one, though it may not be progressive, or only slowly so. This applies to the cases in which the process is not completely resolved, that is, does not disappear. Many cases do apparently recover completely, without sequelae of any kind and without further attacks. However, the number is small by comparison with those who die in the acute phase and those who present alterations in neurological status and behavior.

The behavior disorders associated with epidemic encephalitis have certain outstanding characteristics. They are explosive in quality, and the reaction is total in the sense that it seems to involve the entire organism in an outburst characterized by an almost total lack of inhibitions. Irritability is great, and a minor stimulus will set off a major outburst of temper, an active assault, or a flight reaction. The organism as a whole seems to revert to an all or none type of reaction; that is, the graduation or partialization of response to stimulus which characterizes normal human development seems to disappear. Stealing and lying, often of the pathological type, occur. Ethical standards, which may have been well developed, are lowered or even seem to disappear entirely. Behavior becomes extremely egocentric and hedonistic; lack of consideration for others is outstanding. Sexual activity may be excessive and promiscuous or perverse.

No dementing process has been observed in this disease, in which the chronic lesions are found chiefly in brain areas that do not have to do with the intellect, but it is a frequent finding in children that intellectual development ceases at or about the level reached at the time of the acute attack. A shortened attention span and inability to concentrate are common in the chronic phase, as are general restlessness and talkativeness. Many patients are sullen and morose, or the mood may be very unstable. The children are impulsive to an extreme degree, exhibitionistic and carefree, unless angry. They may be quite suggestible, or, on the contrary, may present a considerable degree of negative suggestibility.

The behavior symptoms may be complicated by organic nervous symptoms. These tend to follow the lines of Parkinson's syndrome, or paralysis agitans. In this disorder there are characteristic tremors of head and hands, a mask-like expression of the face, and disturbance of gait. The tremor of the head is a side-to-side shaking combined with a fine nodding. The most characteristic point about the hand tremor is the way the thumb and first finger tremble in a sort of rubbing fashion, which leads to the name of pill rolling tremor. The gait, in extreme cases, becomes a running one, with torso held forward, even to the extent of being practically parallel with the sidewalk. In earlier stages a visible effort of the entire body is evident as the patient pushes himself forward.

The paralysis is spastic, that is, stiff, and complicated by the tremors. All parts of the body may be involved—face, jaws, hands, arms, legs. A patient in such a state is pitiful to behold. One young man of 23, in a prison hospital, had been committed to prison for stealing $25 to see a doctor who, so the young man had been told, could cure him. He was a helpless, tremulous, spastic paralytic, with jaws hanging open, unable to walk, to feed himself, or to care for his personal needs. Another case, an adolescent with generalized tremors and spasticity, but able to walk, was a constant source of trouble to the school authorities, an object of derision to his schoolmates, an annoyance to his family, and sullen and unhappy. One small girl had, in addition to much impulsive, restless, sexual behavior, a disorder of the respiratory rhythm which involved the entire body in part of the cycle. She could sleep only in a standing position, propped in the corner of a high-walled crib. Cases such as these are obviously in need of hospital care.

In general, hospitalization is rather difficult to arrange because of lack of facilities for the care of such children. It may be necessary to try to arrange admission to a state hospital for mental diseases either by regular commitment or on application of the parents. Neither of these can be arranged where no special laws govern the admission of such cases, unless the courts and hospitals are co-operative, since these patients are usually not psychotic in the ordinary sense of that term. Since few mental hospitals have wards or sections for children, there is need for special consideration from courts and hospitals.

In addition to the danger of personal attacks from these patients, much antisocial behavior occurs. For example, one fourteen-year-old boy would rush out and steal the first available automobile whenever he became angry at home, and go racing through the city streets until he incurred an accident or was arrested for speeding. After this had occurred some half dozen times it was possible to make it clear that, even though not insane in the sense used in criminal law, which is the ability to distinguish between right and wrong, the boy was not responsible for his acts because of an organic brain disease. On the basis of this argument he was committed to a mental hospital indefinitely rather than to a correctional institution for a limited time.* The mental hospital staff does have methods for dealing with the outbursts of individuals which are definitely superior to those used in the average correctional institution. Even today correctional institutions usually rely upon punishment, called discipline, rather than upon clinical understanding and individualized guidance within the limits of its facilities.

If the child is being cared for at home and attending a public school, the family may need assistance in supervision, and the child may need treatment in either a medical or a guidance clinic. Social service is therefore important in the care of such cases.

Depression with suicidal attempts, maniacal states, and paranoid states occasionally occur in association with encephalitis, especially in adults. Only 14 percent of psychotic patients with encephalitis in all state hospitals in 1937 were under age twenty.

Other Forms of Encephalitis and Meningitis

Encephalitis sometimes occurs as a complication of poliomyelitis, or so-called infantile paralysis. In such cases behavior disturbances

---

* It is at least of minor interest to note that following this commitment the state in question provided special wards for such children in the hospital to which this boy was committed.

as well as the characteristic atrophic type of paralysis occur. Also, just as the spinal cord lesions result in a stoppage of growth and development of the affected limb, so the cerebral lesions commonly result in stoppage of intellectual and emotional development at the stage where it is when the disease attacks. The result is a relative acquired intellectual inferiority, perhaps even mental deficiency and psychopathic types of behavior similar to those described in the preceding section. Psychoses may occur in adult cases, or there may be few or no permanent mental symptoms. Similar conditions occur as the result of severe meningitis, where the cortex is considerably involved in a scarring process.

The important point is that these changes in personality and behavior are caused by irreversible losses of nerve cells. Therefore the changes are permanent and influenceable by psychotherapy only to a limited extent. For children, prolonged and individualized training in habits and social relationships represents the best approach to the problems involved.

The nervous system is directly attacked by a number of infections which may be confined to the meninges, or may invade the nervous tissue itself, resulting in a brain abscess. The most common direct infections are caused by a specific meningitis organism, and other types are produced by such diverse microbes as the typhoid bacillus, pneumococcus, gonococcus, other pus-producing organisms, and the tubercle bacillus. The treatment for such infections, obviously, must be directed against the infecting organism. Tuberculous meningitis, unless it involves an isolated tubercle which can be removed by surgery has almost invariably had a fatal result.

In all these cases the mental symptoms are typically delirium and coma. However, in some cases of tubercular meningitis a paranoid state with relatively clear consciousness occurs. Auditory hallucinations are especially threatening in content, and the patients exhibit marked fear reactions together with the depression. Patients attribute both the fear and the depression to the content of their hallucinations.

Degenerative Disorders

Of these, only two will be briefly described. *Paralysis agitans* as ordinarily found, in contrast to that following epidemic encephalitis, is a disorder which develops gradually, without an antecedent acute stage of disease. The neurological characteristics are the same as those already described—the typical tremors of head and hands, mask-like facies, propulsive gait, changes in handwriting. Symptom development may be arrested for long periods; in fact, tremors of head and hands may be the only symptoms for a long time, with little impairment of general functional efficiency. Mental symptoms are comparatively rare. Occasionally paranoid or depressed reactions are found, but it is not clear just how and to what extent these are related to the neurological disorder. Some apparent, perhaps more apparent than real, intellectual deterioration does occur in terminal phases. However, the fact remains that few such cases are admitted to mental hospitals.

Huntington's chorea is an interesting, though not very common, familial disorder which usually develops between the ages of thirty-five and forty-five. Marked choreiform movements and dementia of considerable degree develop fairly rapidly. While the disorder may then remain comparatively stationary for several months to a year or so, the total duration, once symptoms begin to evolve, is not long, ordinarily not more than two or three years. It was first described in some families in West Virginia by Huntington, is of unknown origin, and no effective treatment has been found. Apparently the disorder belongs to a group of hereditary, at least familial, degenerative processes in the nervous system. Another example is familial degeneration of the auditory nerve.

General Comment

The essential characteristic of all these organic disorders is their ultimate irreversibility and permanent loss of nerve cells. If the loss is small, or fairly well circumscribed, resulting disturbances in function may be slight or focal. Treatment, if any, is medical or surgical. In certain cases, when the pathological process has ceased and the extent of personality and other handicaps has become clear, re-educational and rehabilitative measures may become important. Social supervision, interpretation to families of the causal connection between disease process and personality change, training opportunities, and clinical supervision—one or more of these will be important in the individual cases, especially for children.

For adults, hospital care is usually indicated at some stage. In all too many cases is consent only given when the case has reached a terminal stage and after family emotions and finances have suffered seriously. It is here that the social worker may play a valuable role in conserving family integrity and resources; the patient, too, can be helped by stressing the need for early and appropriate treatment, hospitalization, or use of special community resources. In general, it is clear that these are problems for which medical treatment is the most important element.

SENILE PSYCHOSES

The essential feature of the senile psychoses is intellectual deterioration, a dementia characterized by an amnesia for recent events which gradually extends farther and farther back through the life span.

A tendency to "live in the past" is fairly characteristic of old age. Reminiscing, often very detailed and so circumstantial that auditors may have trouble in following the story, has led to a semifacetious dubbing of this period as "anecdotage." In later life a generalized process of involution or devolution usually occurs, affecting physical structure, physiological functioning, and mental operations. The period of old age is variably defined by workers in the field of geriatrics. Common observation shows that there are people who show signs of senile change as early as age forty, while others at seventy or seventy-five show few or no signs of their age. These phenomena are related to such issues as previous disease, endocrine gland functioning and other factors, but not enough is known to lay down a program which will universally either defer senescence or soften its ravages once they begin. The processes start earlier, but we are accustomed to think of old age as beginning at sixty or sixty-five. Retirement policies in public services and industry based on age vary; in different instances the retirement age is sixty, sixty-three, sixty-five, or seventy years.

Senile anatomical changes involve loss of tissue substance, and therefore there is usually loss of weight and height. The latter occurs primarily because of resorption in the vertebrae, with consequent shortening of the spine. Loss of weight leads to wrinkling and cording. All these changes lead to the inelegant terms commonly applied to the old or elderly, such as little and shriveled. Physiological changes involve lessened activity in many ways, including diminished vital force and the need for less sleep. The factor of safety which represents the surplus functional capacity of the organs and organ systems is reduced. There is pathological evidence of differential atrophy in the various organ systems in cases presenting various diseases in this age period. For example, in cases which develop senile dementia there is a greater atrophy in the central nervous system than in cases which do not.

The relative incidence of senile dementia, as measured by first admissions to mental hospitals, has remained about the same through the last several decades (9–10% of first admissions). The number per 100,000 of the general population has also remained about the same. There are numerically more males than females, just as psychotic males (all psychoses) outnumber females. However, the percentage of cases of senile dementia is somewhat higher among female first admissions than among males. About 75 percent of more than 6,000 individuals of both sexes were seventy years of age and over at the time of first admission to hospitals, and 95 percent were sixty years and over. More than half the patients who die in institutions do so within the first year of residence. Only about 14 percent live five or more years in the hospital (figures based on 5,779 deaths of senile dementia cases). The death rate is proportionately very much higher among males during the first hospital year, while a higher proportion of females live five years or more. No valid explanation for these differences between the sexes has been advanced.

The typical case of senile dementia shows little or no clinical evidence of arteriosclerosis. While heart disease is the most common cause of death (51% of 1,052 deaths), arteriosclerosis runs second (35%). The most frequent heart disorder is myocarditis, which is perhaps the least definite of all heart disorders in terms of symptoms and pathological changes. These points are made merely to emphasize the fact that the changes in senile dementia seem primarily due to the processes of aging.

The mental symptoms of senile dementia include more than the typical amnesia previously mentioned. Patients become disoriented for time and place, and this disorientation is extreme. Though there be snow on the ground, they call the month June; immediately after a meal, a patient will complain he has had no food that day, or that he is being starved. Such patients have a tendency to turn night into day, as their need for sleep becomes lessened. They will state their age as many years less than it actually is, and the year is frequently given correctly for the claimed age. It has repeatedly been noted that the life story as given is reasonably correct for the span of life set up by the patient as the one reached.

One complication of considerable social importance is the tendency of many seniles to develop ideas of persecution, especially directed toward members of the family. It is often true that seniles are not too well treated by their families, partly because they can be trying in so many ways and partly due to the fact that the old may be an economic burden. However, when there are actual delusions of persecution, the fact of their fictitious character becomes obvious sooner or later.

Senile dementia cases wander away from home and often pose problems for social agencies in communities other than the one in which they live. They have a tendency to set fires in such inappropriate places as hallways or the parlor floor. This might be interpreted as a reversion to childhood interest in fire, but when it can be discussed with the patient it is usually found that he felt cold and started a fire for warmth. In other words, there seems to be no evidence of pyromania, but a lack of judgment as to appropriate places for fires.

The senile process itself is not reversible. Ultimately, dementia is severe; patients become bedridden and often sink into prolonged coma before death. But one point must be remembered: old people may have recoverable psychoses of other types, such as a manic depressive attack or a delirium because of a toxic infectious process. If the origin is detected and successfully treated, complete recovery without signs of actual dementia can and does occur.

The senescent period is one which often presents medico-legal complications, with special reference to the making and probating of wills. Many suits to break wills are based on allegations of senile dementia in the deceased testator. Testimony by psychiatrists in such cases can only be based on hypothetical questions. This has led to many unjust accusations regarding the integrity of psychiatrists who testify as expert witnesses in such cases. The fact is that hypothetical questions are built by lawyers on opposite sides of a law suit, and materials are selected which tend to prove their respective points. I have seen many hypothetical questions to which the only possible answer could be one that supported the lawyer's contention because of the way in which the question was posed.

Recently a fairly large number of old people are having psychiatric examinations and reports on their mental status before making their wills. This usually occurs when the lawyer or the testator expects there will be a contest to break the will because of some already developed animosities in the family.*

About six thousand people are admitted each year to state hospitals for the first time as cases of senile dementia. The admissions are, as previously noted, predominantly in the age group seventy

---

* The first such case I personally examined was in 1922. A daughter twice tried to have her mother declared incompetent. The daughter was very hostile to both mother and brother, the latter being on good terms with the mother. The will was especially to favor the child of the brother. The old lady was quite normal. The psychiatric report on her mental adequacy prevented two later law suits, one regarding incompetency and the other to break the will.

and over. The percentage rises somewhat in later years, but even so, never reaches a very high percentage or a very high ratio per 100,000 of the same age group. For instance, with a population somewhat in excess of five million who are seventy years of age and over, about 4,500 are admitted in a year to all the state hospitals. These points are brought out because they so sharply emphasize the fact that problems of old age are not primarily problems of gross mental disorder. Even in the oldest groups the percentage who become sufficiently disturbed mentally to require hospital residence is still low. If we combine the arteriosclerotics and seniles of all ages, the incidence per 100,000 of the population is approximately what it is for schizophrenia.

These points have a bearing upon the development of geriatrics, the study and treatment of elderly people, which has lately been devoting more and more attention to the psychological and vocational problems of this group. The outstanding physical disorders of the period are cardiovascular and kidney disturbances, cancer, and organic nervous changes. A whole new development in old age counseling has arisen in the last several years. This promises to take much of the sting of inferiority and being on the down grade out of the process of growing older.

INVOLUTIONAL PSYCHOSES (PRESENILE)

These presenile conditions are included with the organic types primarily as a matter of convenience, not because there is definite proof of an organic or toxic origin. These are psychoses which appear in a period of life when the physical organism is beginning to decline; endocrine changes occur which alter bodily physiology and a number of psychological mechanisms may be disturbed. Several types of involutional psychoses have been described, including certain dementias, but the most frequent form is that called involutional melancholia. This diagnosis is made in approximately 4 percent of psychotic admissions to hospitals for mental disease.

This disorder, if it may be regarded as a unitary one, occurs three times as frequently in the female as it does in the male. The decade of greatest frequency in women is from age forty-five to fifty-four; during this period 55 percent of the cases are admitted to state hospitals. The decade of greatest frequency in men is from age fifty to fifty-nine, comprising 53 percent of hospital admissions.*

Women may develop symptoms of a typical involutional melancholia years after the menopause has been established as judged by the cessation of menses and the ordinary physiological symptoms attending this change; also in the case of men, as judged by the development of physiological impotence. There may be recurrent attacks of the characteristic agitated depression throughout several decades following an initial attack during the obvious physiologically symptomatic menopause, whether in male or female. These cases may have had some attacks of "nervousness" before, or women may have had symptoms at the time of the menstrual period, but nothing that resembled the depression and anxiety of these attacks.

The typical symptom complex of involution melancholia is that of an agitated depression. The dejection is, perhaps, the most painful of any type of depression to the patient and to the observer. The first part of this statement is somewhat uncertain, because of the inhibition of speech and other forms of motor expression in severe depressions without agitation. However, the agitated patients verbalize great psychic pain.

---

* Probably in no other group are the uncertainties of diagnostic standards more clearly shown than in involution melancholia. Many cases formerly so classed are now, on the basis of the case history, recognized as belonging to the manic-depressive group. On the other hand, it is difficult to understand what leads to a diagnosis of an involutional psychosis in the age groups under thirty. Only two possibilities are seen: (1) premature menopause, the diagnosis established by laboratory or other tests, or (2) the diagnosis was based on the clinical picture and would therefore most likely be erroneous. Some 5 to 6 percent of male and female cases were under age forty at the time of their first admission to state hospitals (how long the condition had been in existence prior to admission is not recorded). A considerably larger percentage of women than men were under forty-five, while the figures are reversed for cases age sixty and over. This distribution is to be expected in view of the difference in ages of men and women when the climacteric sets in. The two decades forty to fifty-nine account for 87 percent of the female cases; the decades forty-five to sixty-four account for 84 percent of the males.

The mood is one of extreme dejection, the patient sees nothing worth while in the future or in the present, is convinced of unworthiness, of having committed the unpardonable sin and being eternally damned. Combined with this is motor restlessness and great anxiety. Somatic delusions of a nihilistic type are the rule, and the patient believes that stomach, heart, or intestines are missing or obstructed; that food never reaches the stomach or is not digested; that the blood does not circulate. Some delusions are extremely peculiar, as when one patient asserted that his body was sawed in two and that the halves grated against each other with every motion he made.

The verbal complaints are repetitious to the extent of irritating monotony. The most common form is a repeated moaning and groaning, usually loud and anguished in tone. Other patients repeat their complaints over and over again, while pacing back and forth. Sometimes they shriek repeatedly so that the entire ward is upset. Insomnia, loss of appetite, constipation, and inadequate fluid intake are the rule rather than the exception. The attacks are prolonged; the general outlook is for recovery, but only after two to four years. In some cases deterioration sets in, and a state of dementia is the result. Usually there is only one attack, but sometimes, as already noted, there are recurrences.

Patients are not accessible for psychotherapy during an attack. They are not particularly interested in the procedure after recovery, if this is reasonably complete, even with insight into the nature of the past illness. They then feel that they are safe against further attacks.

Many cases are not severe enough to require hospitalization, at least in the eyes of the family, but such people are unable to work because of the depression, delusions, anxiety, and resulting inability to concentrate. Cases of this kind and those in the early stages frequently yield to vigorous hormone therapy, combined with sedatives when necessary, a wholesome regimen of living, and concurrent psychotherapy. More severe cases have been found especially suitable for both metrazol and electric shock therapy. The attacks are cut short, and the resulting recovery is usually good. It has been reported that in chronic cases the operation of frontal lobotomy has shown good results.

Occasionally the delusions are projected and the psychosis takes on a paranoid cast, with or without depression. Delusions of jealousy are especially likely to occur, particularly in women. In fact, one of the characteristic minor to major problems of the climacteric in women is the development of ideas of infidelity directed against the husband. There may be some insight into the ideas, and treatment may be possible. On the other hand, the menopause may serve as the precipitating factor for a paranoid psychosis.

The period of the menopause is a comparatively stormy one for most women. The development of modern ovarian supportive therapy can ease the situation, even to the extent of preventing severe neurotic and possibly psychotic reactions.

Since women are more commonly affected than men, there is greater disposition to protect them and keep them out of the hospital. At the same time, an irritable, depressed, anxious, nagging wife and mother is likely to be extremely upsetting to the household and its members. Psychiatric advice and treatment are much too frequently not sought until long after the optimum time for treatment.

The social worker should be particularly alert to signs and symptoms of the menopause in women over forty. If there are unusual types of headache, odd feelings in the head, "nervousness," distorted ideas, recognized as such by the patient, "blank" spells, and other unusual symptoms referable to the head and to mental functioning, ovarian dysfunction should be suspected and the client should be persuaded to go to a physician for suitable treatment.

PSYCHOSES OF TOXIC ORIGIN

ENDOGENOUS DISTURBANCES

IN THESE CONDITIONS we have to do with infections localized in the body elsewhere than in the nervous system, which produce psychotic reactions because of a circulating toxin, and with disturbances of metabolism which also produce toxemia. To these may be added the effects of exhaustion, such as that produced by extreme malnutrition.

Delirious and comatose reactions occur in the contagious diseases. These may be due not only to the general toxemia but also, as occurs to some extent in scarlet fever and measles, to an eruption on the meninges. The toxin produced by diphtheria occasionally produces some paralytic phenomena, chiefly in the mouth and throat and occasionally in other areas.

Exhaustion and starvation produce states of delirium and coma, or, as in battle fatigue, neurotic mechanisms may be activated. These usually take the form of anxiety, unreal terrors, even hallucinosis and delusion formation. Amnesia and other suppressions of function may occur in these acute reactions. Visions of food and water are not uncommon in those subjected to starvation or prolonged deprivation of fluids.

Exhaustion and dehydration occur in connection with many physical disorders, producing delirious and excited states either primarily or in combination with toxemia from the physical disorder. Exhaustion and dehydration also occur in the course of many mental diseases and must be guarded against in a hospital nursing program. In former days exhaustion from general paresis was a common statement of the cause of death in paretics. Today, should there be no specific cause of death, such as pneumonia or heart disease, the cause is usually stated only as general paresis.

Of particular interest and importance are the cases of women in whom psychotic states due to toxic-infectious causes occur in relation to childbirth. So-called puerperal psychoses may be schizophrenic, manic depressive, or paranoid, *without* a toxic-infectious factor. In these cases, childbirth is merely a precipitating factor in an already vulnerable personality. Treatment and prognosis are therefore the same as for other cases of the same groups, in which childbirth is not a factor. However, these cases and those due to toxemia of pregnancy or to toxic-infectious states caused by accidents during the puerperium itself, are not always easily distinguishable from the clinical pictures alone. Laboratory and physical examinations will usually clear up the diagnosis, or at least be highly suggestive.

If the post-puerperal state is clearly one of delirium or coma, then toxic-infectious factors will usually be found—damaged kidneys, retained placental fragments, infected uterus, or a metastatic inflammation of the brain substance. Even when these can be and are successfully treated, it sometimes happens that an underlying schizophrenic or other process remains active. Particularly in the case of inflammatory processes in the brain, there may be more or less permanent impairment of mental faculties. To round out the picture of puerperal disturbances, it may be noted that chronic invalidism on a neurotic basis may occur following childbirth, or there may be an acute neurotic upset demanding immediate and intensive treatment.

Personality changes accompany many endocrine disorders, but the incidence of actual psychoses is extremely low, unless all involutional cases are ascribed to gonadotrophic causes. This does not seem justifiable in the present state of knowledge, which includes experiments with therapy.

The best-known psychotic and defect states are those associated with hypothyroidism. If the thyroid is underactive during intra-uterine life and infancy, the resulting condition is known as cretinism, further described in Chapter XII.

When the thyroid becomes underactive in adult life, the result is myxedema, a disorder more common in women than in men. The subcutaneous tissues become infiltrated with a mucin-like substance, giving rise to a peculiar waxy thickening of the skin, which becomes dry and rough. The hair becomes dry and coarse, and there is gain in weight. In the typical psychotic picture, psychomotor activity is lessened, thought processes are slowed, and depression develops. Treatment with thyroid preparations may be successful in relieving myxedema; if it is begun early and kept up long enough, cretinism may also be at least partially relieved.

Hyperthyroidism produces overactivity, sensory hyperacuity, and emotional instability. Minor mental symptoms of other types occur, but actual psychotic states are rare. That the infrequency of psychotic reactions is related to early diagnosis and successful surgical treatment seems probable.

Disturbances in behavior, personality integration, and social adjustment also occur with deviations of pituitary and gonadal functions. These difficulties vary according to whether they occur in the prepubertal or the postpubertal period. Psychotic reactions are rare, at least as direct manifestations of glandular disturbance.

For example, hyperpituitarism in the prepubertal period leads to the condition called gigantism. In the postpubertal period, hyperpituitarism causes acromegaly. Some giants are intellectually retarded and emotionally unstable; longevity is usually not great, and there may be terminal delirium and coma. On the other hand, acromegaly may run a prolonged, often rather stationary, course. For instance, a ticket collector of a commuting train on which I rode showed no perceptible advance in his acromegaly during twenty years. I do not know whether he received any sort of treatment. Aside from psychological reactions to the changes in appearance, mental symptoms of a serious nature are rare. The few cases I have personally seen of psychoses in acromegalics were typical paranoid conditions without any special features indicating that the hyperpituitarism was in any way causative for the mental symptoms. Of course, if there is enlargement of the gland and this enlargement produces intracranial pressure, a brain tumor syndrome, with accompanying mental symptoms of the usual type, may be found.

One acromegalic, in a state hospital because of a paranoid condition, was always willing and co-operative in demonstrations of his condition. Several operations on the pituitary had been attempted, but hemorrhage blocked them. After several years the man developed a left-sided paralysis. It was thought that the pituitary tumor had extended into the right side of the brain. Symptoms of tumor, aside from the hemiparesis, were not marked for more than a year. After his death, autopsy disclosed a slightly enlarged pituitary. There was no extension into the brain, but there was a large tumor of the meninges over the right cerebral hemisphere. Cases such as this show how several processes may be operating at once and result in serious errors in diagnosis. Today, refinements in X-ray procedures, including air encephalography, should obviate such errors.

Hypopituitarism produces recognizable effects chiefly when it operates before puberty and various clinical pictures have been described. Obesity, underdeveloped sexual organs, and hypogonadism are among the most common signs. Children and adults with inadequate pituitary secretion are usually passive, cheerful, inactive, have large appetites, and are not too much disturbed by their condition. Some, however, are overactive and aggressive, a fact which has frequently been overlooked. As adults, these patients are eunuchoid and usually sterile.

Psychoses are uncommon in hypopituitarism, though personality disturbances are frequent. Intelligence levels vary, but there seems to be no specific relationship between the pituitary disturbance and the intelligence level, or with any group of psychotic symptoms.

Patients with chronic mental disorders often develop signs of endocrine dysfunction, usually polyglandular, perhaps after years of hospital residence. There is no particular change in mental symptoms, though physical functioning may be altered in various ways.

Disorders such as diabetes and kidney disease are often accompanied by mental symptoms, especially in terminal stages. The clinical syndrome may be delirium and coma; convulsions are not infrequent. The treatment is medical; specific (insulin) in the case of diabetes, and general in the renal or cardiorenal cases.

ALCOHOL AND DRUGS (EXOGENOUS POISONS)

Psychoses and some defect states are produced by alcohol, by drugs of the opium series, hashish and similar preparations, some sedatives, cocaine, a number of heavy metals, especially lead, and several chemicals in use in modern industry.

Alcoholic Psychoses

Because of the ease of preparation and its accessibility, alcohol enters more largely into the production of abnormal mental states than do any of the other drugs or poisons mentioned. Under average conditions the psychoses appear only in those chronically addicted to alcohol in excessive amounts. There are, however, individuals who react extremely to very small amounts of alcohol. As already noted, this is a frequent finding in persons who have suffered skull fractures. Individual tolerance to alcohol varies within relatively wide limits. But in cases of pathological intoxication, a single drink may be enough to throw the individual into a state of automatic activity, followed by amnesia covering a longer or shorter period. The mechanism whereby these reactions are set up is by no means clear. Under ordinary circumstances these people do not seem to be particularly neurotic, nor do they display such reaction to other drugs or to upsetting realities. Automatic activity, with subsequent amnesia, occurs in many people if they drink enough, even though they do not become comatose or lose motor control.

The problem of the chronic alcoholic must be considered apart from the psychoses. The alcoholic psychoses fall into two groups—the acute and the chronic.

The acute psychoses are delirium tremens and acute hallucinosis. In common practice delirium tremens is not regarded as a psychosis and in some legal provisions for the care of mental disorders, cases of delirium tremens are specifically excluded. At the same time, cases of delirium tremens are admitted to general hospitals, while other types of psychoses, including those of alcoholic origin, usually have not been until fairly recently.

Delirium tremens occurs in chronic drinkers, especially after a prolonged spree during which insufficient food and fluids, other than liquor, are taken. It is typically a delirium with excessive tremor. Visual and extremely frightening hallucinations predominate, and the victims respond with excessive fear. Patients are usually overactive and restless, find it difficult to sleep, are dehydrated, constipated, and have little appetite. After a few days—three to six, as a rule—the hallucinations disappear, the tremors diminish markedly, consciousness becomes clear, there is partial to complete amnesia covering the period of the delirium, appetite returns, and the patient is able to sleep without much difficulty. There is insight into the illness and its proximate cause, i.e., alcohol. Many such cases are spree drinkers and may go for long intervals without drinking. Many, on the other hand, are abstinent for only short intervals, perhaps for a period of days or weeks, after an episode of this sort. Repeated attacks of delirium tremens may occur before alcoholic deterioration sets in, though, as will be shown later, deterioration may occur without such antecedent attacks.

Acute hallucinosis is a quite different type of disorder. Consciousness remains clear; there is no delirium. Hallucinations are vivid, threatening, fear-producing, and chiefly auditory. During the period of the attack patients are convinced of the reality of the threatening voices and the ideas of persecutions based on them. Patients may go to extreme lengths to protect themselves—breaking into churches to avoid a pursuing devil or appealing to police or others for assistance. Rarely do they fix upon some particular person as the source of their difficulties. They may be much excited and very troublesome, both outside and inside hospital.

The disorder runs its course in three to six weeks, and recovery is ordinarily complete, with insight and full memory of the disturbed period. The really distinguishing features are the alcoholic history and the emotional reactions in harmony with the hallucinations. It has been thought that the psychotic reaction represents the blossoming of a particular type of personality, the schizoid type, as a result of the alcoholic toxicity. However, many, if not most, of these cases seem to be of fairly normal personality make-up.

There are several types of chronic psychoses associated with alcoholism. *Simple alcoholic deterioration* is characterized by impairment of memory, judgment, and reasoning, combined with loquacity and a tendency to humor which is often rather strained. When this type of deterioration is combined with delusions, especially of infidelity on the part of the spouse, it constitutes the alcoholic paranoid condition. In this state, hallucinations are not present as a rule. There may or may not have been previous acute attacks of delirium tremens. The delusions may seem to be within the bounds of possibility, but careful questioning will reveal the bizarre nature of the assumed grounds or the distorted reasoning which leads to the conclusions that would be serious if true. Jealousy is always present, and the patient literally tortures the unfortunate spouse with questions, accusations, and even physical assault. The most innocent act may provoke any of these reactions. Paternity of children may be denied; often the patient is impotent, or nearly so, and this factor apparently enters into the psychological mechanism involved.

A more complex picture is that of *Korsakow's syndrome*, polyneuritic delirium. While this syndrome does occur as a result of the action of other toxic substances, both those formed in the body and those introduced from without, it is most commonly a sequel to chronic alcoholism. Inflammation of the peripheral nerves leads to pain and tenderness along the nerve trunks which is sometimes mistaken for rheumatism, relaxation of joints, absence of reflexes,

failure of co-ordination, and often inability to walk. The pathological process in the brain leads to a particular kind of fabricating
delirium. Special senses and speech are not impaired as a rule, so the
patient remains in apparent contact with the environment. There
are usually no hallucinations as such. There is an enormous memory
loss, and the patient fills in the gaps with fabrications. Imaginary
experiences may be suggested, such as a wreck, an accident, or any
other dramatic event, and will be accepted and elaborated, often in
great detail. For weeks on end the patient will tell the same story
each day, using the same tale of experiences, probably representing
his final memories; or he may invent a new story each time. There
is no memory for events of even the few preceding minutes or
hours. In other words, although the patient seems awake and alert
to surroundings, impressibility and therefore memory are practically nil.

Since the pathological changes in the nervous system are severe
and only to a limited extent reversible, few of these cases recover
completely. The usual course is increasing dementia and helpless-
ness and eventual death. In most cases the peripheral nerve disorder
clears up to a considerable degree, but the mental status usually remains one of marked deterioration.

The alcoholic psychoses are not as frequent in mental hospital
admissions as is often thought; nor was there as much reduction
as had been expected in such admissions during the prohibition
years, except for a short period. Six percent of all psychotic first
admissions to mental hospitals in 1937 were alcoholic psychoses,
with a higher proportion in private (8.4%) than in state hospitals
(5.3%). However, among nonpsychotic admissions to the hospitals, 50 percent were for alcoholism. Again the proportion was
higher for private hospitals (60%) than for state institutions
(46.3%). Since no further breakdown is available as to reasons for
admitting these nonpsychotic alcoholics to mental hospitals, it must
be assumed that it was for the purpose of treatment of alcoholism,
either acute or chronic. In many states there are special laws covering the commitment of inebriates, in some instances to special insti-

tutions. Such commitments are usually for three years, shorter terms having generally proved a waste of time. Some states have converted their institutions for inebriates to other purposes, usually to regular mental hospitals. Some states have also abandoned special commitment for inebriates. These changes were made because the results of the special provisions did not seem to justify the measures.

Alcoholism as a Social and Medical Problem

There is no reliable estimate of the number of people in this country who drink intoxicating liquors, but it is known to be very large. Distinctions are drawn between those who drink only socially, in moderation, occasionally, constantly, or to excess. The habitual drunkard, or chronic alcoholic, is ordinarily regarded as a creature apart—a bum, a ne'er-do-well, a weakling, somehow defective, or a pathological personality type. For years there was little or no scientific study of these cases. They were sobered up in general hospitals and discharged as soon as possible. Or they served jail and workhouse sentences of thirty to ninety days or even a year. Anyone who committed a felony while drunk received a prison sentence. The Keely cure was popular for years. Here and there are private hospitals solely for the treatment of alcohol and drug addicts. Most of them treat patients for only a short time and stress the clearing up of physical symptoms and lessening the desire for liquor. The psychological problems are rarely if ever probed.

Lately the problems of chronic alcoholism have become the subject of intensive research from many points of view. There is now a conference group on alcoholism which publishes a quarterly journal. Vitamin deficiencies and their relationship to the reactions of the nervous system to alcohol, allergic reactions to alcohol, emotional conflicts as related to alcoholism, and the way in which they are revealed in the psychoses, methods of treatment and rehabilitation for the alcoholic—these and many other topics are being studied intensively. Various previous theories have been proven; others have been disproven; new ones have been evolved.

Alcoholism in many cases, particularly in that type of spree drinking known as "dipsomania," can be shown to be related to definite disorders of personality. Dipsomania is most frequently associated with difficulties in psychosexual integration—either an unresolved conflict, a strong repressed partial drive such as homosexuality, which is incompletely or inadequately sublimated, or even overt perverse sexual activity. In the latter cases guilt and conflict concerning the activity may be the precipitating factors for the excessive drinking or may be those which perpetuate it.

It has been asserted that all excessive and chronic drinking is rooted in a strong homosexual drive, inadequately repressed, yet not becoming overt in behavior. This assertion is open to serious question; the formula is too simple to cover all the possibilities seen in the psychopathology of these cases. In fact, the essential mechanism in most cases is not known.

Alcohol does remove layers of inhibitions, and repressed mechanisms become operative. A certain amount of insight into basic personality trends may sometimes thus be gained. Some people in their cups become depressed, tearful, self-pitying; others are gay and witty; still others become hostile and belligerent; some become gentler and more suggestible than usual; some display otherwise unsuspected suspiciousness, jealousy, and paranoid trends. Some soon show confusion in thinking, reasoning, and contact with surroundings, while others remain reasonably clear-headed, but develop marked motor inco-ordination.

In many cases alcohol gives a sense of power and security to an individual suffering from marked feelings of inadequacy and insecurity. This more comfortable state is, however, difficult to maintain and calls for more drink. Eventually intoxication ensues and must be slept off, with resultant hangovers and other physical symptoms. As habituation develops, more alcohol may be required, or the individual drinks more and more in order to be continuously in his own variety of dream world. In the end, physical and mental efficiency and social status are impaired. Vitamin imbalance, particularly inadequate amounts of B_1, plays an important role in the development of neuropsychiatric disturbances. It also appears evident that secondary toxemia, originating from the effects of the alcohol on other organs, plays a part.

As a social problem, the use and abuse of alcoholic beverages continues to be, as it has been for centuries, a perplexing problem. All are familiar with the many and varied attempts to control its use by legislation and regulation. There are prohibitions in a number of religious organizations which are apparently well observed, but for the rank and file, nonreligious prohibitions have chiefly been challenges to evade the law.

For example, in New York State the percentage of first admissions with alcoholic psychoses to the state hospitals declined from 10.8 percent in 1909 to 5.2 percent in 1918, the last year before prohibition became effective. There was then a sharp drop to 1.9 percent in 1920, rising to 5.4 percent in 1924, and 7.0 percent in 1927. With small variations, the rate has since remained at about 7 percent, including the years after prohibition. Legal prohibition, therefore, had only a temporary effect in reducing the number of psychotic reactions necessitating hospital care. Another point of interest is that the intemperate use of alcohol among first admissions of all types of psychoses declined from a peak of 38 percent in 1910 to 12 percent in 1921, jumping to 16 percent in 1927. Since then, the figure has remained fairly static in the 15.5–16.5 percent range. Admittedly, these figures are less reliable than those for the alcoholic psychoses, because of the element of judgment involved, but they bear out the previous conclusion.

Among the most interesting developments in the treatment of the alcoholic is the growth of the organization known as "Alcoholics Anonymous." Founded and operated by former alcoholics, this organization is an outstanding success in the field of group therapy as applied by particular types of personalities to each other. While the treatment is not always successful, as is true of all therapies, it does appear that this group attack has achieved better results in salvaging habitual drunkards than has any other method. It is requisite that the individual *must wish* to be rid of the habit, that he face realistically the fact that he *is* a chronic alcoholic, that he admit that for him there is no such thing as taking one drink and stopping. These points are re-enforced by the make-up of the group, all former alcoholics. Some state hospitals have made effective use of such groups in the treatment of their alcoholic patients. Individual psychotherapy is also often effective, and the same principles with regard to facing reality apply if the therapy is to be successful.

Among the many medical approaches which have been made, the recent use of insulin should be mentioned. Combined with psychotherapy, some rather striking successes have been reported. Insulin treatment is also of value in selected cases of drug addiction.

Drug Addiction

Psychotic reactions due to drug addiction are relatively infrequent. That drug addicts are not well integrated as personalities seems quite certain, yet many addicts continue their habit for years without visible signs of physical or mental deterioration. Particularly those addicted to drugs of the opium series seem often to be comparatively free from symptoms of deterioration for many years. If their drug supply is interrupted, they suffer severely from withdrawal symptoms and use any possible means to replenish their supply.

Cocaine addiction, which seems to be relatively uncommon, produces rather marked changes in personality. When a psychosis develops, it is characteristically a paranoid state, with hallucinations of bugs crawling under the skin, fear, and disturbed activity.

Hashish, marijuana, and other preparations of the cannabis indica series, especially marijuana smoked as reefers, have been implicated as serious causes of various types of delinquent behavior. The most detailed studies indicate that the role of marijuana has been overestimated. However, intoxication and even psychoses may result. Characteristically, there is sexual excitement and a loss of proper appreciation of time and space. The dream world is limitless, time floats along, and there are visions of entrancing sexual objects and adventures.

In general, drug addiction is a medical, social, and police problem which has not yet been satisfactorily solved. It is not enough to think of addicts as psychopathic or neurotic individuals. Addiction adds its own problems, of which many sufferers are well aware. They are also aware of the fact that indulgence does not solve their basic problems, but it makes them feel easier, more secure, more competent, and emotionally stabler while they are under the influence of drugs.

Almost any drug which acts as a sedative or narcotic may be habit-forming, though not all lead to addiction in the sense of an extreme or unconquerable craving. Bromides, barbiturates, and other drugs not only may be habit-forming, but may on occasion give rise to psychotic reactions, usually temporary and recoverable. In some instances, however, an acute delirious reaction is followed by deterioration. Finally, the abuse of alcohol and drugs may be only one symptom of a psychosis of some other origin.

Lead poisoning, now comparatively rare, produces defect states and neurological changes. It is sometimes seen in children who eat the paint off their cribs and utensils. States of mental deterioration are produced in adults. Mercury and some other heavy metals occasionally produce neuropsychiatric complications. Similar results are caused by modern solvents and chemicals used in making explosives and in other processes. But as industrial safety measures have developed, fewer neuropsychiatric problems have arisen in this area—at least, fewer patients reach mental hospitals for treatment.

CHAPTER VII

PSYCHODYNAMICS AND
FUNCTIONAL DISORDERS

MENTAL DISEASES without specific pathology or physical etiological factors are ordinarily called functional disorders. They are apparently of psychogenic origin and represent the working out of complexes and conflicts which temporarily or permanently alter or destroy the patient's adequate contact with reality.

Some psychiatrists hold to the theory that there must be some sort of underlying organic pathology in schizophrenia, but there is no agreement as to the type or even concerning which organ or organs may be involved. Many reports have implicated different parts of the brain and several endocrine glands, especially the gonads. Reliable studies have shown that the cardiovascular system is smaller in schizophrenics than in normal controls. The incidence of male secondary sexual characteristics in females and of feminine characteristics in males seems to be higher in schizophrenics than in normals. Several body types have been described in the literature, and it is thought by some that the various types have a relationship to the sort of psychosis which individuals develop. All that can be said concerning this point is that it is not proven. Also, alterations in consistency of the cortex and microscopic changes in the brain cells have been described in schizophrenia, but there is no definite and consistent picture. Similar comment is true concerning the results of physico-chemical research up to the present.

Temperaments having particular characteristics have also been delimited and described. Temperament may be defined as the basic and usual mood or affective reaction and the level of activity peculiar to an individual. Two temperamental types are the cyclothymic and the schizoid, and a number of others have been described by various writers. These are discussed in the sections on the particular disorders with which they seem to have a relationship. It is certain, however, that many people possess strongly marked temperamental characteristics who never develop a psychosis or a neurosis.

It has already been shown that paranoid reactions occur in all sorts of cases with known pathology. The paranoid disorders presently to be described do not have any specific pathology and accordingly are to be regarded as of psychogenic origin.

The borderlines between the several types of psychotic and neurotic reactions to be discussed are not as clear and sharp as the presentation might seem to indicate. However, in typical cases the complete history and the presenting clinical picture leave little question as to the correct diagnosis. Prognosis is also not so definite as was once thought to be true for any of the psychotic reactions described.

To understand the mental mechanisms involved in the evolution of these psychoses and of the neuroses, it is necessary to outline the development and integration of the instinctive drives, especially the psychosexual mechanism.

The instinctive drives to be considered are: (1) self-preservation; (2) ego-maximation; (3) group conformance; and (4) the psychosexual. The first three are essentially drives involving the ego; their development seems to be deeply rooted in biological constitution and greatly influenced by the social nature of man's existence. The sexual drive also has deep constitutional roots and is influenced by the events of living; it seems, however, to be more all-pervasive and subject to more deviations than is true of the ego drives. It is possible to describe the development of the psychosexual mechanism as occurring in fairly well-marked stages, but this is not quite the case with the development of the ego. The evolution of consciousness, memory, associations, judgment, and other aspects of intellectual development seems to flow along in a reasonably orderly course. While these attributes do not constitute the whole of the ego, they do represent ego functions through which the individual maintains contact with reality and with which he tests it.

In ordinary times of peace, threats against the instinctive drive for self-preservation are not continuous, that is, chronic, for any large group of the population in this country, at least at any one time. In peace time the chief threats are hunger, thirst, sickness, accidents, and catastrophies of various sorts. While studies have shown that we do have malnutrition in this country to a greater extent than had been assumed for many years, the fact remains that this country as a whole has been and continues to be the best fed in the world. Peculiarities of diet do exist and not infrequently are related to the production of deficiency diseases. Economic inequalities also play their part in producing threats against self-preservation.

Our accident rate is high, but in general, we as individuals pay little attention to the fact that we may be victims. Illness and death are always with us, but few of us spend our lives worrying about an illness we do not have. Death is a certainty, and a special death instinct has been postulated. There is a period in the life of most children when preoccupation with death is marked, but most adults achieve a reasonably good adjustment to the idea, perhaps by not thinking about it. That would be a way of becoming resigned to an inevitable which is, after all, somewhere in the future.

War brings about a situation in which the drive for self-preservation is continuously threatened for many people. The numbers so affected in the recent war must be counted in the hundreds of millions, both civilians and service people. Anxiety and panic states are among the chief results. Inadequately dealt with by the ego, these may lead into well-developed neuroses of the ordinary types or may even precipitate psychotic reactions.

Fear is the characteristic emotional response to threats against self-preservation. Where it may be freely verbalized and shared with others, it is far less likely to produce a neurosis. It has aptly been said that one of the major issues in the production of so-called war neuroses is the fear of showing fear. That is equivalent to saying that the fear of being called a coward, which certainly no one desires, is an important factor in producing neurotic reactions. In some instances, to be discussed later, this fear may also be an important precipitating factor for psychotic reactions.

Among the many disturbances to emerge in men and women who have served in our armed forces are the neurotic reactions of those who have been wounded, with loss of sight, loss of a limb or limbs or parts of them, or great disfigurement. The same comment applies to many who have acquired some chronic disease. But we must remember that not all the maimed and disfigured display neurotic responses to their plight.

Reactions of the type under consideration also occur in civilian life in relation to the results of accidents, of disorders limiting activities, even though they are not visible to the observer, of crippling disease, and in congenital abnormalities of physical development. The part of the ego involved in such situations, however they arise, is the drive for self-maximation. This drive is involved in all the numerous competitive situations the individual encounters in the course of living. There are competitions for attention, affection, and status at home and at school, in groups of peers, and elsewhere. There are competitions in the intellectual, vocational, and social fields, as well as for love objects. Whatever operates to reduce feelings of personal adequacy in any or all competitive situations will produce feelings of difference, usually spoken of as inferiority, and an emotional conflict and complex will result.

The drive for group conformance and group acceptance is perhaps stronger in children than in adults. At least it is more obvious, and the effects of frustration are both more marked and more directly expressed. It is clear that the drive for self-maximation and that for group conformance are to some degree in conflict, perhaps always and certainly until the individual has achieved a real sense of personal adequacy and a comfortable feeling of belonging to the group. In general terms, both drives are ordinarily at maximum strength during the adolescent period. Then the need for securing emotional independence from the home is at its height, as is the need for support and protection by the group of peers.

Any personal characteristic which departs widely from the average or norm of the groups in which the individual functions may give rise to feelings of difference. This occurs either because of the person's sense of failure to measure up to his own ego ideals or because of the attitudes of his group or of important members of it. Color, race, ugliness, or even beauty, intellectual level, religious, social, and economic status of the family, and so on through a long list of human and social variables, may operate in the production of such an inferiority complex.

The possible reactions to these and other conflicts are comparatively few in number, and may be grouped in the following manner.

1. There may be a natural or an acquired compensation; that is, the feelings of inferiority in one area are balanced by an actual or felt superiority in another field which is acknowledged by others. In many cases the limitations are accepted as part of the person's reality picture, and the individual learns to live with them without particular tensions or difficult behavior manifestations. When a drive which has been repressed has no natural compensation and the energy is diverted to some socially acceptable and personally satisfying outlet, the mechanism is called sublimation.

2. The individual may withdraw from social contacts and retreat more and more into wish-fulfilling fantasies in which power and status are achieved without the need for striving to face and conquer reality. While there are other important mechanisms involved, this is one of the essential features of the withdrawal into a schizoid or schizophrenic state.

3. The reaction may be one of rebellion; the person is unable to accept the imposed limitations, and reacts aggressively. Hostility toward others as well as to the self complicates the aggressive attitude. The aggressive activity may be well controlled, or it may be diffuse and more or less wasted.

4. The individual may submit to his feelings of difference or in-

feriority with feelings of guilt, defeat, and anxiety. There may be no compensating fantasy or rebellion, but a constant state of tension and unpredictable behavior.

Because all these are *reactions to situations*, it seems doubtful that they are essentially determined by the sadism and masochism of the individual, but it is probable that these and other constitutional factors help to determine the type of reaction. According to observations of the behavior of children, rejection by adults—or its semblance—is probably the most important single factor in the production of withdrawing and rebellious reactions in childhood. Once established, the behavior may be carried over into adulthood unless it is resolved by treatment.

This brief sketch must suffice to indicate how the ego functions through certain drives and what happens when there is frustration. All self-regarding ideas and attitudes are functions of the ego; these are constantly tested out against the real or assumed attitudes of the group, as well as against the individual's own ego ideals. Ideals are derived in the first instance from the parental images. The term "images" is used advisedly, since the child translates into his own thinking and feeling his assumptions concerning the high ideals of the parents, their omnipotence, their general superiority, their infinite goodness. In later development, ego ideals are derived from other sources—teachers, neighborhood and national heroes, and the standards and ideals of the group of peers.

The formation of ego ideals does not always proceed smoothly. Parents are inconsistent; their actions and words do not always agree; because of elements of rejection of the child on their part, parents produce an emotional climate which may lead to ambivalence in the child's ideals or even to the formation of negative ones.

Furthermore, a parent, particularly the mother, is the first source of frustration for the child's untrained impulses. Feeding schedules, weaning, and toilet training are essentially functions of the mother or mother substitute, and these training efforts represent the first social pressures exerted against the child's unregulated and to some extent nonrhythmic impulse activities.

Through these and other training pressures designed to assist the child to change from an omnipotent, self-centered, hedonistic being into a socialized individual, the parent represents authority. In the early phases this parental authority stands also for protection and guidance, hence security against unknown and perhaps known dangers. As development proceeds, there is erected within the individual a mechanism, the superego, which performs the same functions of criticism, restraint, and training for the ego that were previously carried out by the adults in the environment. True, the child introjects images of parents and other sources of authority into his own ego. The more severely critical and uncompromising these images are, the more sternly will the child, and later the adult, deal with himself. Guilt feelings and dissatisfactions with his behavior will be correspondingly increased. Such self-criticism assumes abnormal proportions in depressions.

The processes of training and guidance represent essentially deprivation and frustration, and to these is often added punishment. Hence, another ambivalent factor is added. For not only does the child respond to training and guidance out of love for the parent, but fear, resentment, and hostility are also engendered. The hostility is ordinarily repressed into the unconscious, but then strong guilt feelings are evoked. As a rule, these are also unconscious, but add to the torturing conscience. If the repression is adequate and the energy finds satisfactory sublimating outlets, the result is a reasonably well-adjusted personality. If one or both of these mechanisms fail, symptoms of some sort will emerge. The type of symptom will depend largely on the extent to which the hostility becomes conscious and whether it is unconsciously directed against the self or against others, or consciously directed against the original stimulus to the hostility or to a symbolic representative.

As already mentioned, there are several stages in the evolution of psychosexual integration or, in other terminology, the development of the libido. These may be set forth in various ways. The central points have to do with pleasure zones and the search for pleasure, and with the libido as an energy principle.

The early pleasures of the individual occur through the relief of tension. The primitive tensions are: hunger, satisfied by suckling and later by eating and drinking; pressure of feces in the rectum, satisfied by evacuation of the bowel; distension of the bladder, relieved by the expulsion of urine. These functions have psychic values quite different from those of such automatic or nearly automatic functions as breathing, the heartbeat, the rhythmic movements or peristalsis of the intestines, and other vital processes which involve alterations in organ tensions. The oral, anal, and urethral zones not only contribute directly to the pleasure of the individual through the relief of tensions, but each zone becomes linked in its own way to the sexual mechanism. Hence they have erotogenic qualities, as do all general and special senses which also enter into the erotic mechanism.

Oral and anal stages of development are ordinarily separately described, and each plays a somewhat different role in personality development. In the first oral phase the characteristic pleasure-producing activity is suckling. With this there are usually associated movements which often survive in adult life as mannerisms. Finger sucking may occur as a supplementary activity, or it may be pathological; that is, pleasure sucking in the absence of hunger or in a regressive search for comfort in a distressing situation. If suckling is permitted to continue past the time when it should normally cease and the energy be otherwise used, weaning will be difficult and neurotic symptoms may appear. On the other hand, if suckling is suppressed too early, neurotic symptoms based on an unsatisfied need for suckling activity or on rejection of the new method of getting food may appear.

In the second oral stage the characteristic activities are biting and mastication. This brings in the element of pleasurable aggression, or sadism. An ambivalent object relationship is established so that the object which gives pleasure and is therefore loved, is also destroyed by an act of hostility and incorporated into one's own body. Hence this process is spoken of as cannibalism. This term is especially apt in view of the way the baby bites the mother's nipples or other parts of her body and chews all accessible parts of his own body. In addition, the infant is likely to chew and either swallow or eject everything he can get into his mouth.

Mouth activity persists throughout life and is essential to living. Many types of mouth activity other than those of eating develop, most of them socially acceptable, though some are not. Oral tensions may find relief in talking, smoking, gum chewing, drinking, eating, and other mouth activities. Kissing is a type of oral activity which is an essential element of ordinary love-making. Kissing also fulfills other functions in social relationships, such as the expression of friendship, gratitude, or parental and filial affection. Praise and so-called "sweet talk" have the same general functions in love-making and in expressing admiration and affection.

In the early oral and anal stages of development, the individual is in the *narcissistic* phase. The chief love object is the mother or mother substitute, but it seems quite apparent that she is regarded merely as an extension or part of the self, undifferentiated from the self. The factor of nursing would fit into or increase this tendency. In technical terms, narcissism or being in love with the self represents a cathexis of ego and libido. Cathexis is simply a matter of the accumulation of psychic or emotional energy investing an idea or object. In the narcissistic phase the individual is self-sufficient and self-contained, that is, omnipotent. His attitudes are imperatively demanding, and his imperious wants require immediate gratification in primitive, direct ways; he can accept no compromise. In other words, the individual is extremely egocentric and requires prompt gratification without respect to the demands or limitations of reality.

Two special types of personality make-up have been ascribed to the oral character. The first comprises people who attach themselves to others like leeches and are hard to shake off. The second type is carefree, optimistic, and unconcerned. Both types are extremely self-satisfied, though their friends and acquaintances find continuous association with them a considerable strain. Sublimation of the oral erotic drive is said to be shown in ambition to acquire knowledge, in scientific investigation, through the assimilation of observable data and the facts and findings of others.

There are likewise two phases of development with relation to the anal zone, which includes all the digestive tract below the stomach and the surrounding buttocks area. The anal phases are especially marked at ages three and four.

The first stage involves the pleasure and relief of tension secured by expulsion of the residue of undigestible parts of food. In the infant the only regulation involved in expulsion is the physiological level of tension within the bowel. To discharge excrement is, of course, an important self-preservative act, as is the ingestion of aliment. Adults are actively interested in their children's bowel movements, as well as in their own. The interest of the child in his own excretory processes is heightened by the interest and attention given it by the adults. However, the child learns in time that holding back or retention increases the pleasure of the eventual evacuation. Large, well-formed stools seem to be especially of interest, and the value is increased for persons with a fixation at the anal level of development. Regression to the expulsive phase has been demonstrated by psychoanalysis in melancholia and paranoid states.

Expulsion of the stool is also a destructive act, which is pleasurable, but combined with hostility. The excrement may have an identification as a love object, yet a hostile tendency predominates. The emotions are therefore ambivalent; there is positive valuation and the wish to retain, while at the same time there are negative feelings regarding expulsion and concomitant rejection.

Ambivalence implies the simultaneous presence of positive feelings of love or acceptance and negative feelings of hate and rejection. It may be active or passive; there is desire to love and be loved, to look at and be looked at, to beat and be beaten, to eat and so incorporate or possess, and to be eaten or possessed.

In the second anal phase the chief pleasure is in holding back or retention of the feces to increase the pleasure of expulsion. The accumulation of the fecal mass also acquires an independent pleasure-giving function. The stool becomes an important and valuable object, an estimate strengthened by the attitudes of adults. The stool is often presented, as it were, to the adult as a demonstration of love. Training enforces cleanliness and punctuality of bowel movements, as the child is prevented from smearing feces on objects and on himself. The first punishment effort of parents is likely to be directed against soiling, and the first conscious guilt feelings of the child probably arise in connection with some failure to comply regarding bowel movements. Training does not always succeed in completely mastering the pleasure tendencies of retention and evacuation. Some adult psychotics present a regression to smearing and even eating feces.

The child's high valuation of the feces and the urine starts a process which eventually extends to all his possessions, thus assisting toward ultimate social adjustment of anal tendencies. The significance of excrement is often passed on to money and gold.

Fixation in the anal phase leads to neurotic manifestations, as, for example, in neurotic constipation plus a hypochondriacal interest in moving the bowels and in the stool itself. Other examples are the fear of touching objects lest they be contaminated and compulsive washing of the hands which have touched contaminated objects. This phobia and the associated compulsion also occurs in cases with guilt about masturbation. These are instances of defense against the strength of the childhood impulses which have not been adequately incorporated or, perhaps, sublimated.

It is generally regarded that all creative productions, artistic or scientific, are to some extent related to the anal components in personality organization. Orderliness, parsimony, and obstinacy are regarded as anal traits. Sadistic and anal traits combine in orderliness; parsimony is more anal, and obstinacy is more sadistic.

Sadism and masochism flower during this phase of personality development, which comprises the years from two to five. In the first anal phase there is pleasurable aggression against an object. Beating the buttocks is an important pleasurable source of libidinal excitation during this period. Pleasure in beating is sadistic; pleasure in being beaten is masochistic. As perversions, sadism ranges from physical punishment to psychic torture. This is often the chief element in a mutually satisfying sadistic-masochistic physical sexual relationship.

Biting, beating, pricking, burning, scratching, and other punishing activities are forms of sadism, as is domineering over persons, animals, and things and subjecting them to the will of the individual. There are honored and even heroic sadistic acts, such as regulated types of physical combat, political campaigns, and war. In the first phase of anal sadism, smashing and crushing of objects is the typical activity. This is much like the activity of oral destruction. In the second phase the chief pleasure is derived from tormenting, retaining, and mastering the object, whether person, animal, or thing, confining it and restricting its liberty for selfish gratification.

If obedience, humility, and love for suffering are indulged in to an extreme, they are signs of masochism. To a considerable extent, a person is ambivalent in terms of the normal mechanisms of sadism and masochism. It must be emphasized that the oral-anal phases of development and sadism and masochism are normal mechanisms in personality evolution and integration. It is only when one or another mechanism is particularly strong and interferes with the functioning of the total personality, when oral and anal erotism or sadism or masochism become fixated as perversions in adult behavior, that we are justified in calling them abnormal. Anal perversions vary considerably in degree; casual or experimental activity should probably not be classed as perverse.

Particularly in these early phases the anally determined evaluations linked to object relations are carried over to the sexual apparatus. This is the stage of autoerotism, for which the characteristic activity is masturbation. The vagina may be equated, so far as it is thought of at all, with the rectum. Fear of loss of the penis, a castration fear, may be created by the daily bowel movements. Weaning is also a castration threat, since it cuts off part of the introjected self.

So-called infantile masturbation is of value in transferring libido to the genitalia. It presents problems, however, which need to be faced. These are chiefly the anxiety of the parents and, in extreme cases, the threat to the healthy development of the child. The parent should recognize this early genital manipulation as being essential for the child's development and realize that it does not have the same significance as does masturbation or other forms of sexual activity in adults.

Ordinarily the developing child chooses the parent of the opposite sex as a love object, the normal Oedipus situation. If disappointed in the response, hate impulses appear; the child turns to the other parent as an outlet for his need of affection, and thus an inverted Oedipus relationship is created. The Oedipus situation may develop into a pathological complex; in the vast majority of people it is satisfactorily repressed and sublimated. Mother-fixation in boys and father-fixation in girls are the results of an unsatisfactorily managed Oedipus complex. Most frequently this is primarily a fixation of the parents on the offspring, which interferes with normal development.

At about the sixth year the so-called masturbatory activity ceases or greatly diminishes; overt interest in playing with feces decreases or disappears; the Oedipus situation is diluted, and a period of calm, the latency period, sets in and extends to the first stirrings of puberty. Energies thus released are used for adjustment, adaptation, and competition. Actually, I see this as a homosexual type of phase, judged solely by the behavior of the children. During this period, which corresponds with the early school years, there is a very strong tendency to form into groups according to sex, more marked in boys than in girls. The latter often resent being pushed away from the boys, who may freely have accepted the girls as playmates up to this time. Some sexual play of a homoerotic nature does occur, but not very often. When it does, it is usually an older child or an adult who initiates the sex play.

Interest in sexual matters does not disappear, but begins to assume a more adult cast. Sexual intercourse between animals and their birth are likely to be observed and may serve as the basis for questions, but this interest is much more likely to be concealed from adults. It is during this period that children pick up most of the vocabulary of profanity and vulgar sexual terms which so disturbs parents and teachers. There is no lack of sexual curiosity, but the extent varies greatly with different children. Nor is the extent or nature of the curiosity likely to be revealed to adults, especially to parents.

For about two years preceding the definite signs of the establishment of puberty there are indications of increased physical growth, gradual development of adult secondary sexual characteristics, and changes in social attitudes which, taken together, represent the early phase of adolescence. During this period and the pubertal period itself, "crushes" on those of the same sex often occur. Ordinarily they are successfully resolved, even though there may be temporary overt homosexual activity.

Puberty is marked by the onset of menstruation in girls and nocturnal emissions in boys. At about this time heterosexual interests develop, and the object of the love impulses becomes a member of the opposite sex. In terms of age, this occurs earlier in girls than in boys, because girls mature at an earlier chronological age than do boys. Crushes also develop during this and the later adolescent stages, but in the normally evolving psychosexual integration these crushes are transferred to older adults of the opposite sex. This represents an important method of transition from attachments to parental images to the final and most important level of fixation, that is, heterosexual attachment to members of an appropriate age group.

Three important points remain to be emphasized. First, in the normal evolution of the psychosexual mechanism each stage plays its part and is succeeded by others. But no stage is completely repressed or displaced; *partial trends* remain and enter into the organization of the total personality. Oral and anal activity; narcissism and autoerotic activity; parental attachments and sibling rivalry; homosexual trends and heterosexuality—all these exist in the adult individual in varying admixture. Because of the effects of many accidents and incidents of living, there may be regression to an earlier level of integration and behavior patterns. Regression may be partial, temporary, marked, or permanent. The regressions, whether temporary or permanent, are more complete in certain psychoses, while regressions in the neuroses are likely to be less complete, more accessible to treatment, less permanent, and more changeable.

Secondly, the individual may become fixated at any of the several stages of development, however they may be defined. Thus, fixation may occur at the level of narcissism, in the Oedipus situation, on homosexuality, or there may be evidence of bisexuality. Any overt sexual activity will be in accordance with the level of fixation.

Adolescent masturbation may indicate fixation at an autoerotic level, or it may simply represent the only method available for an individual of average heterosexual make-up to discharge sexual tension. Homosexual activity in adults may similarly not be an expression of homosexual fixation, but a matter of opportunity. On the other hand, heterosexual activity, particularly promiscuity, may not represent a real heterosexual organization of personality.

Thirdly, the partial sexual trends, or even fixation at a particular level, may not lead to either regression or overt activity. Instead, the energy may be sublimated into socially acceptable activities. Since sublimation represents successful repression and compensation, conflicts and complexes and neurotic and other symptoms do not appear.

CHAPTER VIII

CYCLOTHYMIC (MANIC DEPRESSIVE) REACTIONS

THE CONCEPT of the manic depressive psychoses represents one of Kraepelin's clinical groupings based primarily on outcome and then carefully differentiated from other psychoses according to early symptomatology. Prior to Kraepelin's delimitation of the manic depressive group there were any number of diagnostic groupings. As has been mentioned, the terms acute melancholia, chronic melancholia, and recurrent melancholia might be applied to the same case in various stages. The same adjectives were used with mania. Then, if a patient had attacks of both mania and melancholia, it became circular insanity. Agitated depressions were called mixed states or simply agitated depressions, but since they were most common at the involution period, they were more likely to be called involution melancholia. Kraepelin brought order into this chaos and showed that the depressions and excitements were integral parts of one and the same total process.

In the cyclothymic reactions the prognosis is always that there will be recovery from the immediate attack but also that there will be further attacks. There is no known underlying pathology: in fact, the brains of manic depressives have been used as normal controls in brain studies in the past. Not only are pathological studies negative in findings, but no specific causative factors are known. Manic depressive psychoses do tend to occur in families and are often spoken of as hereditary. It has been maintained that no diagnosis of manic depressive should be made unless there have been other cases in the family or definite evidence of the presence of the cyclothymic personality in other members of the family.

The clinical pictures of mania and depression may best be described as markedly exaggerated emotional states with harmoniously related activity which otherwise occur as normal reactions. As a consequence, the average person can imagine himself in the patient's state; that is, the empathic index is high. The reverse is usually true in cases of schizophrenia—it is difficult for the average person to put himself in the patient's place. Or, stated in another way, the cyclothymic patient does not seem so odd or so far removed from reality as does the schizophrenic or the paranoid.

Manic depressive psychoses rarely occur under the age of fifteen (there were 19 cases in nearly 69,000 first admissions), but it occurs with more frequency in the fifteen- to nineteen-year-old group (400 cases). The maximum frequency for attacks requiring first hospital admission is the age period thirty to thirty-nine. Certain general rules usually apply. The younger the patient at the time of the first recognizable attack, the shorter the attack is likely to be. Conversely, the older the patient, including first attacks in the involutional period, the longer the attack usually is. With young patients, the interval before a second attack is usually long; after repeated attacks, the tendency is for the attacks to be longer and the free intervals shorter. There are instances in which only one attack occurs. On the other hand, one attack may continue, perhaps with alternating phases, over a period of several years. Chronic mania and chronic melancholia without any particular evidence of deterioration are not especially common, but do occur. The first attack may be of any type. All attacks may be of the same type; more commonly there will be at least one attack of the opposite sort, or the alternation may be more frequent. Apparently first attacks are more often depressive than manic. The disorder is more frequent in women than in men; it is somewhat more frequent among the Jews and the Irish than among other racial groups. Recovery is complete in that the patient develops insight into the fact of having had a mental disorder. However, on recovery the patient does not develop understanding of the psychopathological mechanisms. These are, after all, largely unconscious and quite involved. The patient does have good insight into the nature of the behavior and into the conscious mechanisms. Deterioration sometimes occurs in later life, perhaps from incidental causes.

The onset of the disorder is usually acute; in fact, occasionally it develops in the course of a few hours. Ordinarily there are premonitory symptoms, and through experience with repeated attacks a patient may come to recognize these and either hospitalize himself or seek treatment. Recovery or a shift to the opposite state may also be abrupt. Mixed states, the agitated depressions, are most tenacious and difficult to manage and to treat. At the onset patients have insight, but this is lost at the height of the disorder.

States of depression, or melancholia, are characterized by an emotional tone of dejection; delusions of self-depreciation and self-accusation, frequently somatic delusions; initial retardation of motor activity and executive retardation, constituting a general hypokinesis. Hallucinations occasionally occur, usually auditory and accusatory in content. Insomnia, loss of appetite, refusal to take food and water, constipation, and loss of weight are commonly associated symptoms.

A real danger in all cases of depression is the possibility of suicide, most marked in the early and late phases. At the height of the depression the motor inhibition is so great that the patient cannot carry out the idea, even though it may be strong. Suicidal threats in the early stages usually lead to precautionary measures, even though these sometimes fail to forestall successful or unsuccessful attempts. However, the most dangerous period with reference to suicide is the period when the deep depression has lifted, and the patient's motor activity has become more nearly normal. Enough depression remains so that the suicidal impulse may overcome inhibitions, especially since vigilance is very commonly relaxed. The nurse or companion may leave the patient for a few minutes, thinking the situation safe, and the patient takes advantage of the interval to carry out his impulse.

The depressive state may deepen into a stupor, the patient lying inertly in bed and requiring attention as would a baby. He must be tube fed. There is no loss of consciousness, no cerea flexibilitas or other signs either of an organic-toxic condition or of schizophrenia. He can be prodded into response, which is very slow, weak, and utilizes a minimal expenditure of energy. Efficient nursing care is necessary to keep the stuporous patient from dying of exhaustion. This state seems clearly to be a partial suicide.

When patients are more accessible they respond with the least possible effort and the fewest possible number of words. They express ideas of having committed the unpardonable sin, which usually turns out to be some trivial error. Occasionally the conscious nucleus of the unpardonable sin is some transgression which would be regarded as serious in the patient's family or social group. Usually, however, these major transgressions, while reported and regarded by the patient as evidence of unworthiness, are not given the center of the stage. Patients believe that they should be punished; that they are eternally damned to hell; that the future is entirely black and hopeless; that they can never get well. Ideas of poverty and a future of economic despair are common.

In rare instances the depression takes on a paranoid cast, and the punishments are reported as being meted out by someone the patient has injured or fancies he has injured. Or the patient believes that his hapless plight and depression have been forced on him by the machinations of others, whereas actually it is the patient who has harmed someone else or himself.

Depressions of this type must be differentiated from simple or reactive depressions. In the latter cases the precipitating cause is obvious in external reality and is sufficient to cause any normal person to feel depressed; hence the term reactive. However, the depression is more marked than the cause justifies, is unduly prolonged, or both. Usually there is no initial retardation; executive retardation is not especially prominent. Patients may be self-accusatory with respect to the precipitating events, and some anxiety may be shown. In general, such episodes are short, and the patient usually retains insight into the fact that he is over-reacting, but is unable to shake it off. These patients may also be suicidal.

In recognizable depressions of any type the social worker should not assume entire responsibility for the care of the patient; neither should the family. This should be shared with a psychiatrist, the family physician, or a hospital. The danger of suicide, resulting in guilt feelings for the family and the worker, or family hostility toward the worker, are sufficient reasons for such precautions. Furthermore, as will be shown later, not much can be done by psychotherapy, even of the supportive type, during acute phases of depression; various medical approaches, including hospitalization, nursing, feeding, hydrotherapy, medicines, and shock therapy may be indicated or essential.

In many ways mania is the opposite of melancholia, but it has particular features distinctively its own. Thus, the mood is one of elation, and there is marked overactivity and talkativeness. The train of thought, while connected in ways which can be seen, wanders in accordance with uninhibited inner associations and external distractions, both visual and auditory. This, the well-known flight of ideas, may prevent the patient from completing a train of thought or answering a question. Delusions are of the grandiose type; the ego is exalted. Hallucinations are not common; they are more likely to be visual in manias than in depressions. The patient may eat ravenously, or he may think he is too busy to eat; insomnia is the rule; loss of weight, often considerable, usually occurs. Patients insist that they feel extremely well. They are mischievous, often belligerent and irritable if crossed, though they can usually be distracted from this. They may show strong, though usually temporary, likes and dislikes for people around them. They remain well oriented and in contact with the environment until the mania reaches a considerable height.

This is a reasonably adequate description of hypomania, the most frequent type and the reaction which ushers in all manias. The attack may be maintained at this level, or it may increase in intensity. There is no clear dividing line between hypomania, mania, and furious mania, the names ordinarily applied to the several gradations of intensity. However, the state of activity may become so great that the patient quite completely loses track of his surroundings. His attention can be gained, if it all, only with great difficulty. In these furious states the patient is continuously and violently active, usually covering a wide range of territory; he is denudative, destructive, talkative but often incoherent, and disoriented. There may be considerable amnesia on recovery. The patient injures himself and perhaps others. Unless carefully watched and nursed, death may occur from exhaustion.

At the other end of the scale are states of elation and overactivity so mild that they pass unrecognized as representing any type of abnormal reaction. During such states the patient may do many foolish, grandiose things, such as giving away money, evolving great schemes for becoming wealthy, drinking to excess, showing considerable increase in sexual activity, talkativeness, and showing off. It is only when the number and extent of the items of altered behavior are recognized that the existence of a mild hypomaniacal state is suspected or recognized. There are also mild states of elation, with a feeling of tireless energy, rapid flow of ideas, and some reduction of inhibitions, during which, nevertheless, everything is under control; the individual's activities are co-ordinated, sustained, and effective. With some, this is a continuous state; with others, it is intermittent, being interrupted, perhaps, by periods of mild depression, inertia, inhibition, and inability to get started. With still other people, a gloomy, pessimistic mood is more or less constant.

Such states are characteristic of normal emotional reactions, especially changes in relation to reality factors. If they are marked, or if the alternation is sharply defined, particularly if the external reality cause is slight, we have the classical picture of the cyclothymic personality. This type, marked as it is by sharp swings of mood, is especially likely to develop a cyclothymic psychosis. Bouts of alcoholism may partially or completely replace and obscure the essential cyclothymia.

The mixed psychotic reactions usually take the form of an agitated depression and are particularly likely to occur in relation to the involution period. Inhibited mania is another type of mixed reaction, in which the patient is inert bodily, but may show typical flight of ideas. Or, if there is little speech, the patient may complain of racing thoughts. Attacks occurring in the involutional period tend to be much graver in prognosis than are earlier attacks. The differentiation of a manic depressive psychosis from an involution melancholia is not always easy on the basis of symptomatology, since the delusions, anxiety, insomnia, and repetitive moaning and groaning may be similar. A history of previous attacks or of a definite cyclothymic personality will be the chief differentiating factor in such cases. Differentiation from schizophrenia is frequently difficult, as may be seen by comparing the symptoms in the two disorders. Suicidal attempts in these mixed states are not infrequent and caution should always be exercised.

Perhaps the most important points to be borne in mind regarding manic depressive psychoses are: (1) the life cycle; (2) the extent of recovery; (3) frequency of attacks; (4) duration of attacks; (5) the personality type. These may be briefly recapitulated.

While many patients have only one attack, the rule is for recovery from an individual attack, but the prospect is for recurrence. Recovery is complete, with excellent insight and, in general, no signs of disturbance in mental functioning during the intervals. Attacks in youth tend to be shorter, and the free intervals tend to be longer than in later life. At the involution period first attacks are longer and more severe and frequently tend toward dementia. These may be cases of true involutional melancholia and are not necessarily manic depressive in type. In general, the life cycle of the manic depressive tends to be unstable, in terms of attacks of incapacitating disturbance or because of a cyclothymic personality. The age group with greatest incidence for first admission to hospital is thirty to thirty-nine, though there is high incidence for the disorder in all age groupings from twenty-five to forty-nine.

The readmission rate for manic depressives is higher than it is for all psychoses, but not as high as the readmission rate for schizophrenics. There are obviously different standards for the differential diagnosis of schizophrenia and manic depressive psychoses in different sections of the country, and even in different hospitals in the same region. This serves to emphasize the point that there are few pathognomonic signs and symptoms in psychiatry, so there is ample opportunity for confusion in interpreting symptom pictures in the functional psychoses.

To illustrate, 12.1 percent of first admissions to all state hospitals in the country were diagnosed manic depressive, and 22.9 percent dementia praecox. The combined total is therefore 35 percent. In New York state hospitals 8 percent of the first admissions were diagnosed manic depressive, and 25.4 percent were diagnosed dementia praecox; the combined is 33.4 percent. The difference between this combined total and that for the country as a whole is hardly of significance. Similarly, readmission rates for manic depressives are considerably lower in New York state than in the country as a whole, while the readmission rate for dementia praecox is substantially higher in New York state than for the country as a whole. The combined figures are almost identical.

The typical pre-existing personality types in manic depressive cases are: (1) the depressive, worrying, anxious personality; (2) the cheerful, aggressive, go-getter type; (3) the cyclothymic, alternating between gloom and elation. There is no precise line of demarcation between the normal range of variation and the degree of overemphasis of traits which constitutes psychopathy.

The social worker must always bear in mind the fact that the manic depressive patient is for all practical purposes quite normal in the interval between attacks. There is evidence that a supportive relationship with a social worker or psychiatrist may be useful to the patient at this time in helping him to withstand the stresses and strains of ordinary living which might provoke another attack. Psychoanalysis is the preferred method for treatment if the patient will accept any form of psychotherapy during the interval.

While recovery is complete so far as insight into conscious factors is concerned, strong unconscious hostile and destructive impulses remain. Therefore, some inexplicable swings in mood and unprovoked attacks, verbal or otherwise, may occur.

The psychopathology of depression has been better worked out through psychoanalysis than has the psychopathology of mania. In depression the oral and anal sadistic mechanism is involved. The unconscious hostile and destructive impulses are strong and are diverted from the original objects, the parents, and especially the mother, to the self. In part this is still an attack on the parents as introjected images. Hence, every attempted or actual suicide is in one sense a murder or homicidal assault. In the effort to defend themselves against the unconscious cannibalistic impulses, patients lose their appetite or refuse to eat. The self-reproaches represent in part the reproaches once directed against the patient by the parents and in part those directed against the parents by the patient or by other people of which the patient was aware. Other symptoms represent the working out of repeated disappointments which stimulate many hostile impulses and at the same time leave no love object.

In mania the instinctual impulses break through the restraints of the superego, and contact with reality is broken. There is much oral imagery and behavior. There is an infantile pleasure in activities which in many ways represent a repetition or recall of the Oedipus situation.

It must be repeated that even psychoanalytic investigations have not yet revealed the entire structure of the mechanisms involved in these psychotic states.

CHAPTER IX

SCHIZOPHRENIA (DEMENTIA PRAECOX)

INCLUDED IN this group are a number of psychotic reaction types which at first sight seem to have no very clear relationship to one another. That is, the clinical pictures seem to be quite dissimilar. Following are several examples.

A patient about eighteen years of age wandered aimlessly about the hospital ward, apparently paying attention to no one and to no event. He made no verbal response to questioning or at most responded with a hash of words carrying no meaning. He appeared dazed, as though walking in a dream, often with a silly expression or smile. There were outbursts of crying or laughing for no discernible reason. He ate fairly well sometimes, but often it was necessary to feed him by spoon or tube. He used the toilet spontaneously or when urged. He gave little or no care to his personal appearance or cleanliness. There were short and long periods of excitement, with rather disconnected obscenity, profanity and vulgarity of speech. At such times he smeared feces around and even ate them. Masturbation was openly practiced, and he strongly opposed any efforts at restraint. Stereotyped movements, grimaces, and utterances occurred, and there were evidences in his behavior and speech of delusions and hallucinations, chiefly auditory.

Another patient, age about twenty, lay motionless in bed, eyes closed or staring fixedly at some point. When someone approached his bed, his gaze did not shift to the newcomer, or, if his eyes were closed, there was only a flickering of the eyelids, which did not open. He answered no questions; if an order was given, it was ignored. If there was some slight movement, it was "away from the visitor." When I attempted to move his arm, there was rigid resistance. When the resistance had been overcome, the arm was gradually moved into a position that was awkward and uncomfortable, and there it remained for several minutes. At another time it remained in the same position for hours. Gradually and very slowly, the arm was returned to the original position. This patient voided and defecated in bed. It was necessary to feed him through a stomach tube. His behavior and speech, when there was any, indicated hallucinations in one or more fields.

At another time this same patient was seen standing in the crucifixion attitude which he maintained for an astonishingly long time. On another day he assumed a different constrained and difficult pose. There were outbursts of vituperation. In sudden short surges of activity there were violent assaults upon anyone who happened to be within reach, followed by a relapse into stupor. There were periods of very intense activity, concentrated within a small space and of narrow, repetitive range. Speech at such times was neologistic and confused, and, although words were intelligible, the speech as a whole was usually comparatively meaningless. Delusions were at times expressed; then again a relapse into stupor.

A patient about thirty-five years old was alert and clearly in touch with the environment, though he kept himself rather isolated from others. He entered readily into conversation, was oriented, and showed no particular memory defect. One thing, however, stood out: he was full of delusions and constantly brought any conversation back to his ideas of persecution and of grandeur. Either by his own conversation and behavior or by skillful questioning it was made apparent that he was hallucinated, especially in the auditory and somatic fields. The delusional ideas were usually clearly such and were often bizarre. The delusions and hallucinations were often regarded as extremely unpleasant by the observer, yet the patient seemed unperturbed by them. Emotional reactions to external events were blunted or paradoxical. This patient, too, was assaultive, but always gave a reason that would have been logical had the delusional premises been true. Such a patient will sooner or later decide that some person or organization is responsible for his troubles, and he may start a counter persecution.

A man of fifty was serving a short jail sentence for vagrancy. He seemed indifferent to his surroundings. For the most part he did as he was told, but he complained querulously about things which seemed trifling to others. He was unkempt and untidy. He kept mostly to himself, much of the time reading a small, well-thumbed volume of philosophy. His attitude toward others was one of aloof superiority. He showed some impairment of memory and regarded details about himself as unimportant. The history revealed that as a youth he had been a brilliant student, but in adolescence the quality of his school work began to deteriorate. He became seclusive, less interested in outside matters, unwilling or unable to hold a job, and he was not interested in girls. Although his family was of superior socio-economic status, he drifted away from them and did not avail himself of their social position. He had been a tramp for many years; an unambitious, apathetic, unsocial wanderer, who had been in jail many times as a vagrant or for petty offenses.

These are actual thumbnail sketches of the four main prototypes of the schizophrenic group. These conditions were originally described as separate clinical entities. The first sketch conforms reasonably well to the original description of a condition called hebephrenia; the second sketch, to catatonia. Both of these were first described about 1870. The third sketch corresponds to certain types of paranoid, or "chronic delusional," insanity, with eventual deterioration. The fourth type was originally described as "dementia simplex," and to it was attributed a large variety of types of poor social adjustment, such as vagrancy, prostitution, dependence, and the like. In addition to these fairly well-defined types of disturbance, there were in the many classifications of mental disorders a wide variety of primary and secondary dementias: hebetude, chronic mania, or melancholia with deterioration.

To this chaotic state of affairs Kraepelin turned his attention, publishing the results first in the late 1890's. The net result was that he identified two general groups and their early symptomatology. For one group, characterized by eventual greater or lesser dilapidation of the personality and showing from the beginning alterations in the amount of affectivity or the presence of paradoxical emotional responses, he applied the name dementia praecox. To the second group, characterized by eventual recovery, but a prognosis of future attacks, individual episodes being depressive, maniacal, or mixed in type, he gave the name manic depressive, as already pointed out.

A standard American textbook on nervous and mental diseases (Church and Peterson) published in 1897, gave several classifications of mental diseases and presented the author's ideas under the following headings: (1) Mania; (2) Melancholia; (3) Circular Insanity; (4) Epileptic Insanity; (5) Dementia (primary, secondary, senile); (6) General Paralysis; (7) Paranoia; (8) Idiocy, Imbecility, and Feeblemindedness.

Catatonia was believed by Dr. Peterson to be a type of melancholia; paranoia was a momentous diagnosis, frequently made. "Secondary dementia" was a term applied to deterioration that was "often a sequel to acute insanities like mania and melancholia, and to chronic insanities like circular insanity and paranoia." "Acute or primary dementia" was the term applied to "a form of mental disease characterized in the main from the very beginning by extraordinary psychic enfeeblement."

This brief statement emphasizes the point that in the 1890's there were few pathological concepts and scarcely any etiological ideas entering into the classification of the mental disorders. There has been a tendency to belittle Kraepelin's work on the score that it was not dynamic; that it was merely clinical-descriptive, not etiological. But he did introduce and emphasize a most valuable ordering concept into the attempts to recognize the genera and genetics of mental disease, that of *outcome*. It was a monumental task to make thorough studies of cases of diverse early symptomatology and on the basis of similarities in outcome to trace the essential, prevalent, early symptoms and thus establish common denominators from which studies of etiology might be prosecuted. Not only was it a tremendous job in its own right, but also there was an accumulated inertia of centuries to overcome. While Kraepelin's ideas were not received with unanimous approval, nevertheless the debate was not so much about the existence of the groups he defined as about their limitations and possible causations.

In the eighth edition of his textbook Kraepelin set up fourteen different subgroups of dementia praecox. This elaborate subdivision seems both unnecessary and confusing. At that time he defined dementia praecox in terms of a group of clinical types with a common symptom—"a characteristic destruction of internal associations . . . affecting particularly the emotional and volitional spheres." He also believed that there was increasing conviction that dementia praecox "represents a well-defined disease entity" and that the varied and apparently dissimilar clinical types were manifestations of a single disease process.

In about 1900 some American hospitals began to report cases of "primary dementia with catatonic symptoms." In 1903 at least one American hospital used the terms dementia praecox and manic depressive in its annual report, due undoubtedly to the influence of one staff member who had just returned from study in Germany. In that year the hospital staff classified 27.5 percent of the admissions as dementia praecox and 11.4 percent as manic depressive.

The choice of the name dementia praecox seems to have been based largely on the idea that dementia was characteristic and tended to reveal itself early and that it occurred in young, or at least in not-yet-mature, persons. However, Kraepelin's own work, quickly supplemented by the observations of many others, showed that dementia, at least in the form of irrecoverable intellectual loss, is neither inevitable nor precocious. Nor is the victim always young, at least by the time of his admission to a hospital.

These points are borne out by the 1937 report of the United States Census Bureau. The report shows that dementia praecox (schizophrenia) accounted for 22.8 percent of first admissions to all state hospitals in 1937, or nearly 16,000 cases; about 1,000 more males than females. For those whose ages were known, 9 percent were under age twenty (less than 0.5% under age fifteen); 38.3 percent age twenty to twenty-nine, the peak period being ages twenty-five to twenty-nine, when 20.5 percent of the total admissions occurred; 29.3 percent were thirty to thirty-nine years of age; 15.4 percent were forty to forty-nine years old; 7.8 percent were fifty or over.

Since dementia praecox is a disorder generally characterized by an insidious onset and slow development, these figures tell us nothing of the age of onset or the duration of the psychosis before admission to hospital. They do, however, emphasize the fact that somewhat more than half the cases did not reach the hospital until they were thirty years of age or more. As many patients were seventy years and over as were under fifteen; nearly the same number were fifty to sixty-nine as were fifteen to nineteen. Accordingly, it seems clear that dementia praecox is not specifically a disorder of pubescence or of adolescence. If it has a relationship to this age period, then at least the disturbance only very slowly reaches a level at which hosptial care is needed.

Two further points are relevant. One is that in all age groups, up to and through thirty to thirty-four, there is a definite excess of males, but beginning with age group thirty-five to thirty-nine, females are in excess. The second point is that the paranoid type tends to occur with greatest frequency in the later years, which is also true of the disturbances not classed as schizophrenic, but called paranoid states or conditions. Here the peak of admissions occurs in the age group forty-five to forty-nine, and the decade forty-five to fifty-four accounts for one third of all admissions so diagnosed. It should be noted that there is a general tendency to classify any doubtful paranoid types as schizophrenic if they are young, but as paranoid conditions if they are older.

With regard to the inevitability or the depth of the deterioration, it is reported that nearly 11,000 cases of schizophrenia were discharged from United States state hospitals in 1937, 55 percent of them male. Of these, 14.2 percent were rated as recovered, 70.7 percent as improved, and 14.9 percent as unimproved. These figures, superficially at least, indicate a much more hopeful prognosis than absolute deterioration or even complete chronicity. They do not tell the whole story, which will be discussed in detail a little further on.

There are other indices of chronicity, for example, the record of readmissions. Schizophrenia leads the list of cases readmitted, accounting for nearly one third of all psychotic readmissions; in New York state in 1943 the figure was 39 percent. Second would be the diagnostic classification of all patients resident in hospitals on a given date. On March 31, 1943, in New York, of 82,534 cases on the books, 56.4 percent were cases of dementia praecox. Of the 72,717 cases actually in hospital 64 percent belonged in this group.* Furthermore, at least 90 percent of the patients who had been resident in hospital ten years or more were schizophrenic. Finally, the time of death with reference to the duration of the psychosis is an index of chronicity. Among nearly 32,000 psychotic patients who died throughout the country, 17.2 percent were schizophrenics. Of these 5,641 patients, 13 percent had been in hospital less than a year; 10 percent had been in hospital ten to nineteen years; while 16 percent were in hospital twenty years or more. The largest number of deaths during the year occurred in psychotics with cerebral arteriosclerosis, but 62 percent of these occurred within the first year of hospital residence. There were also many deaths among cases of senile dementia, but again about 55 percent occurred in the first hospital year. Accounting for a large number

* Of the 46,539 cases of dementia praecox on the books, some 91 percent were in hospital, 7 percent were on parole, and the remaining 1 plus percent in family care. The number of cases on the books increased by nearly 6,000 in less than five years.

of cases of dementia praecox, it is found that the average duration of hospital life at the time of death is eighteen to twenty years; the average age at death, fifty-three to fifty-five. This contrasts with an average age of seventy and an average duration of hospital life of less than two years for the arteriosclerotics.

Another point of considerable importance in view of the essential psychopathology of schizophrenia is the marital status of schizophrenic first admissions. Nearly 60 percent were single, the proportion being much greater among the males than among the females. This contrasts sharply with the fact that only one third of the total admissions were single, and the schizophrenics accounted for nearly half of the admissions who were single. If schizophrenics are excluded from both the total admissions and those who were single, only one quarter of all other admissions were single. It also seems significant that among admissions who had been separated and divorced, one fourth were cases of schizophrenia. Separation and divorce and widowhood appear much more frequently among the female admissions than among the male. This is perhaps to be expected in view of the greater incidence of marriage among the females.

From the statistics cited, the following conclusions seem justified: (1) Schizophrenia is predominantly, but not exclusively, a disorder of comparatively early life, some 63 percent of the cases sent to hospitals being admitted before the age of thirty-five. (2) Large numbers are admitted at later, even advanced, ages. (3) It is a chronic, disabling disorder, with a comparatively low recovery rate. (4) It is not a hopeless disorder, since recovery and improvement do occur, there being greater or less improvement in a considerable majority of cases. (5) This improvement is not necessarily permanent, as shown by the high rate of readmission. (6) Whether or not there is improvement, continuous hospital care is necessary for a high percentage of cases, as shown by the hospital census at a given point and by the duration of hospital residence at the time of death.

Partly because of the theoretical and practical objections to the term dementia praecox, but still more because it is important to differentiate the early symptomatology, intensive efforts were made to clarify the psychopathology. A good many emphases emerged, such as intrapsychic ataxia, apathetic emotions, deterioration, blocking, inner absorption, autism, splitting between intellect and affect, and others. Because of the autistic nature of thinking and behavior and the very definite dissociation between the content of thought and the emotions and behavior, Bleuler proposed the use of the term schizophrenia, meaning literally splitmindedness; or better still, in his opinion, the schizophrenias, to cover the group of reactions embraced in the term dementia praecox. In his view the disease was chronic, or it progressed in attacks; it could come to a standstill at any stage, or there might be improvement, but there was never recovery in the fullest sense. Fundamental to the process is a disturbance in associations such that ideas tend to lose their relation to one another, resulting in incoherent thought. Patients lose their contact with external reality in any degree from mild to severe; thinking becomes inconsistent, dream-like, bizarre. The external world may be superficially completely shut out by a behavioristic refusal to accept any sensory impressions from it.

Bleuler's definition of schizophrenia was so applicable to the symptomatology of dementia praecox that the term has been quite generally adopted, except in official classifications, which usually speak of "dementia praecox (schizophrenia)." To all intents and purposes, therefore, the two terms are interchangeable when speaking of a particular type of mental disorder. It should be remembered, however, that the word schizophrenia may also be used to express or to define a symptom or a symptom complex.

CLINICAL TYPES

In the official statistical classification used in this country,* four types of schizophrenia are recognized, and provision is made for

* Classification of the American Psychiatric Association, which may be obtained from the National Committee for Mental Hygiene. The booklet is

"others, to be specified." The diagnosis of schizophrenia itself is based upon the appearance of certain rather general symptoms. Many writers have pointed out the generally unsatisfactory nature of these bases for recognition of the disorder and division into groups. It remains, however, a purely pragmatic matter. Despite intensive research over a period of nearly fifty years, there are no other and surer criteria on which to base differential diagnosis.

The four types officially recognized are hebephrenic, catatonic, paranoid, and simple. Common to all are inner absorption, apathy, and paradoxical responses. The schizophrenic literally lives in a world of his own, one which is penetrated by others only with great difficulty, if at all. Even when the patient is accessible to questioning and is communicative, it is difficult to feel in rapport because the ideas are too unrealistic, the moods are too strange, and the behavior is too silly or too peculiar. The net result is that the observer finds it difficult or impossible to imagine himself in the patient's position. That is, the empathic index is low, by contrast with such conditions as manic-depressive psychoses or neuroses.

The onset of schizophrenia is commonly insidious and gradual. It frequently happens that the changes in personality are so mild and develop so slowly that members of the family and others in close contact with the patient are unaware of the changes, or at least do not see their significance until some rather abrupt happening arrests their attention. This acute event may be almost anything—an outburst of excitement, an assault, a stuporous state, persistent refusal to eat, unexplained absence from home, apparent lack of recognition of the family, a suicidal attempt, blatant sexual activity, an appeal to the police for protection against persecutors, letters to high officials either threatening them or appealing to them for protection, and so on ad infinitum.

It is fairly common, but scarcely universal, to find that these

---

entitled *Statistical Manual for the Use of Hospitals for Mental Diseases.* In addition to the classification itself, there are short descriptions of the conditions included under each heading.

patients have a long history of being odd in various ways. Special stress has been laid on the shut-in type of personality, the unsocial, withdrawn person who has no intimate friends and tends to live within himself in a world of fantasy. The term schizoid personality is used much too freely today; it should be reserved for those who live within themselves and present queer ideas of their relationships with others and to the world at large.

There is no relationship between the level of intelligence and the schizoid personality or the development of schizophrenia. That is, persons of any level of intelligence may develop schizophrenia. Nor have any other factors, physical, mental, or social, a positive correlation. The anatomy, physiology, and chemistry of schizophrenics have been thoroughly studied, but so far no constant and significant changes have been discovered. While physical and mental constitutional types have been differentiated in relation to schizophrenia, it is only fair to say that they also occur in people who never develop the disorder and that individuals do develop schizophrenia who are not of these constitutional types.

In general, the present-day point of view is that schizophrenia is a maladjustment of the total personality to the total situation. From one viewpoint, at least, schizophrenia represents a solution or a cure for an otherwise insoluble intrapersonal problem. Because this is the case, recoveries in schizophrenia *are never complete*, and insight into the nature of the experience as a mental illness is not attained, as it is in manic-depressive psychosis. Even after the resumption of a good general adjustment to life, work, and play and even if the patient no longer sees particular events in the same light, experiences during the height of the psychotic episode will still be interpreted as actual and valid and the patient will deny having had any mental illness. Judging by my daily experience in the practice of psychiatry, this is the most overlooked fact in contemporary psychiatry.

The safest ground at present is to consider schizophrenia not a definite disease based upon definite pathology, either somatic or psychic, but rather a marked personality disorganization, a type of inferior adaptation to stresses and strains, both internal and experiential. It is entirely possible that there is a special predisposition in psychobiological constitution. At least this is the most convenient explanation for the fact that some individuals show an introverted make-up throughout life. And introversion does, in general, characterize the personality make-up of those who develop schizophrenia; more than half the admissions are characterized as being of shut-in type. This is said in the face of the fact that many schizophrenics (20%–25%) are described as having been of normal temperament prior to the onset of the illness. More careful history taking would certainly reveal indications of major deviant make-up in most of them. Excessive shyness, timidity, day dreaming, stubbornness, instability, seclusiveness, and other personality traits may not appear particularly important to the family except in retrospect, and even then may not be revealed in the history because they seem relatively unconnected with the illness. At the same time, it must be granted that there are no precise criteria for determining normality or abnormality of personality make-up. Because of its insidious onset and gradual development, in many cases of schizophrenia it is likewise impossible to say that the disorder began at some particular time. In fact, the early changes are, perhaps, usually recognized only in retrospect.

Many types of admixture of symptoms occur, and classification into groups is not always easy. The predominance of certain symptoms or a particular sort of history will usually indicate the particular group, though there may be transitions.

The essential mechanisms in schizophrenia are, perhaps, best described as regressions to a narcissistic, infantile type of existence. Omnipotence of inner ideas and feeling, anal and oral mechanisms, homosexual ideas, autism and autoeroticism all appear in the symptomatology of different cases in various combinations. The paranoid formula is a denial of a psychosexual fixation, as explained in somewhat more detail in Chapter X.

Hebephrenic Type

This type of schizophrenia tends to develop during the adolescent period. In the prodromal period these patients often express some insight; they complain that their minds do not work right, that there is something wrong. They may ascribe this to some faulty habit, perhaps blaming excessive masturbation. These patients particularly present the seclusive, introverted type of pre-psychotic personality, and excessive masturbation is frequently a manifestation of the essentially narcissistic personality make-up.

The onset of the condition is usually gradual, and the patient progressively withdraws into the self and becomes preoccupied, mute, and inaccessible to questioning, refuses food, and loses interest in personal appearance and cleanliness. The facial expression may be silly; there are sudden and externally unmotivated outbursts of weeping, anger, laughter, and excitement. Early in the development, or when from time to time the inaccessibility can be penetrated, the patient will reveal especially auditory hallucinations and delusions. The latter are usually fragmentary, at least not organized into a system, and while they may determine particular aspects of behavior, they do not control all the life activity. Much of the apparently senseless behavior is in response to the hallucinations and delusions. There are repetitive grimaces, gestures, and more massive movements. There may be frequent repetition of a few phrases or sentences, or the speech may be a hash of words conveying no meaning. Neologisms occur frequently. Sexual ideas color the speech and behavior; masturbation may be openly practiced. Frequently there is preoccupation with feces and urine, and these are sometimes ingested as well as smeared about. If bad news is announced, they may receive it with a laugh or with utter indifference.

Once established, the symptoms tend to remain fixed or to intensify progressively. In perhaps 10 to 15 percent of the hospitalized cases there is sufficient spontaneous recovery so that the patient may leave the hospital and resume work. In a larger group, the symptoms subside or remain stationary at a point at which the patient may become one of the workers in the hospital, perhaps even live in an open ward and have parole of the grounds. Such remissions, which is all they may be called, vary in duration. In such intermissions it will be found that despite the seemingly great withdrawal from reality during the period when symptoms were more marked, the patient has a remarkably good memory for at least the more important happenings. In other words, the inner absorption appeared to be more absolute than was actually the case.

In the intermissions the patient may continue to be hallucinated and deluded, and these factors may control behavior. There is a tendency to be silly and rather uninhibited in actions. The emotional reactions are dulled, the affect is in general indifferent, and the patient tends to remain aloof. Insight is not regained.

Sooner or later the disorder progresses, and the split in the personality becomes even more marked. In the final phases intellectual dilapidation becomes obvious, especially with regard to remembering recent events and the association of ideas. If the patient is at all accessible, the inquirer may find that early memories are fairly well retained.

The usual picture of advanced hebephrenia is of an inert, self-centered, manneristic individual who has regressed to infantile modes of behavior. Death is usually due to some intercurrent disease; pulmonary tuberculosis is particularly common in these cases. This is amply explained by the type of life the patients lead, but it has been ascribed by a number of eminent psychiatrists to a lessened libido of the respiratory tract or to inferiority of the autonomic nervous system, with special reference to this area.

The hebephrenic cases tend to be long-lived, possibly in relation to the relatively early onset. They constitute 15–20 percent of the cases of schizophrenia admitted to hospitals. Many cases with a history of an acute episode of the hebephrenic type improve to a mild stationary dementia and are classed with the simple type in later life.

Catatonic Type

This is the type which is in many ways the most dramatic. The onset of the disorder may be acute; the clinical state may change rapidly; social recovery occurs in 25–30 percent of the cases; the empathic index is higher than for other forms; it is more like manic-depressive psychosis than are the other types of schizophrenia.

Stupor is characteristic. In this state the patient is inert and will lie in one position in bed for long periods. These patients can be aroused and will react to a variety of stimuli, even though the reaction is a negativistic one. Negativism, i.e., doing the reverse of what is expected or commanded, is a prominent symptom. Rigidity, with marked resistiveness to passive motion, and *cerea flexibilitas*, or moldability, are also pronounced; in fact, rigidity gave the condition its original name, *katatonia*, or tension insanity.

In the stuporous phase the patient seems entirely withdrawn. Usually the eyes are closed, at least when the patient is aware of being observed; no indication is given of hearing; the individual does not go to the toilet, but voids and defecates in bed; saliva is not swallowed, but is allowed to accumulate in the mouth and dribble out; the patient does not eat and must be tube fed. This state of suspended animation bears a close resemblance to coma, on the one hand, and to the hysterical trance, on the other, but the resemblance is only superficial. The comatose patient cannot be roused and reacts only slightly, if at all, to painful stimuli, while the hysteric is suggestible and responsive even in the trance. The catatonic gives evidence of being conscious and shows negative suggestibility and waxy flexibility.

Even in the stuporous phase the catatonic may give ample evidence of hallucinations and delusions. While auditory hallucinations predominate, false sensations in other fields are much more common than in the other types of schizophrenia. Visual, olfactory, visceral, and kinesthetic hallucinations are especially frequent. Related to these symptoms are ideas of being gassed, poisoned, and the like. Visual hallucinations are often scenic and so help to determine the fixed poses or attitudes the patient assumes.

Religious ideas color the delusions and help to determine many postures, such as a crucifixion pose or prolonged kneeling as if in prayer. The patient may claim to be Christ or the Virgin Mary, though the verbalization of such ideas is more common in the paranoid.

There is much evidence of anxiety, feelings of guilt, and fear of reprisal not only in the stupor and the supplicating attitudes but also in the way in which the catatonic who is out of bed will sidle away from anyone who approaches, often staying close to the wall as he does so. The latter activity is related to the many anal erotic and homosexual ideas which are present.

A frequently assumed pose, usually long maintained, is that of the fetus *in utero*, with head bowed on the knees which are drawn up, and heels approximating the buttocks. The patient may sit up or lie on his side. The mouth is often strongly pursed (*Schnautz-krampf*), as though to repel oral assault by a penis or to conceal thoughts by making it impossible to speak. These patients are denudative and destroy clothes and bedding with which they are furnished.

Catatonia may be ushered in by depression, stupor, or excitement. Stupor is commonly replaced by excitement, usually sudden and often dangerous to the bystander. This excitement has certain characteristics which tend to differentiate it from a manic state. It is comparatively circumscribed in range. The patient confines the overactivity to the bed or to the room, or there is excessive, often unintelligible, speech and a minimum of general overactivity, or marked physical activity with mutism. Another characteristic is the apparently blind assaultiveness; at any time and without discernible reason or warning the catatonic may launch himself on a passerby.

That anal erotic mechanisms are prominent in catatonia is demonstrated in the olfactory hallucinosis, the ideas of being gassed and poisoned, and in the behavior indicating fear of and protection from anal assault. Many of these and other points indicate also an unresolved homosexual conflict.

Fully developed catatonic stupors are very rare nowadays in well-conducted mental hospitals. As an initial phase they are common enough, but without environmental stimulation the catatonic apparently cannot remain long in a defenseless stupor. As a chronic reaction, the catatonic stupor is now found almost exclusively in training schools for the mentally defective.

Constituting about 25 percent of the schizophrenic group, the catatonics have by far the highest spontaneous recovery rate. Again it must be emphasized that this is a recovery without insight, at least beyond the merest notion that something has been wrong.

One of the most brilliant students I ever had suddenly stood up in class and accused the professor of shooting electric currents through him. In hospital he quickly passed into a stupor, from which he made a recovery sufficiently good so that his family insisted on taking him home. Seven years later he was returned to the hospital, having spent the intervening years as a vagrant. At this time he had many extraordinary delusions, but was characteristically apathetic. At no time had he shown any insight into the nature of his disorder.

Another patient was brought in on a stretcher, having fallen suddenly into a stuporous state during a period of penitential prayer. While the routine examination was being made, a needle was accidentally broken off in his back during the lumbar puncture. Following an operation, with anesthetic, to remove the needle, he was quite lucid and had apparently recovered from his catatonic attack. Allowed to go home, he was returned to hospital some fourteen months later with a fully developed psychosis.

One of the first patients I came to know well in the hospital where I began work was a catatonic who was so dangerous that he was kept in the suicidal ward, where patients were under observation twenty-four hours a day. He was kept there because, although he had been resistive, even stuporous, and had been tube fed for four years, he was likely to assault anyone at any time. As I listened to him and watched him, it was apparent that the people he hated most and was most determined to injure were the married couple who between them took care of him day and night. These people were well aware of his antipathy, but they were also aware of the fact that they could control him if they watched him carefully enough.

About two years later he suddenly improved. Within three months he gained seventy pounds, became quite social within the hospital, and began to talk of going home. At the staff meeting to consider his parole two things stood out. First, and most important, was his denial that he had ever been mentally ill; second, his assertion that the couple who cared for him were actually his persecutors and that he would somehow revenge himself on them. Ultimately he died in the state hospital, after several such remissions.

These cases are cited merely to prove the point that catatonics rather easily make recoveries, some of which are fairly complete from the social viewpoint. The only remnants of the psychosis may be the absence of insight into the nature of the past experience, combined with a general unsociability. Or there may be scattered delusions and a continued hallucinosis, kept under good control. The prognosis is for relapse and progressive deterioration. The stupor may last for long periods, even several years, though this is relatively rare. The excitement is likely to be so intense that the patient becomes exhausted. In both stupor and excitement the motivations are from within; external stimuli are incorporated very little, if at all, and then in terms of delusions.

Paranoid Type

The outstanding symptoms of this variety of schizophrenia are the delusions, fairly to extremely well systematized. Associated with these are hallucinations, most frequently auditory, but not uncommonly involving any or all sensory areas. There are also present the common schizophrenic disturbances of emotional tone, apathetic or paradoxical responses, and negativism. The delusions tend to be changeable, bizarre, and definitely unrealistic.

In the early stages, ideas of reference are common. These eventually become more than ideas, evolving into hallucinations and delusions. Usually the first ideas are painful and threatening, and in the beginning the patient may react appropriately with anger or fear. Ideas of persecution are sooner or later mingled with or replaced by ideas of grandeur. As long as the train of thought can be held together, the patient will speak or write voluminously. The production, however, is stereotyped and repetitive; in the later stages it is disjointed and incoherent.

The paranoid type accounts for about 50 percent of the cases of schizophrenia, and tends to develop later in life than do the other forms. It may develop slowly over many years before some untoward event, such as a period of excitement related to the ideas of persecution, an assault upon an innocent bystander, or some other bit of disordered or antisocial behavior, makes hospitalization imperative. These incubation periods may last for twenty or more years. During such a period, the patient may be regarded as efficient, but queer. An example is an architectural draftsman who had been assigned a room to himself for nearly twenty years simply because his firm appreciated the excellence of his work and knew from experience that he could not work in a room with others. The burden of this man's hallucinations and delusions eventually became so great that in the midst of a snowstorm he ran barefooted and in his night clothes to a police station for protection.

Paranoid cases do not recover completely, although symptoms may subside to a considerable extent. Some patients learn to cover up their delusions and hallucinations and so make a fair social adjustment. This is perhaps especially true if the hallucinations and delusions are focused on some one person or in some particular life area. Avoidance of the person or the area may then permit the paranoid individual to lead a fairly quiet, reasonably socialized existence. In general, remissions are less frequent and less complete than in the other types. Furthermore, the paranoid is always potentially dangerous. The delusions may at any time be fixed upon almost anyone, and assault, with severe injury or even death, may result. This is an especially grave problem, since the paranoid may present little in the way of obviously abnormal behavior.

Simple Type

This diagnosis is made in only 5 percent or less of schizophrenic admissions to state hospitals. In the typical case the whole personality gradually changes, and apathy, irritability, lack of interest, decrease in the power to concentrate, loss of ambition, and diminished activity develop. Criticism has no effect, nor have concern and affection. A dependent role is accepted without question, or, in a minor flash of irritation, the patient may wander away from home. While there is no measurable impairment of the intellect, patients are considered queer and usually can carry out only simple tasks and these under supervision. Many become vagrants, prostitutes, or petty delinquents. They are too absorbed in themselves to carry their drives into competition with others. Nothing in the external world is particularly important.

There may be a short episode in the beginning with some hallucinosis and scattered delusion formation resembling the hebephrenic type. Such episodes are usually transient and do not color the psychosis particularly. Commonly the personality change begins during the teens and for years it may not be regarded as serious. It is only when the early promises are not fulfilled over a long period that friends and relatives can accept the idea that a mental disorder is present.

COURSE, PROGNOSIS, AND TREATMENT

Sufficient has been said to make it clear that the course tends to be chronic, that ultimate personality disorganization is marked, and that the outlook is for more or less permanent hospital care. Actually, schizophrenia is one of our most perplexing public health problems. The high admission and readmission rates, the low recovery rate, and the accumulation of such cases in the hospitals all indicate this. There are apparently more than 250,000 such cases registered on the books of our mental hospitals, and more than 22,000 new cases are being received each year. The cost of their care alone, not to mention the loss of productive capacity, is at least $75,000,000 annually.

Nor is this the worst side of the picture. Perhaps no disease, if this is to be regarded in any sense as a unitary disease process, has been more thoroughly investigated from every conceivable angle of pathology and etiology—anatomical, chemical, bacteriological, and psychological—yet in effect we know no more about the causes today than was known when Kraepelin first synthesized the group. Every conceivable factor has at one time or another been implicated, but none has stood the test of time and further investigation.

Most promising have been various psychopathological leads, especially those showing how partial sexual trends become fixed and operate to produce particular symptoms. These satisfy the observer's need to understand what is transpiring in the psyche of the schizophrenic, but they do not help to bring about recovery. The point is that the trends *are fixed;* they represent a narcissistic, unrealistic solution of a problem insoluble realistically. Accepted as reality by the patient, he shows marked resistance to their removal. Here the patient's absence of insight into the unreality of his symptoms operates as a definite and seemingly final barrier to really effective psychotherapy.

That many patients make a greater or lesser degree of spontaneous recovery under hospital conditions perhaps indicates the best common-sense approach to the problem. In such a protected environment, with a definite routine, there is apparently less pressure on the patient. This gives him an opportunity to organize his defenses so that the need for aggressiveness through symptoms is diminished. Frequently, as already noted, the patient can operate fairly well while in the hospital, but cannot adjust in the outside world.

Every conceivable type of treatment has been tried with the schizophrenic. None, except the several types of shock treatment, have shown any substantially greater success than is achieved through the generalized hospital routine and the efforts of sympathetic doctors and nurses. A recent New York study of 1,128 schizophrenics who received insulin shock therapy at the Brooklyn State Hospital shows that 79.5 percent were able to leave the hospital, and about 55 percent were able to become self-supporting. This is in contrast to the findings in 876 matched cases in other hospitals who did not receive such treatment; in this group, 55.8 percent were able to leave the hospital, and 40.5 percent became useful members of the community. The margin in favor of the shock treatment is therefore nearly one half for those able to leave the hospital and about one third for those able to resume a vocation or select a different one. Furthermore, the length of stay in hospital was appreciably shortened by shock treatment, and the readmission rate was lessened.

Three types of shock therapy are available: insulin; metrazol, which may be used with curare to lessen the violence of the convulsions; and electric current. Up to date the evidence seems to favor insulin for the schizophrenics and metrazol for the cyclothymics. However, electric shock is much simpler to use, less frightening to patients, and has fewer untoward side effects. It yields good results and bids fair to replace the other methods except in refractory cases.

The rationale of the effects of shock therapy has not been satisfactorily worked out. It is most effective in the catatonic and, surprisingly, the paranoid types. The best hypothesis to date to account for its success seems to be that a serious disturbance of memory and association is created, and this affects particularly the more recently acquired or more recently elaborated sets of ideas. Shock therapy is definitely more effective in cases where the psychotic elements in thinking and behavior have been recently developed. It is, of course, particularly striking that the paranoid cases react favorably, since medical treatment, psychotherapy, hydrotherapy, occupational therapy, and the social life of the organized ward have, in general, so little effect on these patients.

It should be noted that in those cases which I have seen in which a social recovery has resulted from shock therapy, there is still an absence of complete insight into the nature of the past disturbance and the effectiveness of the treatment. Patients continue to believe in the former symptoms, but discount them in one way or another.

THE PAROLED PATIENT

As previously noted, large numbers of schizophrenic patients are discharged from hospitals each year—nearly 11,000 in 1937. Almost 15 percent of them were classed as recovered, about 70 percent as improved, and about 15 percent as unimproved and unknown. The discharged cases amounted to 50.7 per 100 cases of schizophrenia admitted. In the same year nearly 6,000 cases of schizophrenia were readmitted to the hospitals, or 52.7 per 100 cases discharged. With about 21,000 first admissions to all types of mental hospitals, some 6,000 readmissions and 11,000 discharges, it appears that movement into and out of the hospitals represents a social phenomenon of considerable moment. It is during the developmental stages and during parole and discharge periods that social service is of the greatest importance.

The extent to which the social worker may be able to help in a supportive relationship with the schizophrenic or by assisting him to find a job, supervising his community relationships, interpreting the patient to his family, friends, and employer will depend to a considerable measure on the degree and nature of the personality disorganization. The paroled patient usually does not show much impairment of intelligence, memory, or the capacity to reason, but there may be mild to marked impairment of habits, of self-regard, of the social sensibilities, and of judgment in practical mat-

ters. If one or more members of the family are genuinely interested and sympathetic yet firm in attempting to socialize the
patient, then a reasonably adequate social adjustment may be maintained for some time. This may, however, be limited to the home
or to some simple routine of occupation with which the patient's
oddities do not interfere.

The difficulty of providing a suitable occupation is one of the
stumbling blocks to successful social adjustment. In the hospital
the patient may do well in occupational therapy or in any one of a
large number of maintenance jobs. There is little pressure in such
tasks, and competition is at a minimum. The schizophrenic often
has impossibly high standards for himself and quickly abandons
effort and withdraws if pressure is great or competition is stren-
uous.

Sheltered workshops have proven of value for some cases, but to
all intents and purposes they are nonexistent for these patients.
Once trained in the routine of an occupation which does not interfere with or reinforce his symptoms, a schizophrenic will faith-
fully perform his tasks for years. Thus, a young schizophrenic who
was constantly reacting to hallucinations and delusions had the job
of cleaning the floors in the administration building of a hospital
and caring for the officers' toilet rooms. He was unconscionably
slow, but very thorough. He rarely seemed to pay attention to anyone he encountered in the course of his duties. Fifteen years later
and twelve years after I had last seen him, he was the first person
I met on a visit to the hospital. Considerably to my surprise, he
greeted me by name and added that he had not seen me for some
time. Despite his excellent memory for names and faces, his behavior showed that he was still reacting to hallucinations and delusions.

In planning for the paroled patient the social worker should be
guided by the medical opinion as to the severity of the disorder and
the prognosis. Since there are no fixed criteria with respect to
these points, the actual course may present considerable variation
from that expected. The worker must therefore adopt a prag-

matic attitude and follow along, be as optimistic as the patient's condition permits, but retain a wholesome pessimism as to future possibilities. Above all, one must guard against overidentification with the patient's interests, especially with his tendency to ascribe his difficulties to hostilities in the immediate environment. To be guarded against also, are two rather contradictory dangers: the development of too great a dependency relationship; and putting so much pressure on the patient to stand alone that he is driven into further withdrawal and a more serious personality split.

Finally, even though it sounds harsh, all who work with these cases would do well to bear in mind the old adage that once a schizophrenic, always a schizophrenic. If this is remembered, untoward developments will not produce too great an emotional effect. The worker will be able to feel a justifiable satisfaction if the patient's remission is long continued, but without taking too much personal credit. It is also worth while to remember that no type of psychotherapy has yet been devised which is wholly effective with the schizophrenic. This awareness will save the worker a great deal of energy which might otherwise be wasted. In other words, one should take advantage of every bit of improvement, but not feel that it is the result of individual effort or the result of any particular type of psychotherapeutic approach.

CHAPTER X

PARANOIA AND PARANOID CONDITIONS

PRIOR TO Kraepelin's reclassification of mental disorders in terms of outcome, there was no more frequently used term in psychiatric literature than "paranoia," of many different types. The plea of innocence based on paranoia was common in criminal cases, especially when murder was involved. Kraepelin and others demonstrated the schizophrenic nature of many cases in which delusion formation dominates the clinical picture. He described one group of paranoid conditions under the name "paraphrenia," but it has never been accepted in this country. At the same time he delimited a very small group of "true" paranoia. These are cases having a single system of delusions, which remains more or less walled off, in which there is little or no disintegration of the personality. Hallucinations are rare and may occur only once or twice in the form of a vision or a communication, often ascribed to God. About subjects other than that on which the patient is "hipped" he may have adequate information, good reasoning powers, and fairly sound judgment.

Within the delusional system of persecution and of grandeur there is impermeability to logic, and all sorts of seemingly unrelated events are woven into the system. In many instances of paranoia the nature of the delusions is such that the fancied persecutions could have occurred and the grandiose ideas might have been true. Analysis of the assigned bases for the ideas will usually, however, reveal the actual lack of logic and valid connections. Such persons are generally regarded as cranks and nuisances. Until they have repeatedly made trouble for certain persons or groups the factor of a really gross mental disturbance is rarely considered.

Furthermore, their reactions to their ideas are consonant with the content of the ideas.

The paranoid states, on the other hand, are chronic delusional conditions, with a wealth of delusions and usually many hallucinations, often in several sensory fields. They represent gradations between paranoia, on the one hand, and the paranoid type of schizophrenia, on the other. Clinical usage seems to differ in the several states, but there appears to be a general trend toward inclusion of the vast majority of the paranoid types with the schizophrenias. In New York state in 1938, for example, the diagnoses paranoia and paranoid conditions accounted for just 1 percent of the admissions and 6.7 percent of all the paranoid types, the schizophrenic accounting for the other 93.3 percent. In general, the term paranoid condition is used for cases which lack some or all of the fundamental symptoms and signs of schizophrenia. It is therefore a diagnosis by exclusion or, perhaps better stated, by negative findings.

There are no precise criteria, in the sense of laboratory tests, for differentiating the paranoid personality at one extreme, paranoia, the paranoid conditions, and paranoid schizophrenia, with its deterioration, at the other. All involve a certain reaction type, a characteristic way of looking at life and one's relationship to it. The development of certain symptoms, such as increases in tension and consequent disturbances in social behavior or the fixation of ideas upon certain people, may tip the balance in favor of one or another diagnosis. Much more important, the presence or absence of behavior-determining symptoms will decide whether the individual may continue to live freely in the community or must be under supervision and treatment; whether he shall be confined in a penal institution or must be hospitalized, perhaps permanently.

In all types of paranoid reaction the basic mechanism is projection. There is a minimum of consciously accepted guilt, anxiety, and awareness of conflict. When with a paranoid person one therefore feels utterly different than when with the anxiety-laden, guilty, and insightful neurotic. Paranoids are suspicious, tense, and often frightened. Whatever occurs in their environment, however little it may actually be related to themselves, is immediately given a highly personal interpretation. Ideas of reference, of being talked about, accused, criticized and blamed, or mild ideas of grandeur, all of which are common enough in the daily experiences of everyone, assume a special, continuous, and over-determined value for the paranoid. Such things happen to him all the time and wherever he is, and anyone and everyone may be responsible. Being talked about, accused, and criticized is never his fault or due to any actions of his own. Instead, all responsibility is projected onto some person, an organization, or a rationalized bit of mysticism, such as fate or the "evil eye."

The paranoid personality is one which is characterized by tenseness, quick suspicion, ready anger, and the inability to maintain a successful personal relationship for any length of time. In addition to blaming others or some untoward situation for their own failures and errors, paranoid persons usually have a very high estimate of their own abilities and understanding. They are prone to pick impractical or unsuitable careers in which failure is inevitable for them. Often they seem to seek advice, but they rarely accept it; failure is only another evidence that the world is against them. Since they frequently lack concentration of attention and persistence in application, they really fritter away a great deal of time. They rapidly become dissatisfied with progress in a job and so tend to make frequent changes, both of jobs and of types of work, or they move to a new community where they believe they will have a better chance.

After only a few days of employment, many of them "know more than the boss." They make ignorant and inept suggestions and have a sense of injury if these are not immediately adopted. They usually feel that whoever is their direct superior is against them and is making every effort to retard their progress or turn others against them. They tend to be constantly involved in petty friction and disputes. As practically everything they complain of can and does happen to almost everyone at some time, the paranoids find sympathizers and followers in crusades "to do something about it." This particular type of paranoid personality often gives the impression of being very social and extroverted. Paranoids are frequently alcoholic and are often less tense and suspicious when drinking moderately than at other times.

The essential points are the repetitiveness of the pattern, the number of people who become involved in the paranoid circle, and the varied situations which do not work out. Many go through the same circuit time after time. There is a new and highly valued friend, or a new position is approached with great enthusiasm and energy, but before long the friend is an enemy, and the position has turned out to be "rotten." So the friend is dropped or even persecuted, and a new position must be found, or the type of work must be changed.

Characteristic of the paranoid psychopath is antagonism to persons in authority. These persons the paranoid cannot accept; they represent some form of restraint, and restraint or being crossed provokes strong reactions. Men in whom these rebellious reactions to authority are strong make poor material for the armed forces. The chances are very great that they will be in constant trouble, spend much time in guardhouse or brig, and probably wind up with court martial or a dishonorable discharge. They foment trouble and keep their outfits in constant turmoil.

Apparently because of differences in total dynamics, some rather paranoid individuals make a good adjustment in the armed services. The security of following a routine and the opportunity to vent hostility in an acceptable fashion, as well as to focus persecutory ideas on a common enemy, would seem to account for this. Such cases seem to be the exception rather than the rule.

It is useless to attempt to argue with a paranoid and worse than useless to try to point out errors in his logic, reasoning, or observation, or to urge him merely to forget or ignore his grievance. It is sometimes possible to inject some elements of doubt as to his certainty by bringing up alternative interpretations, but this must be done carefully and in such a way that he will feel he is still believed in and has the attention, sympathy, and support of the therapist. Of course, if (and it is a very large if) there can be developed in the mind of the milder paranoid some doubt concerning the correctness of his viewpoints, so that he will begin to suspect he is really responsible for his situation, then treatment is possible. But since in many, perhaps in most, cases the paranoid reaction is an ego defense against the admission of weakness and conflict, it is an extremely difficult matter to penetrate the paranoid shell, as many workers have found to their cost.

Paranoid personalities seem to offer one of the best examples of a constitutionally determined deviation and are frequently used to illustrate the thesis that constitution is innate and fixed. The further point is frequently made that some sort of psychopathic predisposition, congenital or hereditary neuropathic instability, or some other "abnormal soil" is necessary as a groundwork on which experiences operate to produce the neuroses and functional psychoses. There is reason to doubt this, at least as a matter of original biological constitution, as was brought out in a preceding chapter.

Paranoid personalities occur in people of all levels of intelligence and from all types of background. There is no particular delusional system; the disturbance is diffuse and unorganized. Other personality factors are also variable. Many are solitary, seclusive types, and when these features are especially prominent, it is called schizoid personality; the paranoid trend is given only secondary importance. A combination of schizoid and paranoid traits is frequently found to exist for a considerable period in many persons who later develop frank paranoid schizophrenia or the less differentiated paranoid conditions.

The true paranoia cases are ordinarily divided into a number of types: persecutory, exalted, religious, erotic, and litigious, to cite one classification. This is not particularly important, however, since these divisions are based more on certain rather superficial resultants of the paranoiac process than on basic mechanisms.

Paranoiacs with marked ideas of persecution are likely to attempt retaliation as soon as they have identified their persecutors.

They present the threat of homicide, but so do those with ideas of grandeur if they become convinced that a particular person stands in their way. The religious type usually reveals himself through ideas of grandeur—he founds a new religion with himself as the Messiah, or is the authentic second Christ, or has been directly invested by God with the gift of prophecy. Many of these individuals are energetic and verbal and gain a considerable following, yet they may act as ruthlessly as do those whose ideas are persecutory, since their divinity or supremeness makes them immune to all laws except their own: "The King can do no evil."

As a practical matter, it should be emphasized that the threats of a recognized paranoiac must be taken seriously. They do not arise out of anger or depression, both of which may be transitory moods which an individual may help to dissipate merely by uttering the threats. On the other hand, the threats of the paranoiac spring from a basis which is logical according to his manner of thinking. Even though he may be indignant or fearful, nevertheless the paranoiac always justifies himself, since he is always the injured party. His acts would be justified or at least condoned *if* the ideas on which they were based were correct and he had in fact been injured or thwarted in the manner which he believes to be true.

The sullen, morose, threatening paranoiac is a dangerous person to be at large. One of the most difficult features lies in the fact that an assault or a homicidal attempt may be suddenly launched against a person with whom there has been no previous contact, or it may be directed against some outstanding public figure. The symbolism of this seems quite obvious. There is little doubt that the assassins and those who have attempted assassination of presidents and other high officials in this country were paranoids of some type, though there have been heated debates as to whether they were insane in the legal sense. This refers, of course, to all those instances in which only a single individual was involved and no cabal or any sort of revolutionary plot was evident.

Some paranoiacs make their attempts at retribution or conduct their crusades for reform only through litigation. They institute suits for what are actually the most trivial reasons, seeking redress for fancied injuries of one or another sort, for fraud, or for other causes. The more suits they lose or have thrown out of court, the more persistently do they enter new ones. Also, as suits are lost or disallowed, the circle of individuals in the plot widens in the paranoiac's mind. It becomes increasingly necessary, therefore, for him to vindicate himself. If countersuits are entered, he meets them with a complete lack of understanding; he is even surprised that his opponents should consider that they have been abused or injured. Some litigious paranoiacs become so involved in suits and countersuits, litigations begun, withdrawn, or altered, that it is impossible for the onlooker to get a clear picture of what is going on. A lawyer or a judge who questions the validity of a suit is promptly placed by the paranoiac on the side of the opponents; he believes they have either been bought off or influenced.

In still other instances the paranoiac wages his warfare verbally. Some of the worst gossip-mongers and reputation-blasters are paranoiacs. This is a way by which they can enhance their own inner feelings of superiority, or, better stated, this is a method of attempting to reduce their unacceptable, conscious feelings of insecurity. Oral assassination of character, known these days as smear, is more common than the written, but paranoiacs are also voluminous writers. In letters—personal and to the editor, in articles, magazines, monographs, and books—the paranoiac pours out his persecutions, his vindications, his prophecies, his claims, and his crusades. In many instances he starts his own weekly or monthly paper. With his own name in the title, and liberal use of italic and boldface type and a plethora of "I's" in the text, the little journal reveals the paranoid personality behind it. The attacks are bitterly phrased, conveying the idea of much more emotion and anxiety concerning the person or situation attacked than the facts or allegations could possibly justify. The logic is confused and wobbly, and there is much retrospective falsification of memory. To be especially noted is the fact that although the attack and the crusade for change may be ostensibly for the good of society, the rationalization is ineffectively carried out, and the sense of personal injury, frustration and aspirations for self-aggrandizement are what really stand out. Arguments are never carried out on an abstract or impersonal level; they are always personal in emphasis, unnecessarily vituperative, and defensive.

Most of the religious, litigious, and verbal paranoiacs are not regarded as insane, at least not during long periods of development and until after much damage has been done. If signs of deterioration develop or the individual becomes too great a nuisance, if his attacks become too absurd or if he commits libel or some other serious legal offense, he may be imprisoned or committed to a hospital. Most paranoiacs are regarded as harmless, though annoying, crackpot members of the lunatic fringe, and nothing is done about them. Since they may continue over long periods to manage their practical affairs with reasonable prudence and foresight, this seems to be legitimate public reaction. Furthermore, it must be admitted that many realistic and worthwhile reforms have been initiated by the complaints and criticisms of paranoid people. Even though their interests were personal and overdetermined, investigation of the complaints uncovered real abuses, stupidities, injustices, and other inequities which clamored for correction as matters of common humanity.

Another manifestation of paranoia is the development of the idea that the subject is loved by some highly placed or distinguished person or by all members of the opposite sex with whom he comes in contact. As a result, demands of many sorts may be made on the supposed lover. The unfortunate victim may be publicly embarrassed and even roundly abused both directly and by mail. Along with this, especially in women, there are frequently ideas that the lover is pursuing and reading and influencing the thoughts of the paranoiac. He influences her to have sexual dreams and sexual desires while awake, and by remote control causes various symbolic events to occur, even though the two are miles apart and never see each other. Such a state may exist for years without the occurrence of hallucinations or a splitting away from everyday reality. That is, the paranoiac may continue to hold a position effectively, and the only things about which he complains to his employers and his family and the only unusual conditions noticed by them are "nervousness" and perhaps some irritability and emotional instability. This, then, is a matter of rationalization by projection of impulses, emotions, and inner experiences which the patient does accept as validly unrelated to outside influences.

At times the inner tension may become so great that a state of panic or an attack of nerves or a nervous breakdown will occur. These acute emotional states may clear up rather quickly, and the patient be regarded as having recovered. In many instances during such an acute state the patient reveals his ideas for the first time. This may permit a therapeutic approach. If the nervous attack clears up, the patient's rigid personality is usually resumed without much alteration, though there may be more tenseness and suspiciousness. In many instances the panic state marks the beginning of an elaboration of the psychotic picture. This is in no wise remarkable, since tension has been building up over a long period and the panic states represent a point at which the ego defenses have been broached on a large scale. New symptoms appear, or it may happen for the first time that the paranoid reveals the extent of his hallucinatory experiences, the wealth and systematization of his delusions, and the degree to which he is emotionally disturbed. As previously noted, once a psychotic level of elaboration has been reached, only a small percentage of paranoids remain at the comparatively simple level of true paranoia. It is probably true that most cases of true paranoia are not committed to mental hospitals, but even so, their number is very small, indeed, by comparison with the number of schizophrenic and other paranoid types.

It should be noted here that paranoid reactions occur in every one of the major groups of the psychoses, in the psychoneuroses, and in the psychopathic personalities. These are discusssed in their appropriate chapters. However, it is important to remember, since the treatment procedure and the prognosis will vary according to the basic diagnosis, that the acute alcoholic paranoid state known as acute alcoholic hallucinosis, requires treatment which differs from that for paranoid schizophrenia or the chronic alcoholic paranoid state. It also has a more favorable prognosis.

Paranoid ideas may take almost any direction and have as content any sort of suspicion. Intense jealousy, conviction that the spouse is unfaithful, and ideas of persecution, grandeur, or superiority may all occur in relation to a person or group or some large segment of the social order. The patient's attention and effort may be absorbed in working out a new philosophy or an invention which would put Rube Goldberg to shame, perfecting a perpetual motion machine, or some other idea equally absurd, except that the patient takes it seriously.

These points are repeated because they give some clues to the probable underlying mechanisms in the paranoid conditions. Freud was the first to develop the idea that these states were based on an inversion and projection of a homosexual mechanism. The fundamental feature of the paranoid is fixation at an early stage of psychosexual development, with particular reference to the following points: (1) an unresolved incomplete Oedipus complex, which means, in effect, failure to identify with the parent of the same sex and transform the affectional relationship with the other. (2) An essentially narcissistic fixation. In some sense, at least, the homosexuality represents a projection of the narcissism. Because of the special make-up of the paranoid, this is unacceptable as an impulse arising within the personality and so must be projected onto those in the environment. (3) Diminished genitalized libido for which there is ample evidence; the sexuality is expressed in ideas, particularly the delusional systems, rather than in action. Perverse types of actual sexual gratification are common, related to the weakness of the sexual impulse. (4) Weak ego structure, making it difficult to adapt to and surmount reality, explains in part the inability to deal with the partial sex trend and the fixation at early levels of psychosexual development. (5) Hostility and rivalry also tend to remain fixed at an infantile level. (6) Bisexuality is a common symptom, explained on the basis of the conscious rejection of homosexuality and an effort to achieve the socially accepted goal of heterosexuality. But the heterosexuality is usually comparatively feeble, with the result that the sexual relationship is rarely adequate from the standpoint of the sexual partner.

The essential mechanism in paranoid states is the negation of the homosexual wish or drive. Thus, the original "I love him (or her)" is unacceptable and becomes transformed into "I hate him (or her)." This, too, is unacceptable, and so it is projected, becoming "he (or she) hates and persecutes me." The patient then feels free to hate in return, because of the persecution. Delusions of being loved by many of the opposite sex are also a defense against the unconscious homosexual wish or the fear of impotence. The same is true of delusional jealousy and ideas of infidelity; the homosexual drive is negated by projecting it onto the spouse—"I do not love him (or them); she (he) loves them." Accusations and repeated questions then follow.

We must, of course, always bear in mind the important fact that infidelity does occur and that in many situations suspicion and jealousy are perfectly normal reactions. In such situations the patient can and does produce evidence which is coherent, logical, well-connected, and possible. On the other hand, when the ideas are delusional they lack some or all of these characteristics; particularly the bases for the accusation of infidelity, which are illogical, unsubstantial, and often unrealistic in the extreme.

The social worker must be on the alert for indications of delusional trends, of fixed ideation, of logic-tight compartments, of tense, constant suspiciousness. The mere presence of such mechanisms, however, should not be overinterpreted since they occur in everyone, but only as transitory emotional states. In the paranoid person the states are permanent and the mechanisms tend to pervade all social relationships and attitudes. Many paranoids are reasonably innocuous in the community, even though they may need financial assistance and social supervision. When the worker suspects the existence of a paranoid state, or when such a state is obvious, a psychiatrist should be consulted with reference to further procedure. Because the patient may be dangerous, or potentially so, the worker should not attempt to carry all the responsibility, but share it with or transfer it to the psychiatrist. It was with reference to a paranoid person that a noted alienist once said that he always shared the responsibility for such patients with the court.

If the worker constantly remembers that paranoids show many reactions at an immature level, the attitudes to be exhibited toward patients who remain in the community under supervision will be clear. The worker's approach to the paranoid includes sympathy, patient listening, direct advice, even orders at times, and acceptance of his ideas so far as may be possible. It is not wise to try to oppose the ideas directly, but they may be questioned, though this may cause rejection of the worker by the patient. If there is any reason to believe that the patient cannot tolerate even the slightest doubt of the correctness of his paranoid ideas, it is better to be silent concerning one's own views, since expressing them might lead to unnecessary and unprofitable explosions. Some paranoids will maintain a good working relationship with one person over a long period, usually because of a dependency situation which is acceptable to them. For reasons obvious in the mechanisms, this is more likely to develop when worker and patient are of opposite sexes. Most commonly the paranoid does not develop a sustained relationship with any worker, but must keep changing.

It is noteworthy that these paranoid conditions, which hitherto have been notoriously untreatable, yield a high percentage of favorable results with shock treatment. This appears to be true with both insulin and electroshock. The present general practice seems to be to use electroshock first; then, if the results are inadequate, to use insulin, especially for schizophrenics.

CHAPTER XI

THE CONVULSIVE DISORDERS

CONVULSIONS appear as symptoms in relation to many conditions. They occur in toxic and organic conditions affecting the nervous system, in hysteria, in endocrine disorders, in temper tantrums, and even during the teething period. Among the organic-toxic conditions which may produce convulsions either during the course of the disease or in the terminal state are: alcoholism, acute infections, cardiac conditions, renal disease, diabetes, general paresis, brain tumor, and skull fractures.

Convulsions with such specifically related etiology cannot be considered in the same way as cases in which convulsions are the chief feature and no specific causative pathological conditions are to be found. The distinguishing feature of *idiopathic epilepsy* is the convulsion. Epilepsy is a disease of unknown causation, as the term idiopathic implies, and there are usually no clinical signs of organic disease. At autopsy, however, many cases show pathology of the brain in areas which do not produce clinical evidence of brain damage. Epilepsy is variable in its course and severity. Three classical types of seizure have been described: the grand mal, petit mal, and the Jacksonian or focal. The latter type of seizure begins in a specific area, such as a hand or one side of the face, and progresses in a regular march until the entire body is involved. There may or may not be associated loss of consciousness, and the attacks can often be checked by a sharp slap. Surgical intervention is the preferred method of treatment, since there is usually a localized lesion and focal signs to indicate its location.

The grand mal and petit mal types of seizure characterize idiopathic epilepsy. The seizures may be replaced by psychic equivalents, such as a dream state with automatic activity or marked excitement, the epileptic *furore*. These equivalent states are succeeded by amnesia, which is often doubted by the observer, especially if some crime has been committed during the period. Specifically in the furore, crimes of extreme violence and unnecessary brutality may occur. In fact, when atrocious crimes are perpetrated, an epileptic state in the criminal should be suspected. Other symptoms and syndromes are also apparently associated with epilepsy, although the manifestations may never reach the seizure stage. Migraine, narcolepsy, and some mild episodic phenomena of the type of a vaso-motor crisis are examples of this and are frequently found in the collateral relatives of epileptics.

While it is estimated that there are three hundred thousand to five hundred thousand epileptics in this country, only about twenty thousand are in specialized institutions. Several factors characterize the institutionalized epileptic. In one large group psychotic symptoms predominate in the picture which leads to commitment. For example, about the same number of cases are admitted each year to the New York state hospitals and diagnosed "psychoses with convulsive disorders" as are admitted to Craig Colony for Epileptics, which is for nonpsychotic cases. Furthermore, there were 1,693 psychotic epileptics in the state hospitals on March 31, 1943, by comparison with 2,485 patients in the Colony or on parole therefrom on the same date. Three times as many epileptics with psychosis were admitted to all the mental institutions in the United States in 1937 as of epileptics without psychosis to the same institutions. Those with psychosis represented 2 percent of psychotic admissions; those without psychosis, 3.4 percent of the nonpsychotic.

A second factor of importance in the institutionalized group is the prevalence of an associated mental deficiency. Thus, 80 percent of nearly 500 admissions to Craig Colony were classed as subnormal, 50 percent of them definitely of feebleminded level and classified as idiot, imbecile, or moron.

Another point, of uncertain significance, is the relative age of admission to Craig Colony and to state hospitals. For the Colony,

21 percent were under ten years of age; approximately 80 percent of the admissions were under age thirty, while two thirds were under age twenty. By contrast, the age groupings of patients admitted for the first time to state hospitals for "psychoses with convulsive disorders" sharply reverse these figures. Whether the 1,600 admissions to all state hospitals in the United States for 1937 are considered, or whether one uses New York figures alone (350) for the same years as the Colony figures, makes only a slight difference. Only 15–16 percent of the psychotic cases were under twenty years of age; 52–57 percent were over thirty years of age.

This serves to bring out an important fact regarding the epilepsies as a social problem. Easily recognized epilepsies of some severity are or tend to be institutionalized early. Those less easily recognized and less severe, or possibly more amenable to treatment, or because of some other variable, tend not to require, or at least to receive, hospitalization until a psychosis or deterioration becomes part of the picture. This means that it is possible for epilepsy to exist as a medical and social problem for a long time, perhaps for life, without symptoms necessitating hospitalization. In such cases an intelligent combination of medical treatment and social case work may be very important in keeping the patient out of hospital and at work. This point is emphasized by the known duration of the epilepsy before admission to Craig Colony. In approximately 31 percent of the cases the disorder had been in existence less than five years; in about 32 percent the duration was five to nine years; while in 36 percent the disease had been in existence ten years or more.

In occasional cases the convulsions occur only during the night, and patients lose no time from work. Thus, one patient was known to have had convulsions for sixteen years, but during this period only one occurred in the daytime, and he continued successfully in business. Because of his condition, he did not marry and lived a quiet, rather retired social life. Then he developed a continuous series of convulsions, the *status epilepticus*, which occurred both during the day and at night. This state and the ensuing period of confusion and delirium lasted for about a week. He developed a series of superficial infections, which required some six weeks to heal. When he was about ready for discharge from the hospital, another status developed and it was necessary to commit him to a hospital for prolonged care.

As a general rule, however, grand mal convulsions occur at any time, day or night. The nocturnal cases may be difficult to diagnose, since the convulsions may not be observed. In fact, such cases have been known to exist for years before they were finally diagnosed as epilepsy. Suspicious symptoms are: fatigue on awaking with sore and aching muscles; bitten tongue, often with flecks of blood on the mouth and on the pillow; bed wetting and even defecating in bed during the night. These are episodic and may occur either very rarely or with considerable frequency.

Sooner or later the process known as epileptic deterioration may appear. This is a typical intellectual and emotional dementia, with no specific signs except that the amnesia is more patchy than with other types. If dementia occurs it may become extremely marked. Delusions and hallucinations may appear, perhaps persecutory in character, or with a strong religious cast. Irritability and egocentricity are outstanding characteristics of such psychotic states.

Dementia and other grave psychic phenomena are apparently greatly reduced in cases that are properly treated in private practice. Many common statements regarding the gravity of the prognosis and the apparent inevitability of deterioration are based upon studies of hospitalized cases. These are admittedly the more serious cases, often improperly or inadequately treated, or perhaps not even diagnosed until irreparable personality damage has occurred.

Acute clouded states also occur, preceding, replacing, or following convulsive attacks. Patients are confused, usually actively hallucinated especially in the visual field, are fearful, and may be violent. The religious content of the hallucinations and delusions is marked and there may be moods of great exaltation. These acute states may clear up to approximately the level of functioning prior to the attack, or they may issue in a chronic state which, in turn, may be progressive.

The petit mal type of seizure resembles nothing so much as a momentary state of suspended animation. The patient stops what he is doing or saying; he may change color, usually turning pale. After five or ten seconds, sometimes a little longer, he resumes activity as though there had been no interruption. These cases may present difficult problems in diagnosis. In many instances the diagnosis becomes clear only when a typical convulsion occurs. It is often asserted that the petit mal type leads to earlier and more complete deterioration than the grand mal type, but is less frequently associated with mental deficiency. However, this so-called mental deficiency may actually be a very early deterioration associated with epilepsy in small children. There is good reason to doubt the gloomy prognosis in cases with only petit mal attacks.

About one third of the cases admitted to Craig Colony are attributed to definite organic brain disease or some toxemic process and are classed in the symptomatic group; the other two thirds are classed as idiopathic. In physicians' private practice the proportion of idiopathic cases is higher. In either group, unless the somatic process is in and of itself remediable, treatment must be directed to the epilepsy.

Probably no disease process has been more exploited by the sellers of patent and fake remedies. This is a particularly vicious racket, since false promises of cure are believed, resulting in the disillusionment of the sufferer and unfortunate delay in beginning proper treatment. Such remedies as are of any palliative value usually turn out to be very expensive bromide or phenobarbital mixtures. Bromides, phenobarbital, dilantin and mesantoin are the drugs which have proved most effective in controlling seizures in legitimate treatment. Triodine has proven effective with petit mal, which is often resistant to other treatment.

Some babies have a few convulsions during periods of developmental stress, and thereafter remain free from them. The prognosis is better if epileptic manifestations begin after puberty than if they begin before. The prognosis is especially poor if they are definitely established before the age of five.

A convulsion is usually preceded by premonitory symptoms, the warning or aura. This may be sensory, referred to the abdomen, the limbs, the special senses, or it may be thoughts and emotions. Many patients realize what is to come when they experience the aura and lie down or otherwise dispose themselves as protection against injury.

Following the aura by a few seconds, loss of consciousness supervenes. The patient falls, stiffens out in the tonic stage, and in a few seconds the convulsive movements of the clonic stage ensue. The face turns purple from anoxemia as the breathing becomes heavy and gasping, the condition of stertor. The tongue may be bitten until blood comes, sometimes so severely that stitches are required. There is usually involuntary urination and defecation. After a short time, perhaps one to three minutes, the convulsion subsides, and the patient goes into a deep sleep from which he can usually not be roused at once. After an hour or more he wakes in a state of confusion, which may last up to twelve hours or longer.

Sometimes there are premonitory emotional signs of irritability and behavior suited to the irritation, including assaults, over a period of one or more days. An *epileptic temperament* has been described as compounded of irritability, some irregularities in intellectual functioning, a shallow religiosity, and more or less pronounced ideas of grandeur. Surliness and a tendency to irregular depression mark the social behavior.

Epileptic equivalents sometimes replace the convulsions. There may be running attacks, automatic activity with the assumption of an alternate personality, even delinquent and criminal acts. For all these activities there is subsequent amnesia, which may raise important medico-legal problems, since the amnesia may not be accepted as real, but considered as malingering.

In one case a man developed epilepsy following a severe head trauma in the frontal area. At the time of examination there was a deep depression in the right forehead, indicating marked loss of brain substance. His convulsions caused very little disturbance in his work life, which consisted of comparatively simple tasks. At home, one night, he beat his mother to death most brutally. There was no doubt of the epilepsy or of the amnesia for events prior to, during, and after the murder. The man was committed to hospital as an insane criminal. As is usual, this meant that he could be brought to trial for his crime if he was ever classified as recovered.

In another case of undoubted epilepsy small quantities of alcohol would bring on an equivalent state. This young man would assume an alternate personality and travel long distances, find a job, and establish himself in another community. After several weeks to six or even more months, he would suddenly recover his proper identity, with complete amnesia for the preceding confused period. At least once he found himself engaged to marry a girl whom he did not even recognize when he regained his usual identity. He had many patches of amnesia, from a few days to several months. Fugues such as the one just described and dream states occur particularly in hysteria. In one case I saw, fugues apparently replaced manic depressive attacks.

There are theories of a psychogenic origin for epilepsy. It is true that sudden emotional upsets caused by external reality may precipitate an attack, but in general, the psychogenic theories do not explain all the findings in epilepsy. Alcohol, intestinal stasis, and heavy protein diets all play a part at one time or another. Therefore, the diet and elimination of the epileptic require special attention, along with proper medication.

The electroencephalogram is a particularly important aid in the diagnosis of doubtful cases. The test must be made, and, particularly, it must be interpreted by an expert in its use.

Many lines of employment, such as truck or car driving and work with machinery involving special hazards, are unsuitable for most epileptics. Clerical work and most types of farm work are satisfactory.

Some sort of social supervision, preferably rather unobtrusive, is usually essential once the diagnosis of epilepsy has been established. Medical treatment and supervision usually need to be continuous. With proper treatment the spells may become infrequent or disappear, and there may be little or no interference with normal living. This is certainly true for about one half the cases.

Though epilepsy is not considered hereditary as such, epileptics should be generally advised not to have children. Familial types do occur, and the descendants may be subject to migraine or other phenomena of a like order.

CHAPTER XII

MENTAL DEFICIENCY

TWO GRADES of mental defect, idiocy and imbecility, have been recognized for many years. In early times the terms idiot and idiocy applied to all grades of recognized defectives. The higher grade of feeblemindedness was named moron and properly classified only within the present century, following the development and standardization of mental tests. Previously, and until the present time in England, these higher grades were simply called feebleminded, whereas in this country the term feebleminded is used to cover all grades of defectiveness. Mental deficiency is also called amentia, hypophrenia, and oligophrenia. The terms in most common use are feebleminded and mental defect.

There is a popular misconception that mental deficiency is always or usually hereditary, or at the least, familial, but this is by no means the case. The most modern estimates are that only about one third to at most one half of the mental defectives are familial cases. These for the most part are morons and high-grade imbeciles. Idiots and low-grade imbeciles are more likely to present signs of organic causes for defective brain development.

Mental deficiency is defined as a state existing from birth or early childhood, by contrast with dementia, which develops later in life, after there has been normal or average mental development. Mental defect is characterized by delay in physical development, such as teething, in motor development—holding up the head, sitting up, creeping, walking, and talking—in formation of such habits as toilet behavior, learning to dress and undress, self-feeding, and table manners. Retardation in the learning process in school subjects, defective reasoning and judgment, often heightened suggestibility or excessive stubbornness and self-will are also characteristic.

The causes of mental deficiency vary. Prenatal pathology may occur in a number of ways, such as the transfer of infections from mother to fetus, endocrine disturbances and toxic states in the mother, anomalies of development, and from other causes. Birth injuries account for some cases; infections and toxic states in early infancy account for still others.

Several types present distinctive anatomical characteristics, among them the microcephalic and macrocephalic (or hydrocephalic) idiots and sometimes low-grade imbeciles. Mongolian types, either idiots or imbeciles, resemble each other more closely than brothers and sisters usually do, even though they are born into different families. They are called mongolian because of the slant eyes, thick, wrinkled tongue, very short incurved little finger. Mongolians are usually short; they tend to be timid, though temper tantrums may be regular features of their behavior.

Many theories have been advanced to explain mongolism, but none covers all the observed facts. The favorite theory was the degeneration of the germ plasm, since it was observed that in many instances the mongol was the last of a number of children in a family, when the parents were advanced in age. However, many children born to elderly parents are not mongols; the first child of young parents may be a mongol. Two successive pregnancies may rarely result in mongolians. A few cases of mongolian twins have been reported, but the most complicated situation is that in which one dissimilar twin is mongolian, while the other is not. In a recent case of this sort that I examined, the boy was definitely mongoloid, while the girl had distinctly superior intelligence.

One theory of causation implicates pituitary, thyroid, and thymus glands. Some cases treated with pituitary and thyroid have shown real improvement, but the method has not proved itself in the hands of most psychiatrists.

Cretinism, a form of general physical and mental stunting, is due to early deficiency of thyroid secretion. Early diagnosis and thyroid replacement therapy sometimes yield excellent results.

There are various anomalies of brain development and prenatal agenesias. These show physical signs of organic nervous disease as well as intellectual defect of a severe grade.

In addition to the organic and familial types, mental defectives without evidence of specific organic causative factors occur as "sports," in the Mendelian sense, in families with an otherwise clear hereditary record concerning mental disease and defect. There may be factors as yet unrecognized which affect an individual pregnancy and produce such results.

The higher the grade of mental defect, the more usual the physical appearance. High-grade morons are often deceptively normal in appearance; they often verbalize so readily that the presence of the defect may not be suspected until repeated school or vocational failures arouse suspicion. Morons of stable personality make-up may be trained for many industrial and other vocations. It has been said that the stable moron is the backbone of the industrial world. While this is, perhaps, an exaggeration, it is true that many morons are quiet, self-sustaining citizens who do not get into trouble or become dependent.

Idiots are usually abnormal in appearance; imbeciles are also peculiar in appearance, awkward and poorly co-ordinated. Stigmata of degeneration are common in these grades and occur to some extent among morons, but not, in general, to a marked degree among the highest grades.

Since mental tests have been so widely used, there has been a tendency to rely upon the results of these tests for detecting the feebleminded and classifying them as idiots, imbeciles, and morons. As noted in Chapter II, this practice cannot be justified. Many other data enter into the diagnosis of feeblemindedness. Necessary information includes the family history, a record of development, the medical history, school progress, employment records and economic efficiency, social relationships and behavior, and psychiatric and physical examination findings. These are essentially the fields of inquiry which Dr. Walter Fernald insisted must be studied in order to arrive at a correct diagnosis.

As for the results of intelligence tests, idiots score mental ages under three years, with IQ's 0 to 20. It is obvious that only rudimentary habit formation and little or no speech may be expected. Idiots constitute about 12 percent of the residents in state schools and about the same proportion of first admissions.

Adult imbeciles score mental ages of three to seven; children show IQ's from 20 to 40. They are trainable to a limited degree; for example, they can be taught to dress themselves and to read a few simple words. They may be able to carry out simple tasks, but always require supervision. They cannot apply past experience to new situations, nor do they become self-supporting. About 40 percent of institutional inmates are imbeciles, though the admission rate is somewhat less than this figure. There is, accordingly, some accumulation of imbeciles in the institutions.

Adult morons score mental ages between seven and eleven; in children, the IQ range is 40 to 70. Morons usually progress not farther than the fourth or fifth grade in school. They constitute nearly half the cases in training schools, though the admission rate is higher. This means that morons are discharged into the community as partially or completely capable of self-support, and there is no accumulation in institutions as with imbeciles, or maintenance of a fairly steady number, due to deaths among inmates, as with the idiots.

Mentally defective persons may develop such marked psychotic reactions that care in a hospital rather than in a training school is indicated. In one period New York state hospitals admitted for the first time about one fifth as many cases of "psychoses with mental deficiency" as the training schools admitted of mental defectives without psychosis. That these psychoses are not all acute reactions which clear up to the previous level of functioning is shown by the census in New York state hospitals. About 3.5 percent of the cases were diagnosed as psychoses with mental deficiency. Furthermore, the state hospitals had about one sixth as many cases of defectives with psychosis as the training schools had without psychosis.

Defectives may develop any of the usual types of psychosis. When the symptoms are clear, it is the practice to classify such cases as manic depressive, arteriosclerotic, senile, or other types of psychosis.

Those who are classified as "psychosis with mental deficiency" are not otherwise classifiable. The typical states are acute excitement, often with delusions and hallucinations, and there may be confusion or semi-delirium.

Defectives are susceptible to the usual physical diseases. For many types the span of life is short. In general, among institutionalized cases, about 60 percent have died before reaching the age of thirty, and slightly more than half have been in the institutions less than seven years. What the facts are regarding longevity of those in the community who are never institutionalized is unknown.

The number of feebleminded in this country is not actually known. Estimates vary, but a conservative figure would seem to be about one percent of the population. Two major types of social provision have been developed. One is institutional care in state and private training schools for defectives. All such institutions exercise a custodial function for untrainables and in addition train those who can profit by training. In New York state there were more than 18,000 in training schools at the end of 1945; the total for the country was 115,600. In states where county poor farms and infirmaries are operated, such institutions care for many of the feebleminded as well as for quiet chronic psychotics.

A few states have special institutions for defective delinquents, in recognition of the fact that the defective who is also delinquent requires special treatment. Formerly, in using intelligence tests for the study of delinquents, very high percentages of so-called feeblemindedness were found. These diagnoses were false in a very high proportion of cases. Actually, the best studies, especially those of Tulchin,* indicate that there is about the same proportion of feeblemindedness among delinquents and criminals as in similar cross sections of the general population. Or, more accurately stated, it has been found that the curve of intelligence distribution from high to low is approximately the same for delinquents and criminals confined in or entering correctional institutions as it is for groups of nondelinquent males of comparable age and origin.

The other major type of social provision for defectives is that of special or ungraded classes in public school systems, now available in all larger city systems. These classes share in special state aid, since the cost per pupil is two to three times as great as for pupils of similar age in the regular grades. Usually the law provides that these ungraded classes shall be available to those who are retarded a certain number of years in school, are of chronological age for third grade or more, and have an IQ between 50 and 70. These children are, of course, the more educable group of morons. As it happens, many of them can be more effectively trained in institutions because of social and economic conditions at home or because of personality deviations.

The education of trainable feebleminded children is primarily in terms of motor skills. It is usually assumed that these children are defective in transfer learning and are superior in direct or motor learning. When this is true, it is only relatively so; that is, individuals of inferior general intelligence are usually inferior on performance tests also, even though they may rate higher on performance than on tests of general intelligence. In general, however, it is true that defectives are best trained through motor activities and associated kinesthesis.

In clinical demonstrations of the feebleminded it is customary to present groups of dissimilar chronological age and physical development who are of similar mental ages. Thus, groups of idiots or imbeciles may be presented together, although they may range in actual age from a few years to adults. These cases may present a

* The comparisons in Tulchin's study were made between inmates of Illinois institutions and the Illinois draft army of the First World War.

wide range of neurological disorders and macrocephaly and microcephaly, while some may present only minor abnormalities of appearance.

Another favorite way to demonstrate, for teaching purposes, the feebleminded in institutions is to present a series of individuals of the same chronological age, but of different mental ages. Still another method is to present a family of feebleminded individuals of varied ages and usually somewhat different IQ's. To find such a family in an institution is not too common, but it does occur.

Perhaps it is well to remember that all infants, even the normal and the superior, are "idiots" at birth and that in the course of normal development they pass through stages comparable to those of the imbecile and the moron. The difference is, of course, that the normal individual *passes through these stages at the proper time* and goes on to an average or superior maturity. Not so those with defective or inferior intelligence; they may or may not pass through the various stages of physical development at a reasonably normal pace, but the lag in intellectual development usually becomes evident fairly early. At the same time, it must be remembered that lags in the development of social reactions may be due to emotional causes related to the family or social situation rather than to intellectual deficiency.

Many individuals in whom schizophrenia occurred in early childhood find their way into the training schools for the feebleminded. As adults, these patients show rather typical end stages of schizophrenic deterioration. Recently I arranged a series of clinical demonstrations for social workers in psychopathic and state hospitals and in training schools. Despite earnest search, no hospital could produce a case of typical catatonic stupor, whereas several cases were seen in the one training school we visited.

One situation related to the problems of mental defectiveness has not yet been squarely admitted and faced in our system of democratic, universal education—the question of educational procedure for children of inferior, but not defective, intelligence— those with IQ 70–90 (or 65–85). These children fall between the provisions for those of definitely defective intelligence and the ordinary curriculum designed for children of average or superior intelligence. The inferior children are usually better at direct, or motor, learning than at transfer, or book, learning, but manual training is not available, as a rule, to any but defectives until the seventh grade is reached. Yet children with IQ 70–90 have great difficulty in reaching this grade, so the educational procedure is largely wasted on them. Meantime, much money is also wasted in futile attempts to educate them. The worst of it is that continued failure creates feelings of inadequacy and insecurity. Rebellion may ensue, resulting in several types of asocial and antisocial behavior. Hence many become delinquent and are subjects for correctional institutions.

Defectives are often sexually delinquent. Not infrequently it is attributed to being "oversexed," but this is a moot question. It is impossible to define what is meant by the term oversexed, aside from the occasional cases of nymphomania and satyriasis. These are specific abnormal states and present other signs which prove the existence of a definite mental disturbance to account for the sexual overactivity. There is no reason to assume that those of inferior intelligence differ from the general run of the population with reference to the strength of the sexual drive. This tends to follow the usual curve of all mensurable attributes, from those with little or no evidence of sexual interest to those who show great interest and activity. But there are no positive criteria as to what may be normal or average.

The fact is that individuals of inferior intelligence have fewer sources of pleasure than do their more intelligent brethren, yet like all people, they seek to find pleasure and avoid pain. Their capacity to enjoy literature, music, art, sports, and other forms of recreation, all of which may and do represent ways of sublimating sexual energy, is distinctly limited, so that the libido is much more likely to find satisfaction in direct fashion. In other words, sexual activity is one of the few pleasures easily accessible to the defective. There is nothing to show that it is more pleasurable to them than it is to others. An additional point is that, because of inferiority and consequent lack of success, defectives are particularly susceptible to flattery. This is especially true when the individual has been the subject of much criticism or unfavorable comparisons and therefore has experienced real or apparent dislike from members of the family. It is often stated and may be true that defectives are generally more suggestible than are people of average or superior intelligence. If true, this is probably in relation to the factors just mentioned—the need for affection and approval.

With regard to illicit sexual relationships and illegitimate births, it must be remembered that the feebleminded are likely to be incapable of understanding and applying moral codes. Not only that, but having barely the most elementary ideas of the physiology of conception and the course of pregnancy, illegitimate conception and offspring would be more likely to occur in this group. This is not to say that either illicit relationships or illegitimacy stand in any direct relationship to defective intelligence. In fact, there is evidence that the reproductive rate among defectives is less than was formerly assumed.

Eugenic sterilization has been proposed and bitterly debated, especially for the feebleminded, some psychotics, and for criminals. Permissive laws have been passed in some states, and sterilization has been practiced to some extent. Very little evidence has been produced to show that sterilization would in any way influence the incidence of mental deficiency, for reasons already given.

The social worker must be alert to signs of defective intelligence in order to meet the client's needs most effectively. Perhaps the most important point to remember is that no amount of training, diet, vitamins, or other forms of treatment so far devised will increase the actual amount of intelligence in the true defective. Knowledge and experience may or may not increase the capacity to survive successfully, but the most the social worker can offer is friendly and consistent supervision and support. It must also be remembered that the defective learns slowly and through many repetitions, but once habits of working and living are learned, they are persistent. Training therefore requires a long-time program. Certainly for the very defective, institutional training presents the best opportunity for permanent results. Many institutions operate colonies or board out individuals who can work effectively with a minimum of intensive supervision. These are, in general, older inmates who have been well trained to carry out the tasks for which they are fitted.

Mental or intellectual defectives also present in some cases marked abnormalities of personality organization which are similar in type to the cases of psychopathic personality who are not intellectually defective. Defective intelligence occurs in about 10 percent of psychotic cases with other diagnoses. Of these, nearly 70 percent are classified as having borderline intelligence. The main point remains clear: those with defective and inferior intelligence may have abnormal personalities or develop specific types of psychoses not apparently directly related to the intellectual inferiority. Schizophrenia shows a higher percentage of cases with inferior intelligence than is true for manic depressive psychoses, but the significance of this is by no means clear.

A word should be said about "constitutional inferiority" as I conceive it. This term should be reserved for those who show signs of physical inferiority, such as stigmata of degeneration, undersize, unusual susceptibility to disease, poor physique, and the like. They also present inferior, but not defective, intelligence, poor emotional adjustment, and inadequate control of impulses. Such cases, in other words, combine features of several types of inferiority. They require special training, special physical care, and special social regimes. They, too, present a need for long-range planning and training, which all too often they do not get. They cannot be wished into normality, nor can they be trained further than their capacities permit.

CHAPTER XIII

THE NEUROSES (PSYCHO-NEUROSES)

AS PREVIOUSLY EMPHASIZED, the neuroses comprise the group of disorders in which psychogenic origins are most clearly demonstrable. Neither neurological, endocrinological, nor any physical causative factors need be called upon to account for individual symptoms or the total picture of the neuroses. It has been brought out that the neurotic knows he is ill, even though the real nature of his illness may be masked from him. Some other points of difference between neurotic and psychotic reactions require emphasis at this point. The chief comparisons to be made are related to variations in reaction to reality situations and in the maintenance of social relationships.

The psychotic person is detached from reality to a marked degree, often completely or nearly so. This is not true of the neurotic, except perhaps for intervals in dream states or fugues, or possibly concerning some elements assumed by him to be causative for his condition. The neurotic is puzzled by the failure of his hypotheses to explain his condition or help to alleviate it, but the psychotic rejects or ignores any discrepancies in his notions as to what is wrong and remains fixed upon any explanation which satisfies his inner psychic needs.

The psychoses are characterized by an inner absorption in which there is an interweaving of internally determined and developed ideas and emotions. There is marked endopsychic distortion of external events, brought about by the overwhelming strength of the autistically derived constellations of ideas and impressions. There is no sustained and consecutive interest in environmental happenings; instead, there is a repetitive, unrelated pattern of behavior reactions and verbal production. This observation holds true even in those conditions in which the psychotic patient is oriented, displays reaction to people and to the physical environment, has a good memory, and shows emotional responses consonant with many external stimuli. Nevertheless, the elaboration of ideas, the development of emotional sets, and the attitudes toward a variety of situations affecting the self or even impersonal ones are all determined by unrealistic, uncritical, and often bizarre formulations which arise within the psyche. The capacity for criticism of his own ideas and behavior tends to disappear completely. Since the constellations are endopsychic, they are influenced or determined by internal conflicts and imperfectly resolved drives which were evolved earlier. As such, they are not influenced by inner inhibitory processes, are not amenable to reason and logic, and cannot be influenced by the arguments or example of others.

The behavior toward people or in social situations is largely or entirely determined by the inner sets, which are not adequately differentiated from external reality. The psychotic can and does deny the validity of external events, especially in their possible application to himself. He lives in a world of his own and ascribes to it all those aspects and qualities of reality which may be necessary for him to remain on a plane of integration satisfying to all those complicated needs which he cannot meet realistically. Because the realities in situations are ignored, misinterpreted or falsified, social relations are misconstrued and adjustment to the usual social amenities is abolished. The verities of life cannot be adequately tested, since at all points the inner mechanisms and the magic world created by them dominate the scene.

The development of a psychotic picture may aptly be described as a process of personality disintegration. The particular sectors of personality which undergo the greatest distortion will vary in accordance with etiological factors, as already illustrated in discussing the several psychoses. The disintegration may be temporary or permanent, depending upon the malignancy of the process

and its reversibility or irreversibility. Even in the more benign reactions, personality disintegration is marked during the height of
the attack, though there may be complete reintegration later. A
classical example of marked detachment from external reality, the
individual living in and reacting to his own inner world, yet with
ultimately complete recovery, may be found in the delirious states.
In organic dementias the inner absorption has its own peculiar
characteristics, dependent to a considerable extent upon the limitations resulting from the destructive, irreversible process. Similar
points may be made respecting the functional psychoses, with
reference to malignancy and reversibility. The more complicated
the mechanism and the greater the difficulty of satisfying the
inner drives through ordinary modes of behavior, the more malig-
nant the process and the farther removed the patient gets from
reality.

By contrast, the neurotic shows no such disturbances either in
degree or in kind. Even in states of fugue or amnesia, social orientation of a particular sort is retained. There is no especial retreat
into a world conditioned only by inner experience and psychic
constellations. The ego is not impaired, though it may be restricted;
the neurotic remains in contact with reality and can test himself
in relationship to it. He does not deny reality, though he does try
to manipulate the environment and may invest some aspects of it
with exaggerated emotional values. However, there is no attempt
to substitute an internally created world for the external one. It
follows that the general social adjustment is not impaired, unless
it be in some limited way, such as invalidism. Responsibility, fear,
hostility, anxiety, and guilt are not projected, but remain as part
of the torturing insight. Personality integrity is retained; the individual is sick and realizes it, though unaware of the essential nature of the illness.

There is no clear dividing line between the neuroses and the
states we regard as normal. For this reason the empathic index is
high, while at the same time members of the family often express
impatience with the neurotic because of his apparent general nor-

mality. Some neurotic traits may be expected in everyone, but this does not justify the frequent use of the term neurotic to apply to anything and everything someone does with which we happen to disagree. The separation of the neuroses into the several types presented here is recognized to be somewhat artificial and unsatisfactory. However, it is necessary to provide some definitions and to bring out variations in mechanisms and treatment. It seems most effective to present these points in relation to the groups which have the weight of clinical tradition behind them.

In the usual classification of the neuroses there are six groups: hysteria, neurasthenia, psychasthenia, anxiety states, hypochondriasis, and mixed neurosis.* To these have been added, for convenience in this exposition, the psychosomatic disorders. From a clinical viewpoint the neuroses may be divided, according to another principle, into two groups. The first would comprise all cases in which the complaints expressed by the patient are chiefly or entirely in the physical field. Included would be conversion hysteria, neurasthenia, hypochondria, tics, and habit spasms; also some actual physical disorders, such as gastric ulcer, some cases of hypertension, suppression of menses in certain instances, and some types of disturbances of cardiac function, such as rapid pulse or intermittent bradycardia and tachycardia. These physical disorders are among the types of reaction now included among the psychosomatic disturbances. In the second group set up according to the principle stated above would be included all cases in which the symptoms are chiefly psychic: the obsessional-compulsive states, officially classed as psychasthenia, some cases of hysteria, the anxiety states, and conditions such as psychic impotence.

We must also distinguish between neurotic traits which do not interfere with reasonably adequate adjustment, the neurotic personality, and the fully developed neuroses. The first two are not particularly incapacitating, while those suffering from neuroses are likely to be seriously handicapped in some or all of their activities.

* The classification adopted by the American Psychiatric Association lists these and certain others under the official designation "psychoneuroses."

Estimates of the incidence of neurosis, in the total population vary greatly, and the number has never been determined. Functional or psychosomatic disturbances are described in all systematic presentations of organ diseases and their treatment. Physicians have reported in the literature and have stated to me personally that 40 to 70 percent of their patients present emotional problems either as a primary focus for treatment or as complications of their physical disorders. It is usually accepted that about 10 percent of the adult population suffers from frank neuroses, but only a small fraction of the neurotics ever reach mental hospitals. About 3 to 4 percent of first admissions to such hospitals are classed as psychoneurotics, and they are included among the groups with psychosis.

About one third of the hospitalized cases are admitted to private hospitals. The discharge rate per one hundred admissions is high, but only one third are discharged as recovered. It seems clear that the hospitalized cases present the most severe pictures, often serious enough to require commitment.

Both pre-Oedipal and Oedipal mechanisms are involved in the production of the neuroses. Hostility, anxiety, anal and oral mechanisms, suppressions, distortions of object love, guilt, fear, repetition compulsions, doubts, and other evidences of emotional instability appear in various combinations.

HYSTERIA

Hysteria was recognized, described, and named in remote antiquity. It was originally thought to occur only in women and to be related to uterine disturbance. Hence the name, from the Greek word for womb, *hyster*. It is now known that hysteria occurs in both male and female and that it is based on a disturbance in the psychosexual mechanism involving particularly the Oedipus complex. The dissociated energy of the repressed wishes, guilt, hostility, and anxiety finds symbolic expression in the symptoms. Patients are as a general rule quite unaware of the symbolic meaning.

The syndrome is commonly called conversion hysteria, since the unsuccessfully repressed conflict is translated into physical symptoms. It must be emphasized that the result of this conversion of affect is a *suppression of function* in some sensory or motor field. There may be hysterical blindness, deafness, loss of sense of smell or taste, anesthesia, hypesthesia, and paresthesia. There are two distinguishing characteristics of these losses or changes in sensory functioning. In the first place, there are no associated signs and symptoms, such as reflex changes, to point to a general or local organic disease or to localized lesions of the central or peripheral nervous system. The eyegrounds are normal in cases of amblyopia (blindness); no lesions are detectable in ear, nose, and mouth in cases of anacusia (deafness), anosmia (defective sense of smell), and ageusia (loss of taste). There are also likely to be irregularities in these losses which would not be present in organic cases.

The second distinguishing characteristic is that the losses, particularly those affecting skin sensibility, are not located in the areas in which actual neurological lesions usually occur. Anesthesia, instead of running the length of arms and legs or overlapping the midline in hemianesthesia involving the torso, follows the lines which are popularly supposed to represent the segments of sensation. So the hysterical anesthesia affects hands and wrists, feet and ankles. This is the glove and stocking anesthesia, which may extend to elbows and knees or above. In hemianesthesia of the trunk, the anesthesia stops sharply at the midline, which is not true of organic lesions.

In the motor field, symptoms such as paralysis of one or more limbs or other muscle groups, mutism, tics, and tremors occur. In the case of paralysis of both legs, paraplegia, the patient is unable to walk and is commonly bed-ridden. Paralyzed limbs may be held in one position so long that contractures result. In some cases an abnormal, bent posture of the trunk, called camptocormia, is developed and seriously limits activity. But whatever the type of motor disability, the reflexes remain normal, and the expected associated disturbances in other related functional fields are absent.

Suppression in the field of consciousness, a partial or complete amnesia, also occurs. There may be transformation of personality, sometimes with alternation of the Jekyll and Hyde type. Dream states with automatic activity occur, as do trances which closely resemble stupor. Perhaps more common are situations in which the individual loses all sense of personal identity and memory of his past life and does not recognize relatives, friends, and former familiar surroundings. All these reactions represent suppression of some particularly painful conflict or complex, carrying along associated material.

Convulsions do occur, most commonly during the trance state. Similarly, the grand arc, with the patient resting rigidly on head and heels, occurs in association with the trance. Abdominal symptoms of various types occur, so that appendicitis, pregnancy, and so forth may be erroneously diagnosed. Operations are sometimes performed, and symptoms are temporarily relieved. I have seen a patient who, on the basis of hysterical symptoms, had undergone seven abdominal operations with negligible anatomical findings. The chief point about these hysterical simulations of organic disease is that the complaints are wholly subjective, and no real objective physical signs are elicited. Patient complains of severe headaches, often described as a feeling of something sharp being driven into the brain. The symptoms are protean and may simulate almost any real disorder.

The hysteric personality presents many signs of immaturity, emotional instability, egocentricity, and marked suggestibility. Violent likes and dislikes characterize interpersonal relationships; strong liking for a person rapidly changes to marked hatred with no discernible reason. The patient will circulate vicious rumors about a former friend, send poison pen letters, and make other efforts to blacken the reputation of the erstwhile friend. Much deceit and lying is also practiced.

The suggestibility of patients is such that they easily adopt symptoms from other patients or evolve symptoms on the basis of some casual comment or reaction of the physician. At the same time, this suggestibility makes it especially easy to rid the patient of particular symptoms. These are the cases in which miracle cures occur so frequently. Electricity and any other type of staged show will remove symptoms, but they return or others replace them. In other words, the real nucleus of the disorder is not reached by such purely symptomatic treatment. Hysterical patients are easily accessible by hypnosis.

In one case a man became suddenly blind when he read he had succeeded in passing the bar examinations after having failed five times. Pressure on the eyeballs associated with suggestion relieved this symptom. On regaining his sight, he fitted up an elaborate law office. When he was to go to court to try his first case, he suddenly became mute. He was sent to a sanitarium for treatment, where he became acquainted with a lady who spent a good deal of time talking with him while he put his thoughts into writing. One day he wrote that if she would kiss him, he believed he would be able to talk. She did kiss him, and he promptly began to speak. He left the sanitarium as cured. About eighteen months later he lost an important case, whereupon his sense of personal identity failed. He went to another city, and was there picked up by the police and sent to a psychopathic hospital as a case of amnesia. When he recovered his identity, he was transferred to a psychopathic hospital in his native city. After a few days of observation he was discharged, with a diagnosis of hysteria.

In ordinary civilian life hysteria is much more common among women than among men. War strain, however, brings out many hysterical reactions in men, as do many types of accident in civil life. In fact, most traumatic neuroses are hysterical; at least they have many hysterical symptoms. One man whom I saw in consultation was being treated as a total permanent disability as the result of a bullet wound supposed to have been received in war and to have severed the spinal cord. Both legs were paralyzed; he spent his time in bed, and a nurse was supplied to care for him. On examination, it was found that there was no atrophy of leg muscles, reflexes were normal, there were no abnormal reflexes or anesthesia; bowel and bladder control were normal. There was no scar from the wound, and the indications were that he had really been kicked by a mule. Persuaded to stand up, he was placed far enough away from the bed so that he had to walk a few steps to return to it, which he succeeded in doing.

This case also illustrates an important point about many, perhaps most, neurotics. That is, there are secondary gains from the neurosis which may set up and maintain an unconscious desire not to get well or, at the very least, produce resistance to recovery. The patient may have a conscious, verbalized drive to be rid of his troublesome symptoms, but the secondary gains inhibit full effort and co-operation. This and other resistances are shown in many ways, such as refusal to accept treatment, breaking appointments, keeping to trivial matters in therapy interviews, rejecting interpretations and treatment plans, or developing a negative transfer.

Especially the neurotics who resist treatment and recovery, but even some with what seems to be genuine wish for help, carry their troubles to all sorts of healers and cultists, as well as to physicians and surgeons. One of several things may happen. The patients may be told by physicians that they are organically sound and to go home and forget it, or a special regime of treatment may be instituted which may have merit as a method for treating some disorders, but does not meet the neurotic's needs. The treatment may follow a magic formula and consist of placebos or some type of manipulation, including operations, which temporarily alleviate one or more symptoms. Quackery flourishes at the neurotic's expense, and it is little wonder that some eventually come to the cynical conclusion that no one understands their condition—indeed, that no one seems to try to understand.

Many neurotics seek the magical cure which will relieve them of their distressing symptoms, but do not wish to undertake any type of treatment which will reveal underlying mechanisms, require effort on their part, or cause them to make any personality readjustment which might be painful. These patients promptly take up any new treatment fad, run from doctor to doctor, from clinic to clinic, or seek any other cure of which they may hear. It is characteristic of such patients that if a treatment procedure begins to show results, they quickly abandon it, and criticism is heaped on the doctor or the clinic. These are the patients who have no real desire to recover; as said before, they are to be found in the ranks of all types of neurotic.

One of the important factors in the maintenance of a neurotic reaction is to be found in the desire for economic gain and less need for competitive striving. The soldier cited above had been a village blacksmith before he was called into service. As a civilian he had never earned more than $30 per week. As a war casualty, he received around $180 per month, plus the services of a nurse. He led a life of pampered ease, with much attention. Where, then, was the external incentive to recovery? Nor was there an internal incentive; the ego structure of this particular patient was too weak to operate as a driving force for recovery and assumption of an adult status. This does not mean that such a mechanism is peculiar to or common in service men.

Similar explanations are true for many cases of accidental injury. The results of the injury may be objectively real enough, but the whole traumatic episode becomes invested with a secondary neurotic complex. In some accident cases there may be no actual physical injury and the disability may be a "traumatic neurosis" from the beginning. In both cases the experience of industrial compensation boards and their physicians has conclusively shown that weekly compensation only prolongs illness. It may, indeed, tend to fixate the neurotic process to such an extent that some patients become chronic and untreatable. As a result of these findings the principle of lump-sum payment in cases of traumatic neurosis has been rather generally adopted.

In the treatment of hysteria two general procedures may be employed. The first is to relieve the immediate symptoms, commonly a fairly simple task, but, as already emphasized, this is not enough. In fact, this step may often best be eliminated and only the second procedure employed, which involves thoroughgoing psychotherapy, preferably a full psychoanalysis. Hypnoanalysis is a combination of hypnosis and psychoanalytic interpretations and further analytic exploration based on material revealed during the hypnotic trance as well as during the conscious state. It is being used at the present time, but it is not yet clear that this method shortens the time of treatment or is actually superior to regular analysis without hypnosis.

The essential psychopathological mechanisms in hysteria revolve around the Oedipus complex; that is, the neurosis is at the genital level, and unacceptable wishes find expression in symptoms which in general are symbolic of punishment for the offensive thoughts or wishes. The actual content of the ideas may not be sexual, but the associated emotional reaction activates or reactivates the sexual conflict which originally sprang from the internal and external taboos that are attached to sexuality.

NEURASTHENIA AND HYPOCHONDRIASIS

When neurasthenia was first described, many pathological states were included and it became a sort of universal waste basket. Gradually, however, various groups were separated, and neurasthenia was established as a separate disorder having particular characteristics. It is obvious from the name that neurological ideas dominated the delimitation of this group of reactions. Asthenia means "weakness, tending to exhaustion," in this instance an exhausting process affecting nerves or nerve centers. The symptoms are such that the name "fatigue neurosis" has been suggested as being more accurate than neurasthenia.

Several etiological theories have been advanced. The one which has achieved the greatest credence is that an emotional conflict concerning masturbation is the essential mechanism. It is certainly true that most neurasthenics display a great deal of conscious guilt and anxiety about masturbation. The great majority are male, and they almost invariably complain of impotence in heterosexual relations which they ascribe to excessive masturbation in the past.

The neurasthenic complains of pains along the spine, where there are associated areas of tenderness, inability to concentrate, irritability, some degree of depression, easy fatigability, and excessive fatigue reactions to any sustained exertion; he complains of insomnia and various other hypochondriacal symptoms. Some anxiety symptoms involving the cardiovascular and digestive systems may occur. Although the neurasthenic laments the loss of appetite and insomnia, he usually eats well and maintains his weight and an outward appearance of sound health. Careful observation shows that he also sleeps well, or at least a great deal more than he believes. The impotence, or relative impotence, is real, as attested by the mate.

Because of the physical symptoms, these patients seek medical assistance. Since no actual physical disease process can be discovered even by the most elaborate examinations, they are often told to go home and forget it. This only serves to reinforce the patient's opinion of the importance of his symptoms. He believes his illness to be such that it baffles even the trained and experienced physician. It was especially to neurasthenic cases that the "rest cure" was applied. This worked fairly well with many, as did sea voyages, trips for recreational purposes, and the various recommended therapeutic resorts such as spas. We now know that the reasons for the success lay in one or both of two factors—the transference relationship between patient and physician, and the patient's isolation or removal from the usual environment. These factors were not recognized earlier, and the dietary and other regimes were given credit for what were, in essence, purely psychological factors in the improvement or the so-called cure.

It has been my experience that most of these patients do not react too favorably in analysis. They are impatient for an immediate cure and because they become fixated on a physical explanation for what seem to them physical symptoms, they are reluctant to accept a psychological explanation or a psychotherapeutic approach. However, if they do accept these viewpoints or can be persuaded of their validity, analysis is the method preferred for therapy. At present, data are insufficient to be entirely reliable, but there are what seem to be good grounds for believing that cases belonging in this category will react favorably in psychotherapeutic groups.

It must be remembered that these patients are resistant to all types of treatment because of their essentially narcissistic personality structure. As has been stated, this always operates to interfere with therapeutic procedures of any type. It is for such patients with their hypochondriacal ideas, that the use of placebos has been most advocated. This sugar pill type of medication has unquestionably helped many neurasthenics to adjust to their disabilities.

So far as practical therapy is concerned, and the practical of today is not necessarily the obsolete of tomorrow, the point of adjusting to a disability and making the best of it is often quite as important for the neurotic as it is for one who has a physical disability. Many neurotics should *not* have psychotherapy; the resulting upset of a partial sublimation could be too devastating. In all such cases a supportive relationship with a social worker, physician, or some other person emotionally important in the patient's life may serve as the needed crutch to help him accept and adjust to his difficulties.

PSYCHASTHENIA: PHOBIAS, OBSESSIONS, COMPULSIONS

The obsessive-compulsive neuroses are perhaps the most frequent of all. They are also impressive because of the nature of the symptomatology and the insight shown by the patient, who realizes that his fears and compulsions are utterly foolish and that he makes himself ridiculous, yet feels completely baffled as to how to cope with them.

The fears displayed may refer to almost any everyday and necessary activity. As a rule, they are not the ordinary fears which all of us experience at some time, especially as children. Fear of the dark, of animals, of strange people, of heights, and of small enclosed places are so common that in and of themselves they cannot be regarded as neurotic. Such fears may be neurotic under certain circumstances, and when this is the case it is made clear by associated symptoms.

These neurotic fears or *phobias* are legion; one small dictionary lists seventy-six. A few of the more common are mentioned here, chiefly to show the base from which the names are formed. Claustrophobia is the fear of being in narrow or enclosed spaces, while agoraphobia is the fear of being in wide open spaces. Mono- or auto-phobia is a morbid dread of being alone; pantophobia is the fear aroused by being in crowds; xenophobia refers to being in the presence of strangers. Acrophobia is the fear of being in high places or aloft in the air; while fears of being in tunnels, basements, etc., constitute one type of claustrophobia, often complicated by nyctophobia, which is fear of darkness or of night. There are morbid aversions to or fears of being in the company of men or of women, andro- and gyne-phobias. Mysophobia is the fear of contamination or dirt; coprophobia is repugnance to filth or the act of defecation. Nosophobia is fear of illness, especially of some specific disease. Similar names are given to morbid fears of dogs and of contracting rabies; to aversion to assuming responsibility and to work; to fear of red, of blushing, or of showing embarrassment; to dread of new things or situations; to aversion to cold, and so forth through a long list.

The important point is that these fears are *morbid;* that is, they are far in excess of any normal reaction to the situation in which they appear, are accompanied by some or all of the physical manifestations of fear, and occur repetitively whenever the phobic situation is encountered. The sufferer recognizes intellectually that the fear is unnecessary or unduly intense and that the reaction is excessive in degree and duration. Nevertheless, he feels unable to control his emotional upset and cannot explain the fears, which he recognizes as abnormal, to the satisfaction of himself or others. The reason for this is simply that the external situation which is feared is only symbolic of the real fears, which are buried in the unconscious. This is essentially the meaning of the patient's in-

sistent statements that he cannot understand why he has these reactions, which he knows are unnecessary and unconstructive.
There is, in other words, a realization of the fact that the fear
really belongs to something else which is unknown to the conscious
self.

Compulsions follow along the lines of the fears, though there are
some rituals which have no relation to specific phobias. Such is the
ritual of dressing, which may take hours before the individual is
ready to leave the bedroom. Stockings are put on and taken off; so
are shoes, underclothes, and outerclothes, until half the day may
have passed. Even then the individual has as many doubts and indecisions about leaving the room or attempting the ordinary routine
of living as he had about clothing himself.

Of the many such compulsions, one of the commonest is that
of cleansing. This usually involves washing the hands, though it
may also involve other parts of the body or the body as a whole.
While the patient recognizes the stupidity of the activity, it is
nevertheless kept up even to the point of painful abrasion. He
protests against the activity, but is compelled to persist in it.
Doubts, indecision, and anxiety complicate the picture. The
washing is a symbolic attempt to cleanse the unconscious guilt associated with anal interests, masturbation, or similar anxiety-producing situations.

In the phobic situation there may be marked physical symptoms,
such as sweating, palpitation, pallor, and tremor, which cause the
patient to make frantic efforts to get out of the fear-provoking
spot. He will strenuously try to avoid getting into the same set-up
and waste an enormous amount of time and effort in his attempt to
evade the pain-producing situation.

The obsessive-compulsive personality is characterized by over-
scrupulousness, rigidity, formality, adherence to rituals, asceticism,
expiations and atonements, inhibitions, extreme orderliness, and
even minor phobias. This personality type may never develop
clear-cut neurotic symptoms.

The preferred treatment for the psychasthenic case is psychoanalysis, even though it is difficult and usually prolonged. The fears and rituals serve as such strong protection against the irruption into consciousness of the underlying mechanisms that the unconscious resistance is high. The unconscious content has to do with sexual fantasies and conflicts, guilt over masturbation, incestuous ideas, hostility, and sadistic impulses. These are magically projected into the external world, which explains the patient's recognition of the absurdity of his ideas and behavior. Even though he cannot verbalize it, there is some realization that the problems are intrapsychic and that the ideas and behavior are symbolic masks. Doubts, indecisions, and preoccupation with unanswerable questions are often defenses against dealing with the inner problems. It is obvious that anal-sadistic factors are operative and that the earliest attachment to parents is involved. Shock treatment has been used for obsessional-compulsion neuroses with a moderate degree of success where the symptoms have existed only a short time. In more advanced cases, however, the value of such treatment is very dubious.

Compulsive symptoms are fairly common in children of six to twelve years of age. Usually the symptoms are few in number, they do not dominate the psyche, and they are evanescent. In some cases, however, a true neurosis develops.

ANXIETY STATES

While anxiety appears to some degree and at some time in all people, there is a special group of neurotic cases in which anxiety, with associated physical symptoms, dominates the clinical picture. In these cases, as they appear in civil life, there are no specific phobias, though there are vague, unformulated fears, best denominated as apprehensiveness. In the individual attacks, apprehensiveness may reach an intensity best designated as panic.

In the anxiety attack, physical symptoms of sweating, generalized tremors, pallor, chilliness, palpitation, feelings of pressure in chest and head, butterflies in the stomach, and other feelings occur. A feeling of impending death also adds to the patient's terror. Such attacks occur at almost any time, and no specific precipitating external factors may appear to be involved. It is this point which differentiates the anxiety states from phobias with associated anxiety symptoms.

Attacks of anxiety were originally described as affecting women. They were ascribed to the repeated building up of sexual tension not adequately discharged by normal sexual relations. It was later found, particularly in neuroses in males originating during combat, that ego mechanisms are also involved. Hostility, guilt, and infantile sexual mechanisms are reactivated, with the production of marked anxiety.

In acute attacks of anxiety, sedation may be necessary. Shock therapy has been employed with some success in milder cases. A combination of drug-induced narcosis and psychoanalytic interpretation, called narcosynthesis, has been employed with considerable success in acute anxiety states arising in combat. The results with this method have been especially impressive when carried out within a few hours or days, and near the battle lines. Under narcosis the anxiety-producing or anxiety-releasing situation is likely to be re-enacted, with discharge of affect and subsequent release of tension. Group psychotherapy has been found of value in many cases. Psychoanalysis, however, is the method of choice for the treatment of cases of longer standing. Almost all cases arising in civil life have reached a chronic stage in terms of the duration of symptomatology and disability by the time they are referred to or consult the psychiatrist.

PSYCHOSOMATIC CONDITIONS

A brief discussion of the general relationships between emotional tensions and bodily changes, with particular reference to psychopathological elements in somatic illness, is all that will be attempted here. The outline is, in the main, adapted from Franz Alexander's contributions to the subject.

The autonomic nervous system, also designated as vegetative, sympathetic, or involuntary, mediates the interaction of psychological and somatic factors. This rather primitive organization of nervous tissue has direct connections with the mid- and hind-brain and with the spinal cord. Peripherally, it is distributed to smooth or involuntary muscle, the cardiovascular system, the viscera and the secretory glands; in general it regulates the involuntary or vegetative activities of the body. The autonomic system is composed of two mutually antagonistic arrangements of neurones, commonly designated as the sympathetic and parasympathetic systems, which act as inhibitors for each other.

Behavior reactions such as laughter, weeping, or even sexual activity directly express or relieve specific emotional tensions. The behavior has no utilitarian goals, but represents a discharge phenomenon which is a direct concomitant of the emotional state. In a somewhat different type of reaction, there are modifications in functions mediated by the autonomic system which permit the organism to respond to changing conditions. If danger threatens, flight or fighting is made possible by elevation of blood pressure, acceleration of heart beat, changes in the distribution of blood, mobilization of carbohydrates, release of adrenalin, and so forth. These physiological changes are definite constituents of rage or fear, which are not expressed or relieved by the changes, yet could not be discharged unless these alterations took place. The two types of reaction outlined differ considerably from voluntary behavior, which is integrated and adapted to the achievement of conscious and more or less practical goals.

When there is an imbalance or disharmony between emotional states and vegetative functioning, a psychosomatic problem results. For the most part, such conditions appear in people who are frustrated, disturbed, and unhappy in interpersonal relationships. The resultant tension and anxiety upset physiological balances so that a long list of somatic symptoms may ensue. These are not always associated with definite signs of physical pathology in the clinical and laboratory examinations. In other cases the symptoms are greatly in excess of expectations in view of the actual pathology. Careful history taking, especially discriminative listening to the spontaneous outpouring of frustrations, often reveals the particular situational factors and emotional tensions which are directly related to the original appearance of symptoms, or to exacerbations. In any case, it has been amply demonstrated that organic diseases may develop as an end result of chronic functional disturbances.

Chronic emotional tensions, such as anxiety, hostility, guilt, discontent, or a longing for dependency, result from continued repression or inhibition of the normal expression of emotions. The tensions operate in the unconscious and through the autonomic system find expression in constellations of somatic symptoms in people who would seem to have some predisposition to them. The psychopathology is that of chronic inadequacy of emotional expression; somatic pathology is a result.

The basic psychosomatic orientation is, accordingly, to study the total personality in relation to disturbances in the total configuration of physiological processes. This should ideally yield a concept of disease very different from that of isolated local processes. It is reasonably argued that all diseases have a psychosomatic component; resistance to infection, for example, depends in part upon the emotional state of the patient. Disturbances in the vegetative functions are related to a variety of etiological factors, organic and emotional. The psychosomatic approach involves simultaneous study and treatment of psychological and somatic factors and their interrelationships.

Some psychiatrists hold that there is a specific relationship between the particular unrelieved emotional configuration and the vegetative organ system in which symptoms appear. According to this view, the emotional background differs with different diseases —hypertension or asthma or gastric ulcer. There is a considerable body of evidence to support this thesis, but conflicting observations indicate that the relationships are not so specific.

Without going into detail, it may be stated that certain cardiovascular, gastrointestinal, respiratory, gynecological, and endocrine disturbances have been correlated as psychosomatic reactions. This is also true for some rheumatic and rheumatoid cases, and particularly for accident-prone people. The fact that many cases of pathological conditions are psychological in origin does not *ipso facto* mean that all such cases are; the possibility of physical etiology has already been stated.

Three final points deserve passing mention. In the first place, emotions, endocrine glands, and autonomic nervous system form a sort of closed circle, such that activity in any one stimulates the others. In many cases it is extraordinarily difficult to determine whether endocrine over- or under-activity is responsible for particular emotional sets, or whether the reverse is true. Decision as to initial therapeutic approach may need to be based on practical considerations as to which symptoms are most serious; at other times, there must be empirical testing of possibilities.

The second point concerns the differences in physiology and psychodynamics for the physical symptoms of conversion hysteria and those of disturbances of vegetative functions. Hysterical symptoms, as Alexander states, are symbolic or substitute expressions of emotional conflict restricted to the voluntary motor and sensory systems, although the attempt at relief of emotional tension is not voluntarily initiated or controlled. Psychosomatic symptoms, on the contrary, do not represent symbolic expressions of a frustrated emotion. Instead, an organ is involved in the direct expression of emotion and, because of the chronicity of stimulation from tension, symptoms are produced.

The third point will merely serve as a reminder that acute and chronic organic diseases frequently have important effects upon mental attitudes and emotional reactions. Psychological effects may be more important and more permanent than are the physical. Particular attention should be given to the meaning of a disease process, a disability, or disorders of even minor significance in those organs considered by the patient to be especially important. It is in this area that professional people are sometimes extraordinarily careless in what they say to the patient or in his hearing regarding his disease, its possible after-effects, or his chances of survival. As a result, the patient may experience unnecessary panic respecting death or permanent disability, brood over the seemingly hostile attitude of doctors and others, or resort to compensatory aggression.

Psychosomatic reactions have long been known and dealt with after a fashion, but they were not systematically studied and correlated until they were brought together under the unifying psychosomatic concept. One result of this should be a firm integration of psychiatric concepts and approaches with those of general medicine, leading to a final erasure of those artificial distinctions between soma and psyche which have so markedly handicapped many aspects of the practice of medicine and, it may be added, of social work.

SOCIAL WORK WITH NEUROTICS

Many neurotic clients apply to social agencies for help with various issues. When the client's personality problems are such that a fully developed neurosis seems to be indicated, the worker would do well to enlist the services of a psychiatrist immediately. In many cases, however, there are only neurotic trends or mild or very few actual symptoms of neurosis. Or the client may have developed a satisfactory compensatory way of living with his personality difficulty, in which circumstance the social worker is justified in establishing a supportive relationship. It is extremely difficult to draw any hard and fast lines with reference either to the patients who should be selected or the lengths to which the worker should go in treatment. The only safe rule is, when in doubt do nothing until it is possible to consult with a more experienced person.

CHAPTER XIV

PSYCHOPATHIC PERSONALITY

THE TERM psychopathic personality is used to designate a group of people who appear, up to a point, normal—not psychotic, feebleminded, epileptic, or neurotic—but whose social behavior and character sets are deviant. In preceding chapters the personality types associated with the psychoses and neuroses have already been discussed—the hysterical, the epileptic, the schizoid, the cyclothymic, the paranoid, and the neurotic.

In the present chapter we are concerned with a group of abnormal personality types which have no specific relationship to any of the psychoses or neuroses; that is, they are not "miniature" psychoses or neuroses. These psychopathic personalities are not too well delimited, and apparently there is considerable disagreement among psychiatrists concerning the exact definition of the term and just how inclusive or exclusive the group really is. The important point is that psychiatrists agree there is such a group of abnormal personalities, by whatever term they may be called, and regardless of the precise limits of inclusion or the theories advanced to explain the abnormalities in behavior.

The earliest terms applied to this group were "moral insanity" (or derangement), and "moral imbecility." The concepts underlying these designations were that there was no intellectual defect or impairment, but that the "moral senses" were perverted or depraved. As a result, the individual was unable to conduct himself with propriety and decency. The feelings and temper were regarded as subject to morbid perversion. Another way of putting this was that it was like a blind, instinctive, irresistible impulse, with a special propensity to destroy. Some psychiatrists tended to include all recidivist delinquents in this group, but others maintained that there were many delinquents who were neither moral imbeciles nor morally insane.

The term moral imbecility especially connoted the idea that the condition was innate and thus probably hereditary. As more careful studies were made, particularly better individual case studies, the conclusion was finally reached and sustained that probably all so-called moral imbeciles were mentally abnormal in some way but were not actually devoid of moral feeling.

The terms psychopathic personality and constitutional psychopathic inferiority than came into vogue. The majority of psychiatrists and practically all statistical reports use the former appellation. The term constitutional psychopathic inferiority is still in use despite its unfortunate and misleading connotations. Thus, the term implies an inferiority which is not necessarily present. Certainly, if the inferiority is supposed to have any relationship to physical make-up, intelligence, sensitiveness, or creative ability, then for many cases the concept is entirely erroneous. Many patients present considerable superiority in some or all of these fields. Their difficulties are in the quality *and excess* of responses rather than in inferiorities. Secondly, on the basis of our present knowledge constitutional factors are not believed to play the dominant role in the production of these disorders. Observations of the effects of pathological and traumatic life situations during the early months and years of life show very definitely that particular types of character deviation ensue. In fact, children who are reared during the first months of life in even the best of infants' homes emerge with an isolation type of personality structure which seems to be permanent. Children who are openly rejected and those who are excessively overindulged, often to conceal an underlying parental rejection, also show pathological characters.

Because the symptoms of psychopathy are manifested in the field of social behavior, the term "sociopath" has also been proposed to designate this group, but has not achieved popularity, probably because the specifically important symptoms are embedded in the personality structure. The latest term proposed is "neurotic character." Distinctions are made between the neurotic personality, in which a neurosis may or may not develop, the neuroses, and the neurotic character.

The neurotic personality displays a variety of neurotic traits which do not ordinarily interfere with fairly adequate adjustment. In the neuroses the conflict is expressed by symptoms of illness which are socially acceptable, at least no social harm results, whereas the neurotic character represents a condition in which there are no symbolizations in the form of symptoms, but the primitive impulses are externalized in direct action. Even though their actions injure others and are prejudicial to society, there is an inner but unconscious condemnation that also makes them injure themselves in some way. The neurotic character is said to begin during the latency period, as the result of inadequate resolution of the Oedipus conflict. The psychological content is alike in the neuroses and in the neurotic character, but the dynamics of the expression of the conflict differ in the two conditions. Studies of psychopathic states with these concepts in mind have enriched our understanding of these conditions, even though therapeutic affectiveness has not as yet been particularly increased.

Many attempts have been made to establish a classification or grouping of psychopaths. Most ventures were based on clinical descriptions, and only one or two have essayed to group these deviant personalities according to etiological factors. Actually, classification into types is not especially important. Since the boundaries of the group as a whole are indefinite, it is often a matter of individual judgment as to whether the deviation in a particular personality is sufficient to justify calling it pathological, that is, psychopathic.

One of the earliest classifications was that of Kraepelin, who set up seven groups; Herman Adler proposed four groups, while Eugen Kahn described sixteen. In these groupings and in others similarly based on clinical descriptions, it must be emphasized that there is a core of symptoms common to all, but the presence in marked degree of certain behavior reactions leads to the group designations. For our purpose the character traits which are more or less common to all are more important to understand than is any grouping. Karpman has delimited two groups of anethopaths, as he prefers to designate the psychopaths. One group, which includes about 85 percent of the total number, comprises those whose behavior is psychopathic but is really symptomatic of some type of psychogenetic conditioning. This is revealed by careful study of socio-psychiatric material which reveals adequate and understandable reasons for the reactions. The second group, comprising about 15 percent of the total, is the idiopathic, in which the behavior cannot be traced to psychogenetic factors. These cases Karpman divides into two subgroups, the aggressive-predatory and the passive-parasitic types.

The character traits and behavior reactions of the psychopath are, at least to some degree, common to all people at some stage of development. This accounts for some of the difficulties in establishing precise criteria for differentiating psychopathic conduct from behavior which falls within the normal range of variation. Furthermore, except in certain instances of characteristic types of response and excesses of reaction, it is difficult to be sure whether a child is psychopathic or whether the behavior and apparent character set will be successfully modified or replaced in subsequent development and growth. In children, therefore, it is a wise rule to undertake a therapeutic test before concluding that the behavior which is psychopathic in type is really evidence of psychopathic personality.

This brings out the first point with regard to adolescent and adult psychopaths, that of essential untreatability. This is linked with one of the most important points about the psychopathic character; namely, the inability to learn by experience even though intelligence is adequate. That this is related to the compulsive nature of the behavior seems clear, but the compulsion is deeply buried in the unconscious. The result is that the patient really tells the truth when he says "I do not know" why a particular act or series of acts were committed.

Another striking point about the psychopath is the absence of conscious guilt feelings and anxiety concerning the socially objectionable behavior. This, of course, contrasts sharply with the anxiety and guilt of the neurotic. The psychopath may say "I'm sorry" and promise not to repeat the behavior, but the words are meaningless, as shown by the subsequent, often immediate, repetition. There is no real feeling behind the verbalization. It is this which leads to the commonly made assertion that the affect of the psychopath is flattened or impoverished. This is only partially true, since the psychopath is likely to be extremely emotional about matters which affect him or his safety, but cold-blooded or indifferent about the ills or misfortune of others. He is likely to be particularly so if his actions are responsible for the sufferings of other people. "He has no feelings" is perhaps one of the commonest criticisms of relatives and friends. The psychopath usually finds some rationalization for his behavior and does not even say he is sorry. Instead, he puts emphasis on some situation as the provocation of his behavior or stresses the responsibility of other people. In other words, he blames anything or anyone except himself for his difficulties.

One of the striking defects of the psychopathic personality is the inability to form adequate object-love relationships. This is due to marked egocentricity. The psychopath demands much love, attention, and praise, but can give little or none in return, even though he may appear to do so. He cannot tolerate frustration or criticism, but himself freely and harshly frustrates and criticizes others. Because many are superficially attractive, outgoing, flattering, and charming in manner, psychopaths make a good first impression and are quickly accepted by people of intelligence and consequence. But the emotions and attitudes are basically egocentric, and the contacts so established are quickly turned to selfish ends. The result is that the ultimate outcome is the bilking of the new friends in one way or another. This pattern is repeated over and over. Much the same comment applies to sexual and love relationships; the psychopath demands much, gives little, and rapidly and cold-bloodedly passes from one relationship to another.

This relative inability to form an adequate relationship with another person also accounts for the fact that it is usually impossible to establish an effective treatment relationship. Because the therapeutic situation is ordinarily a permissive one, a relationship on a superficial level is easily set up. In fact, the very facility with which the relationship is established is an important danger signal. Most children, for example, if they are asked in the first interview, "Whom do you love best in all the world?" will name one or more members of the family. But the psychopathic child will answer, "You," and give the same answer to the next person who asks the question. In some instances the child may even answer, "Me," and, so far as one can ascertain, mean it.

The relationship established in the permissive therapeutic situation is tenuous and commonly lasts only until the psychopath is out of his immediate difficulty or until the therapist or the therapeutic situation necessarily produces some frustration, or appears to the patient to do so. Attention is called to these points because of the deceptive façade of interest and responsiveness, even apparent insight into treatment possibilities, which these patients present in the first contacts. When the contact is seemingly so easy it is wise to review the patient's entire history, preferably a factual one obtained from outside sources, in order to determine whether the response is genuine or only a psychopathic manifestation. If it is the latter, a repetitive pattern of this type of behavior will appear very clearly.

When the childhood history of the psychopath is reviewed, it will usually reveal the existence of many abnormal traits and failure to develop the socially aceptable behavior to be expected at different stages of development. Behavior which is normal for a given stage of development will be excessive or inhibited in the psychopath. It may be prolonged far past the time when it has served a useful purpose and is ordinarily replaced by progressively more integrated personal and social reactions. Persuasion, punishment, and demonstrations of love are powerless to prevent the recurrence of the behavior.

As children, psychopaths tend to show many behavior traits, such as aggressive demands, temper tantrums, anger, running away from home, enuresis, cruelty, stealing, and destructiveness far in excess of such manifestations in normal children. These same traits continue into adolescent and adult life. The psychopaths are stubborn, sensitive, morose, boastful, erratic, shameless, wily, arrant liars, and deceitful. Many are sexually precocious, and sexual curiosity, early sex play, and masturbation to excess are common.

In adolescence the normal rebellion against family ties is multiplied many times. There is lag in emotional development and control, with increasing lack of adjustment between personal instinctive drives and social mores. Foresight and critical judgment are inadequate. Among other juvenile traits, the foregoing of an immediate pleasure for a future goal is never learned by the psychopath. Hence much adult psychopathic behavior is called impulsive and thoughtless, and objectives remain in the confused state so characteristic of adolescence.

The psychopath is restless, without knowing exactly why. Routine is difficult to tolerate, and marked vocational instability is shown. Enthusiasm for a new situation or a new job runs high, but only for a short time. Then there is increasing dissatisfaction and tension, often ending in an explosive departure. The psychopath is not content to learn a vocation and strive upward in it; he wants to be top man immediately. Despite obvious lack of knowledge and efficiency, he is always sure of his ability to manage other people, organizations, or any situation. In fact, he is usually content only where he can be dominant.

Rebellion against home authority is extreme and is carried over to all other forms of authority, including political and social organizations. Psychopaths who have a drive to create in music, literature, and the arts are contemptuous of all existing and preexisting art forms. They boast of the new modes they will originate, but their actual effort is scattered, and the results are negligible. They "talk" great plans and ideas, but always for the future; meanwhile they fritter away their time in various sorts of dissipation. When they do produce some ineffective piece of work, they bitterly resent its nonacceptance. Their attitude then is that people are too ignorant to understand, and they launch barrages of violent criticism against persons who actually have superior knowledge and skill.

The psychopath adopts many methods to escape his own unconscious motivations. He may resort to alcohol, which often causes him to be belligerent and destructive. Prolonged and violent sprees may still further complicate his problems. Sexual activity, extravagant spending, and various sorts of antisocial behavior may emerge.

The social adjustment of the psychopath is, from all this evidence, clearly inadequate. It ranges from eccentricity to definitely antisocial, delinquent, and criminal behavior. Cranks, extremists, unstable, excitable, inadequate, and socially misfit people are to be found in this group. Many recidivist criminals are psychopaths. It is necessary to emphasize the fact that not all delinquents and criminals are psychopathic and that many psychopathic personalities are not delinquent or criminal. The diagnosis should *never be based on behavior alone;* it must be based on the demonstration of psychological mechanisms which are directly related to the behavior exhibited. Nor should the diagnosis ever be based on the occurrence of single symptoms or occasional apparent deviations. It is the combination of symptoms and the frequency of their appearance which makes diagnosis possible.

Three groups deserve some special discussion: (1) the pathological liars and swindlers; (2) the antisocial; (3) the sexual psychopaths. The pathological liars and swindlers are among the most interesting examples of the so-called charming scamps. They are extremely imaginative and champion tellers of tall tales, in which they invariably play the leading role. They make social contacts easily and build up their stories by proper accessories, such as accents, uniforms, forged documentary evidence, and other items. From time to time newspapers report the exposure of a bogus nobleman, officer, diplomatic agent, or some other impostor. Their activity sometimes takes the form of sexual conquests, and they may obtain money under false pretenses, either on the promise of marriage or after a bigamous marriage.

Unable to accept responsibility and routine work, which they regard as drudgery, they live in an unreal world of fantasy in which there is great ego-maximation. The fantasies are wishfulfilling; similar to those which normally occur in childhood, but are ordinarily superseded as the ability to live with and accept reality develops. In the psychopathic adult fantasies are much elaborated and take in many social situations which the child does not encounter. When detected, psychopaths often insist that their stories are real; sometimes they claim amnesia for particular episodes. Psychopaths are usually intelligent, but feelings of inferiority, of sibling rivalry, jealousy, and rejection are common. Repeated exposures and punishments are ordinarily ineffective in controlling the false and unsuccessful attempts to satisfy the intrapsychic problems.

The antisocial personality is characterized by a marked lack of feeling for others, arrogance, lack of a sense of honor or loyalty, and socially destructive behavior. These are the recidivist criminal types; the gangsters who exhibit a sadistic delight in torture and murder; those who proudly defy law and order. They usually feel justified in their actions and resent punishment, which, accordingly, does not act as a deterrent. On the other hand, in many cases punishment such as penal incarceration apparently relieves any possible sense of debt to society that they may have accumulated and so acts as a stimulus to further crime. There are more and more such cases among the repeaters in admissions to penal institutions.

Sexual psychopathy is an intricate subject of large proportions. Masturbation and homosexual relationships in adults are only to be regarded as psychopathic when they are not due to lack of opportunity for other relationships, but represent the methods of choice for the satisfaction of the sexual drive when other methods are available. There are many forms of deviation from the normal sexual impulse, most of which represent fixations on partial sexual trends. Frigidity and its opposite, hypererotism, are usually neurotic in origin and therefore susceptible of treatment.

Perversions of the sexual drive are less amenable to treatment and are founded either in biological or psychological factors or in both. Sadism, masochism, fetishism, and exhibitionism are particularly based on psychological factors and represent failure to develop beyond early stages of psychosexual integration. Fixation at these levels usually depends upon experiences which reinforce the mechanisms operative at the particular stage of development. Oral and anal erotism may also become fixated for either homosexual or heterosexual activities. A particularly difficult complication is the fixation of adults of either sex on children of either sex as sexual objects.

Judging by the reactions of the public, the most important problems in sexual activity seem to be masturbation and homosexuality. Viewpoints on both have been changing gradually during recent years. Formerly, masturbation was viewed as an activity which would stunt growth and create mental inferiority or even insanity. Actually, some form of masturbatory activity occurs in practically all individuals at some stage of development and in most of the mammalian species. The usual psychological reactions in the human are feelings of guilt and degradation, fears of the consequences of the activity, and resentment because of inability to control the impulse. The social reaction is usually one of condemnation. None of these reactions are likely to appear in psychopaths to whom masturbation is the only acceptable form of sexual activity. Such psychopaths are the narcissists who are unable to form sustained relationships of any type with others, while imagery associated with masturbation is usually rich enough to be entirely satisfying. Aside from a withdrawn, egocentric, and somewhat negativistic personality, narcissists who are not definitely psychopathic may function fairly efficiently.

Homosexuality presents many problems to society. Most accounts of homosexuality stress only the masculine or active type of female homosexual and the feminine or passive type of male homosexual. It seems to be forgotten that every active lesbian requires a passive female partner, just as every passive male homosexual requires an active partner. Actives of either sex do not mate with actives, nor do passives mate with passives. A complication in understanding homosexual relationships has to do with the mode of activity. This may involve mutual masturbation or oral, anal, and other methods.

Transvestitism, the wearing of clothes of the opposite sex or clothes modeled on them, is common. Boys may express a desire to be girls and are interested in essentially feminine occupations. Much more common is the wish of girls to be boys and the openly expressed resentment that they are not. It is an interesting and important point that girls more easily surrender their wish to be boys and accept femininity than do boys who wish to be girls accept their masculinity. In the vast majority of people, homosexual drives, even though they may be strong, are suppressed, replaced by heterosexual drives, or sublimated along socially acceptable lines.

Biologically the human race is bisexual; psychologically, this is also often true. In the course of normal development masculine factors come to predominate in males, and female factors in females. However, in many instances the physical make-up indicates a deficit of male biological factors in males, with an excess of female factors; the situation is reversed for women. These biological points indicate one line of treatment which may be successful if employed in the prepubertal or pubertal period. If there are definite indications of gonadal insufficiency, endocrine therapy may be of considerable service and even curative. Where no special indications of physiological imbalance are obvious, but a psychological fixation at the homosexual level exists, endocrine therapy is of no value and psychotherapy is difficult. In the majority of cases of homosexuality an adjustment is made such that a reasonably successful life is carried on, the homosexuality remaining in the background as a matter of private interest.

The psychopath, however, is not so successful in organizing his life, and homosexuality openly dominates his or her activities. This brings the psychopath into conflict with social opinion and with the law, which defines homosexual activity as illegal. Punishment by prison sentence is, however, ineffective. Treatment is also difficult and may only be attempted if anxiety and guilt lead the patient to seek it. The consciousness of social disapproval or feelings of guilt aroused by being detected in the activity may sometimes lead a patient to seek help, but this is not usually true of the psychopath. It is much more common to find repressed and unconscious homosexual drives operating to produce neurotic symptoms, which in turn cause the patient to apply for treatment.

Some of the sexual psychopathies are socially dangerous. Sexually perverse drives in the psychopath may lead to rape and sadistic murder, often centering on children. Exhibitionism of the purely sexual, not sublimated, type, and voyeurism, or peeping, are likely to be perverting, especially to children, and may lead to criminal acts. These are all classed as legal offenses.

Up to this time no satisfactory techniques for the treatment of psychopaths have been evolved. The absence of genuine insight, the self-satisfaction, and the inability to establish and sustain object-relationships are ordinarily insuperable obstacles. If the therapist becomes the source of ego-ideals for the patient, as sometimes occurs, a transfer and a transference neurosis may be developed which can be successfully used in treatment. If guilt and anxiety can be brought into consciousness, treatment is possible.

The chief point the social worker should bear in mind in connection with this group of cases is to guard against becoming too optimistic about the possibility of treatment on the basis of early contacts. Nor should the worker become too upset when the early promise of treatability is not fulfilled. Even so, he should not fail to attempt supportive treatment in such cases, at least tentatively, on the chance that the diagnosis is wrong or that the case may turn out to be one in which sufficient anxiety may develop to permit effective treatment.

CHAPTER XV

BEHAVIOR AND ITS DISORDERS

SO FAR, we have presented the personal and social maladaptations dependent upon well-defined psychopathological states, especially in adults. Treatment in these conditions is primarily directed at the disease process at work in the individual patient. Hospitalization, medical and surgical procedures, psychotherapy, special education, and social supervision may be required, either singly or in combination. These matters were presented first because they constitute the background of knowledge essential to a discussion of behavior disorders in children. The study and treatment of children's problems is the essence of preventive psychiatry; that is to say, orthopsychiatry.

Properly to understand the problems in behavior which arise out of the nexus of interpersonal relationships that so strongly affect the growth and development of the child, it is first necessary to clarify what is meant by normal, abnormal, and problem behavior. Adaptive behavior is both a biological and a social function of the organism; normal and abnormal variations arise in either functional field.

ORIGINS OF BEHAVIOR

Behavior, whether broadly or narrowly defined, is the sum total of reactions by an individual to stimuli or situations that result in physiological tension, the energy of which is discharged by the reactions. These stimuli or situations may be external or internal and they undergo elaboration, modification, or interpretation within the individual. Such changes in the nature or intensity of stimuli are related to past experiences, conscious and unconscious. As a result of the combination of present stimulus and past experience, however this may come about and whatever the theoretical explanation, a reaction is initiated and either carried through or inhibited.

The resulting behavior reaction may be external, in which case it is directly observable as it affects the individual himself and as it affects the person or group to which it is exhibited. The reaction may also be only internal, with no manifestations that can be perceived by others. Finally, the reactions may be both internal and external. In this case there is no necessary similarity between the two sets of reactions; in general, we interpret the internal reaction, made up of feelings and thoughts, by the externalized behavior. This is always a delicate task, especially if there is partial to complete voluntary suppression or distortion of external reactions, even in situations where emotions are acute. As examples, people weep for joy as well as for sorrow; some redden and some pale with anger; cursing and calling names may be hostile or, under certain circumstances, friendly.

It is obvious that from this viewpoint any and all changes in the dynamic equilibrium of the individual are to be called behavior. Some aspects of behavior are social; they occur in reaction to and react upon the social group. Other aspects or types of behavior are more purely personal, since their effects are chiefly within or upon the individual himself.

Because the organism is always in a state of dynamic, unstable equilibrium biologically and psychologically, the behavior in response to a given stimulus may constantly be modified, at least to some degree, on repetition. At the same time, there is a marked tendency toward the establishment of fixed modes or patterns of response to a repeated stimulus through the continuous process of conditioning, and the innate trend toward the establishment of automatic reaction patterns.

All behavior is purposive in the sense that through the changes involved in action of any sort there is an alteration in the tensions involved in the production of the reaction. This is true of the behavior of the amoeba in reacting to a food particle, of the behavior of the heart in its function, or that of the total human being in the various situations to which he reacts.

Biologically, behavior in some situations is early correlated into automatic types of reaction. Examples of this are the heartbeat, intestinal peristalsis, and expulsion of urine from the ureters. This type of behavior is characterized by rhythmicity and is not subject to conscious, voluntary, control. It is to be noted that these automatic activities are under the control of the vegetative nervous system, though they may be stimulated by emotions aroused by external events. In certain other types of automatic activity the surface of the body is involved, as in respiration, urination, and defecation. Here a certain degree of voluntary control enters in, so that automaticity may to some degree be altered—to a lesser extent with respiration, and more so with excretory functions. Rhythm is still an important part of the reactions. Specific sexual activity, though to some extent rhythmical, is much more under voluntary control than are any of the others mentioned.

Automatic and reflex reactions have a quite different relationship to mental life and processes than do reactions and associations related to external situations. This is because they are direct biological responses to immediate protoplasmic needs, and so do not enter particularly into the stream of consciousness. It is also true that we are more conscious of functions, however rhythmical, if they involve the surface of the body, as is especially true of the excretory functions. These are the first to be subject to external social pressure to bring them under conscious control. The functions then acquire quite different emotional values for the individual than do the more purely automatic ones.

One type of internal stimulus may be described in terms of memories of previous experiences. These are significant in direct ratio to the ease with which the earlier situations may be recalled. They act either to condition or to modify reactions to new situations or to reprecipitate an older form of response that may be less suitable and so interfere with a desirable or necessary response.

It is obvious that external situations are important as stimuli to internal, external, and social behavior. In addition, since previous impressions are retained, they act as conditioning or modifying factors for reactions to later situations. This points up the continuity of mental life, since no experience occurring after consciousness and memory are physiologically possible is ever completely lost unless a deteriorating process develops. During development definite patterns of behavior appear as more complex integrations of simpler reactions, and many tend to become automatic under ordinary conditions. Walking and speech are outstanding examples of this tendency toward the formation of action patterns which become more or less automatic.

Enough has been said to make it clear that some kinds of external behavior are related solely to internal mechanisms, while others are produced or modified in accordance with environmental stimuli and pressures. We are confronted with a dynamic organism, subject to laws of growth and relationship to the physical environment, and constantly changing its adjustment to stable or changeable external factors. Furthermore, it is clear that there is no such thing as a fixed, static, unitary environment. Instead, we have to do with a series of environments, each with its own dynamics, modifications, progressions, and recessions. Within any environment the most important factors are the personalities; it is the persons, and the use they make of the physical environment, who determine the nature of the stimulations and repressions which act upon the individual. And in so acting, especially in the early years, these people, the dynamic organisms, profoundly influence the direction of development of the personality of the growing child.

What has been presented also illustrates another very important point, namely, that human behavior is not determined by innate biological constitution, the heredity, alone, or solely by environmental influences. Instead, behavior and personality are clearly produced by interaction between constitutional factors on the one hand, especially the innate capacities to respond in various ways, and the driving, modifying, and repressing stimuli from the environment on the other. If we include, as I think we should, physical disease among the environmental or acquired factors, then even the capacity to respond may be directly and biologically varied by the action of the environment.

The influence of social pressures operates primarily through the impact of other personalities, singly and in groups. That the nature of personality is affected by such physical features of the environment as climate, food, vocational and recreational possibilities, geographical and other features, is not to be denied. These factors operate not only in terms of stimulation or retardation of physical growth, but also in terms of their influence on intellectual and emotional growth. Attitudes, outlook, and disposition or mood may be determined by such variations. Even though stunting or the release of growth energy may be determined by variations in the physical environment, the fact remains that the extent to which development or use will occur in the psychological quantums of, for example, intelligence and emotions, will depend upon the impact of other personalities. Human nature, broadly speaking, is the same the world over. What seem to be qualitative variations are really variations in quantitative relationships of the many elements entering into personality make-up.

All humans are endowed with potentialities, among them the capacity to think, to love, to hate, to fear, to be curious, and to react, but the original strength of these capacities may vary. Furthermore, one or another capacity may be underdeveloped or overdeveloped, while others may be inhibited.

The nature of social behavior will also vary in accordance with culture which, after all, is merely the sum total of the blended responses of groups of people to their environment. A culture may become stagnant and yet be eminently satisfying to its members. Or a culture may be progressive and achieve great material and even intellectual advantages, what we rather loosely call civilization, at the expense of large sections of the populace.

If we clearly recognize that what happens in personality development is related both to innate capacities to respond, and to environmental situations in which native potentials are developed, we shall have a working basis from which to proceed with formulations respecting normal or abnormal, healthy or unhealthy, and satisfying or unsatisfying behavior for the individual and for the group.

From this point of view the physical environment is chiefly of importance with respect to any limitation of possible functioning which it imposes. In this concept of the environment the period of embryonic and fetal life should be included. Throughout the generations the races of mankind have acquired fairly stable features of color, appearance, size, and other characteristics. Many of these are easily modified by crossbreeding, and some may be modified by transfer to a more favorable environment, even in one generation.

With regard to physical environments, it is the *attitudes* shown by the people who use or inhabit the environments which make for the variations in behavior shown in different settings. Thus, it is the use to which people put houses, schools, stores, churches, offices, theaters, etc., that makes for differences in behavior in these edifices, rather than their architectural variations. Many items of physical equipment and of the physical environment in general may be put to a variety of uses, dependent entirely upon human manipulation.

From earliest infancy until death we are reacting to people, to their behavior, their expressed or surmised attitudes, their approval or disapproval, their love or hate, their dominance or submission. Perhaps the most significant data demonstrated over and over again during the past twenty-five years have to do with the enormous influence on the development of personality and behavior patterns of an individual's relations with people, especially those of the own family and during the first few years of life. It cannot be too often stressed that it is in the details of the relationships rather than in mere factual statements or diagnostic categories that the fundamental points are to be found.

Confronted with an actually psychotic adult, one could conceivably determine only whether there are other cases of nervous and mental disease in the family, and if so, of what types. But certainly for the functional psychoses, many toxic-organic types, the neuroses, and psychopathic states much more knowledge is needed regarding the actual dynamic relationships between personalities during the formative period if the abnormal state and its development is to be understood. A neurosis or a delinquent career can never be understood or treated on the basis of factual data alone.

Nowhere are these points more clearly demonstrated than in the study and treatment of behavior problems. At the risk of seeming to elaborate the obvious, it must be emphasized that problem behavior is only behavior to which a particular person or group objects. Some types of problem behavior are regarded as more serious than others, and social objections are crystallized in legal codes. Some transgressions are regarded as particularly serious and classified as felonies, and punishments are assessed in graded severity all the way from imprisonment for shorter or longer terms up to execution. Other infractions of the legal code are classed as misdemeanors and carry less social and legal stigma and punishment, such as fines and short terms of detention or imprisonment.

There are also codes of manners and morals, less crystallized, more variable, and more easily changed from time to time and from community to community than are the legal codes. Infractions of social mores also carry more variable penalties, less well-defined and usually more realized in the rejecting attitudes of individuals or groups than through punishment. There have been times, and this is still true for some groups, in which infractions of the codes of manners were viewed much more seriously than were infractions of the law. Indeed, with some extremely unpopular laws, such as the prohibition amendment, it may be regarded as an infraction of the codes of manners and morals for some groups *not* to break the law.

Manners and morals vary from time to time for large sections of the world and from place to place at the same time. So do legal codes, though less widely and, in general, less rapidly. The law is notably conservative and slow to change. When changes are made in any code, they are likely to be extreme, often resulting in considerable confusion. It will bear repetition that there are so many prohibitions imbedded in the multitude of local, state, and federal laws that one can hardly go from home to office without breaking a few.

It is interesting and enlightening with respect to our attitudes toward behavior that all our codes are much more concerned with "thou shalt not" than they are with emphasis on "thou shalt." The attitude seems to be to restrain the other fellow from interfering with our peace and comfort, while we proceed with our activities and aggressions. Nowhere is this more clearly seen than in the ordinary course of so-called child training. I venture the assertion that despite all the efforts of the past fifty years, almost the entire period during which the child has been accorded some degree of status and rights, more children are still brought up in this country under a barrage of "don't," "no," "mustn't," and prohibitions and punishments than are reared with an intelligently used balancing of "do's" and approval. Note the use of the phrase "intelligently used balancing." There *are* things which must be prohibited and disapproved, but for healthy personality development the prohibitions and disapprovals must be balanced by substituted activities as outlets for energy and curiosity and by affection and approval as a means of establishing inner security and self-confidence.

The extensive use of prohibitions and punishments has, in one sense, a valid foundation. This lies in the original essentially egocentric, hedonistic make-up of the infant, which is only gradually transformed into one that permits the social relationship of give and take. Many people have recognized the stifling effects of too many prohibitions and have attempted to "set the children entirely free." This, too, has proved to be a mistake, not only because of the possible perpetuation of the early personality, but also because many children feel that all support has been taken from them. Since they really need support, they feel bereft when it is lacking. As a result, anxiety is generated and wildly overcompensatory behavior is developed. This in turn makes for difficulties in social living. These points are elaborated to the extent consonant with the purposes of this book in the sections which follow.

GROUPING OF BEHAVIOR DISORDERS

It is always an objective in medicine to arrive at an etiological diagnosis. As previously pointed out, disease entities are usually first established on a basis of clinical signs and symptoms; the second step is to establish the pathology; and the final step, if possible, is to ascertain and prove the causative factor or factors involved. In psychiatry the major etiological factors are known for only about half the psychotic cases, and the situation is similar with respect to behavior disorders. The official psychiatric statistical classification in this country has a major category designated as "without psychosis." * Included under this are conditions such as epilepsy, alcoholism, drug addiction, mental deficiency, psychopathic personality, and primary behavior disorders. The grouping of primary behavior disorders includes simple adult maladjustment and primary behavior disorders in children.

Simple adult maladjustment is described as follows in the manual:

Under this heading are to be classified those cases which, without evidence of psychosis, or without a history of symptoms of psychopathic personality, appear nevertheless to be maladjusted, particularly to specific situations such as marriage, the home and occupation. Adaptation seems limited and such persons may be dependent more or less chronically on others for their support.

Primary behavior disorders in children are classified in three groups: habit disturbance, conduct disturbance, and neurotic traits. These are further subdivided in the official classification as follows:

Habit disturbance. Indicate symptomatic manifestations, e.g.: nail biting, thumb sucking, enuresis, masturbation, tantrums.
Conduct disturbance. Indicate symptomatic manifestations, e.g.: truancy, quarrelsomeness, disobedience, untruthfulness, stealing, forgery,

* American Psychiatric Association, *Statistical Manual.*

setting fires, destructiveness, use of alcohol, use of drugs, cruelty, sex offenses, vagrancy.

Neurotic traits. Indicate symptomatic manifestations, e.g.: tics, habit spasm, somnambulism, stammering, overactivity, fears.

The manual contains the following comment on primary behavior disorders in children.

Under this heading attempt is made in the sub-groups to classify various disturbances seen in children which are *primary* and *not secondary to disease or defect of the nervous system or other organic pathological states.* One of the purposes of this classification is to separate them from the group "without psychosis" under which they had been previously classified, particularly in institutions and clinics.

Cases showing definite clinical pictures of psychoneuroses, dementia praecox or manic-depressive reactions or other reaction types elsewhere classified, are to be placed under the appropriate headings in this classification and not under the present heading. It is expected therefore, that *the group of so-called "problem children" who do not show definite symptomatology of recognized groups of mental disorders will be classified here.*

It is obvious that there may be some overlapping in any one case of the symptoms of the various sub-groups but the cases should be classified according to the predominant behavior symptoms. [Italics mine throughout.]

The above has been presented in such detail because it is representative of the confusion which is developed when attempts are made to set up a classification scheme to cover the behavior disorders. This particular classification may be of value for the statistical accounting of cases in institutions, and it would therefore be useful in institutional clinics, since it would permit direct comparison of the symptom pictures of persons admitted with those of persons not admitted to hospitals. Unfortunately, there would not be general agreement that the three categories—habit disturbance, conduct disturbance, neurotic traits—are on the same level of symptomatic designation. Nor would there be general agreement regarding the distribution of particular symptomatic manifestations into the three categories. The designation of these disorders as primary is also misleading to the nonmedical reader.

Strictly speaking, all disorders of behavior, certainly all those listed above as examples of symptomatic manifestations, are *secondary* to *something*, even if we do not know exactly what that something is. The concept of "primary" here is strictly medical; it means disturbances *not* due to "definite symptomatology of recognized groups of mental diseases" and, accordingly, not secondary to individual disease, defect, or organic pathology. Since no disease or defect of the individual exists, such maladjustments are primary; that is, in a strictly medical interpretation, they are of unknown causation.

With this point of view one must sharply disagree. As I have tried to make clear in the preceding section, the individual organism, whether diseased or healthy, is only one part of the equation which results in social adaptation or social maladjustment. In all cases of maladjustment, factors can be found in personal-social relationships which determine or influence the behavior disturbances. It is imperative to recognize that by primary behavior disorders is really meant *reactive behavior disorders*. Invariably in these cases environmental factors of sufficient intensity to cause the undesirable behavior are to be found. These factors may be rejection, overprotection, or any of many well-recognized environmental situations. The children involved are essentially normal, as the classification indicates, and the causes for their difficulties must be sought outside themselves; the maladjustment is reactive. Internalized psychopathology may develop as a result of the disturbances in interpersonal relationships, and such cases may be stubbornly resistive to treatment, or even untreatable. Even though they originate as reactive manifestations, these conditions would then presumably be classified as psychogenic and placed in diagnostic categories appropriate to the symptomatology.

It is perhaps unfortunate that no better classification than the above can be offered. As it happens, there is very little to be gained by attempting to apply diagnostic labels to children who present behavior problems. These may be redefined as behavior manifestations which are socially unacceptable at home, in school, or to the community. Some represent the continuance of behavior, once useful, past the time when it should normally be replaced by physiologically and psychologically better integrated reactions. In other instances there is regression to an earlier type of behavior which had been "outgrown." Other problems occur as manifestations of hostile aggression or of its suppression, or as a result of guilt, anxiety, and so forth.

The symptoms do not appear as unitary manifestations. Many are merely exaggerated forms of behavior common to all children at some time or other. It is possible to recognize neurotic symptoms as usually defined in many of the cases, and in others neurotic conflicts may be discerned which have produced symptomatic behavior rather than symptoms of illness. If the conduct disorders bring the youngster into conflict with the law, we have delinquency. It should be noted that much delinquent or illegal behavior does not result in police or court action; the individuals showing such behavior may not be delinquent in a technical sense, but their actions are delinquent.

Study of Behavior Disorders

In the clinical study of problem children we must investigate the social milieu, with special reference to the dynamic interplay between the individuals who compose it and a particular child. It is not enough merely to catalogue particular items, such as broken homes, insanity in the family, nervous mother, and the like, although very nice statistical tables may be made in this way and totally unwarranted conclusions may be drawn from them. The child himself must be studied from the standpoint of physical status and functioning, intellectual status and functioning, the emotional and instinctive status and functioning; in other words, the total personality of the child. Once in possession of these data, a diagnostic synthesis may be made of the total personality functioning in a total setting. Causative factors may be demonstrated or inferred, and the particular mental mechanisms operating in the individual ascertained. The underlying motivations may be complex, and the behavior pattern simple, or the reverse may be true. What emerges is not a diagnostic label, but a synthesis; not a simple, direct response to the behavior, but a comprehensive idea of the necessary treatment procedures. That it may be impossible to carry out some of the indicated treatment lays a burden upon the ingenuity of the clinician to find effective substitutes.

There are various ways of accumulating the necessary information. The original method in clinics was to have the studies made in sequence, beginning with the social data regarding the problems stated in the original interview. Then, either at this time or in subsequent interviews, the history is secured from one or more adults important in the child's daily life. This is followed in rapid succession by physical and psychometric examinations and, when all other data are at hand, by the psychiatric examination. In addition to making his own observations, the psychiatrist brings together all data to arrive at a dynamic interpretation of the child's total personality, the environment, and the interactions. The psychiatrist may or may not do the physical and neurological examinations.

The usual procedure in child guidance clinics then calls for a conference of all the workers involved in the case study. On the basis of free discussion, tentative diagnostic formulations are set up and a general outline of treatment is established, including the allocation of roles for the different workers. Customarily, the roles are flexible and interchangeable, so that any worker may treat child or parent in accordance with needs. Contact with schools, social agencies, and others is usually the responsibility of the social worker, though the psychologist may assist with school programming and in work with teachers. The psychologist generally assumes responsibility for remedial tutoring, vocational guidance, and curricular planning, but also does direct psychotherapy in individual cases in accordance with his training and experience. The psychiatrist usually does not assume responsibility for any indicated physical therapy, but refers cases needing such treatment to physicians or clinics according to the economic status of the family. He does assume responsibility for direct psychotherapy of child or parent in accordance with indicated needs, and supervises or follows closely the work of other members of the clinical unit. The social worker, in addition to using more purely social manipulative treatment, also applies direct psychotherapy to parent or child within the limits indicated by the distribution of functions between herself and the psychiatrist.

This traditional child guidance procedure demands the collaboration of at least three people representing the four disciplines, psychiatry, internal medicine, psychology, and social work. The psychiatrist is the leader of the team, but all members have their own unique responsibilities and contributions to make. Repeated conferences are necessary to maintain an integrated view of developments in the case, which, it must be emphasized, always includes several people and situations in addition to the child.

Objection has been made that this formula is too static, that it places too much stress on elaborate and detailed histories and examinations and too little on the dynamics of the treatment process. The answer to this objection is that it is not the formula which is at fault, but the tendency of those who use it to fall into a rut and feel that having made a study according to an outline, something real has been accomplished.

Anything that tends to break down the imaginary barrier between examination and treatment is certainly to be welcomed. Anything that shortens the period between first contact and the beginning of effective treatment is doubly welcome. But—and this applies to beginners and to the experienced alike—nothing can be taken for granted in this complex field of interpersonal relationships. The sequence in which the data are secured is unimportant, but they must all be secured sooner or later. Less experienced workers must actually get data by examination and questioning. Workers with much experience may correctly deduce many facts, but, even so, they will usually need the pragmatic test of checking. Examination for examination's sake and history for history's sake are at best empty gestures. At the same time, there is no substitute for the painstaking collection of data on which to build a complete clinical picture if the dynamics of the situation are to be thoroughly understood and adequate treatment is to be carried through.

The best term I can apply to a more flexible type of approach is "differential treatment." This proceeds on the basic assumption that a problem has been recognized and enough insight developed by some one, the parent let us say, so that treatment is sought. As every psychotherapist knows, this is the first and most difficult step in treatment, and the very first contact is therefore fraught with many possibilities for later success or failure. In the first interview, problems not seen by the parent, but clear to the worker, may be so prominent that now one and now another study or treatment approach must be concentrated on; the ordinary routine procedure may be set entirely aside. The essential problems for which treatment is needed may appear very definitely in the first interview or may not become clear until many interviews have been held and many data secured.

In a differential approach, those who are working with the case proceed in accordance with the needs revealed as the case itself unfolds, varying the tempo and sequence as indicated. Obviously this is not a safe procedure for the inexperienced worker to follow. It requires the greatest of skill to make correct clinical inferences from incomplete data. Much experience is required to insure reasonably correct, at least not dangerously incorrect, interpretations of the dynamics of situations. It requires considerable openmindedness and inner security on the part of the worker to accept the fact that an erroneous interpretation has been made, if one should occur, and to change not only interpretation but also tactics accordingly.

SOME ASPECTS OF TREATMENT

In the treatment of children there is one extremely important point to consider. The child, especially the young child, is usually *brought for treatment*. Usually, too, he sees no problem, or perhaps sees that he has been "bad" and is to undergo a new, unknown, and therefore terrifying type of punishment. Or he may see his problems in a different light from that in which his parents see them. Often he must be induced to accept treatment, though this may be unnecessary if from the beginning of his contact with the clinic he recognizes the workers as sympathetic and interested in him and in his problems *as he sees them.*

It is an intricate and difficult procedure when the child sees no problem or sees his problem only in terms of punishment, or has been conditioned to fear all adults as untruthful and inconsistently brutal. Conditions are made still worse if he has been called dumb or crazy and threatened with being sent to a clinic or a psychiatrist. Still greater difficulties are encountered if the child has heard from his family, his teachers, or his jeering companions that a psychiatrist "is for crazy people," and because of some such phraseology he develops the idea that he must be crazy and the psychiatrist a sort of ogre. Some children are so frightened that they cannot cooperate; others will be on the defensive throughout, so that no results are valid; still others will assume a belligerent attitude, which may effectively bar the establishment of rapport.

Some opinions to the contrary notwithstanding, most children with problems who are brought for study have experienced a great deal of rejection by parents, siblings, teachers, companions, and others. Or, if the rejection was not overt, there has been a considerable amount of unfavorable comparison, scolding, or punishment, which the child interprets as rejection by those who are important to him. Therefore, to be brought to a clinic is yet another evidence of rejection, possibly the last step in being sent away to some mysterious and presumably horrible place.

Another point is increasingly important in the treatment of children's problems. During the past twenty-five years major emphasis has been on the treatment of the child in his usual environments. If there are no specific indications that adequate treatment requires a specialized set-up of some kind, it is clear that there must be alterations in the dynamic environment if healthy development in the child is to occur and be maintained. In fact, for very young children it is generally more important to change the attitudes of key persons in the environment than to apply direct therapy, whereas direct treatment for adolescents is usually far more important than attempts to treat their parents.

It is increasingly seen to be essential to treat both parent and child, especially in dealing with children from about age four or five to the postpubescent period. In the early days of child guidance the parent was supposed to need advice and education rather than treatment. It was quickly found, however, that this was an inadequate approach. Parents, too, had problems which required working through if their attitudes were not to continue to cause disturbances in interpersonal relationships and so affect the behavior and personality development of the child. It was therefore decided that treatment for parents was necessary, focused in the beginning on the parent-child relationship, but extending into other parental relationships as well, especially into the childhood relationships of the parents. Because mothers play a more active role with children and because they are more available than the fathers, the treatment of parents and their problems is usually focused on the mothers. Any treatment program for the problems of the average youngster in an average home necessarily involves treatment of both mother and child if effective results are to be obtained. Finally, more and more fathers are being drawn into the treatment picture. In fact, in the past few years many fathers have themselves referred the problem situation to clinics, psychiatrists, and social agencies and have participated in the treatment program on their own initiative.

CHAPTER XVI

MENTAL DISORDERS IN THE YOUNG

THE DEVELOPMENT and progressive integration of personality throughout the formative years of childhood and youth is a dynamic process, dependent upon the interaction of relatively mobile and often antagonistic forces. From the nature of the unstable equilibrium involved it follows that the process is vulnerable at many points. Unfavorable circumstances produce a variety of difficulties and failures in those adaptive mechanisms which are essential for personality growth and the constantly expanding demands of social adjustment. In general, the signs indicative of maladjustment are evinced in the conduct of the individual. The disorders of behavior may take such forms as deficiencies of function, learning difficulties, overactivity, emotional instability, retention of infantile or other outmoded habits of reaction, asocial or antisocial patterns of conduct, and so forth. Or, particular constellations of symptoms related to disease and defect states may be the outstanding features.

Two major groups of causes for behavior disorders in children are to be discerned, with some overlapping instances. The first of these two groups is composed of cases in which the disturbances are directly related to the presence of specific mental disorders and their accompanying internalized pathology. In the second group the behavior symptoms appear as reactions to disturbed interpersonal relationships, which, in turn, often develop because of a distinctly pathological environment.

The first category of behavior disorders with internal pathology includes those which are primarily due to the existence of a psychosis, epilepsy, mental deficiency, psychopathic personality, or a

neurosis. Available statistics * are not especially revealing with regard to the importance of these disorders in the causation of behavior difficulties, but some points may be made.

The only index of the relative significance of the psychoses in
the age periods under consideration here is found in the statistics
of hospital admissions. The 1945 Census Report already cited shows
that one half of one percent of nearly 113,000 psychotic first admissions were under fifteen years of age. An additional 4 percent
were age fifteen to nineteen, bringing the total group under age
twenty to 4.5 percent. To these may be added the 8.2 percent of
admissions without psychosis who were under age twenty. Altogether, 986 children under the age of fifteen were admitted to the
hospitals; 64 percent were males; approximately one half of the
total number were psychotic. It is of some importance to ascertain
the conditions which led to the commitment of these children, both
the psychotic and the nonpsychotic.

The largest diagnostic category was mental deficiency without
psychosis; the second largest was psychosis with mental deficiency.
Approximately one third of all cases under age fifteen presented a
basis of mental deficiency, to which had been added a psychotic
reaction or some behavior manifestations believed to indicate a
psychosis. This is presumed to be true, since most states make provision for the care and training of the feebleminded without psychosis, and mental defectives are usually not committed to state
hospitals unless a psychosis is present or suspected.

Next in order of frequency among admissions to the mental
hospitals were the primary behavior disorders. It may be pointed
out that in 1945 New York state hospitals admitted a total of 196

* From the 1943 report of the New York State Department of Mental Hygiene it is found that there were nearly 11,000 first admissions to state hospitals,
state training schools, and the colony for epileptics. Of these, 13 percent were
under twenty years of age. Five percent of the admissions to hospitals, 82
percent of those admitted to the training schools, and 60 percent of those
sent to the Colony were under age twenty. No figures are available on the
extent of problem behavior leading to court appearances and commitment to
correctional institutions for juveniles. It is known that arrest rates for those
under age twenty are high, as reported by the FBI.

patients of all ages without psychosis. Of these, 62 were under the age of fifteen; and the total New York admissions in this age group, including psychotic cases (122), represented about one fifth of the admissions under age fifteen to hospitals for the entire United States.

A point to be emphasized is the extreme variation in number of admissions of children under age fifteen in the several states. This is fairly directly related to the extent of provisions made for the reception of children in this age group. Thus, New York has made special provision for the care of cases suffering from personality disorders due to epidemic encephalitis and, in addition, has a special unit for children of average intelligence presenting behavior problems not due to organic causes; that is, the primary behavior disorders. For the most part, admission in this group is restricted to children under age twelve.

The ten states * having the largest number of first admissions to state hospitals in 1937 admitted approximately 55 percent of the United States total. Of these, 10 percent were without psychosis, but numbers varied greatly in the several states, as did the rate per 100,000 (24.3 to 98.0). Wide variations in practice in the different states account for the marked discrepancies. New York, Pennsylvania, and Virginia had the highest percentage admission rates. The ten states also admitted 61 percent of all cases of primary behavior disorders in the United States in that year. They admitted proportionately fewer children under age fifteen and a relatively greater number of cases diagnosed as primary behavior disorders than were admitted in the country at large.

The New York figures are striking. Despite a very small number of cases of all ages without psychosis, the number of children under age fifteen was comparatively high; a third of the not psychotic group was in this age range. Similarly, the diagnosis of primary behavior disorder was made more frequently in New York than in any

* New York, 12,566; Illinois, 6,645; California, 5,129; Massachusetts, 3,731; Ohio, 3,158; Virginia, 2,651; Pennsylvania, 2,474; New Jersey, 2,359; Michigan, 2,159; Texas, 1,939; total for the United States, 78,217, or 60.5 per 100,000 population.

other state, and the cases represented more than a third of the total for all states. This is interpreted as indicating that as soon as provisions are made to meet particular needs, they are utilized. Many states have special state organizations and institutions for the study and treatment of children with behavior problems, and these may take the load from the state hospitals. For instance, New York has several institutions for defective delinquents, mostly older, and practically all states have training schools for delinquent boys and girls. Illinois has the Institute for Juvenile Research, Ohio has its Bureau, and so forth; several states have private institutions.

The fact remains that psychoses are relatively infrequent in children under age fifteen. As has been stated, the largest group is that of psychoses with mental deficiency. The implication is that all symptoms occurring in the mentally defective are not necessarily those of mental deficiency alone. It is also clear that mental defectives often exhibit temporary outbursts of behavior which are regarded as evidences of psychosis, when actually, it is inability to control the emotions. These are the nonpsychotic cases committed to hospitals.

The next largest groups—schizophrenia, psychoses with convulsive disorders, and congenital syphilis with a clinical picture of general paresis or with other disorders of the nervous system—follow in the order given.

Only about one third of the cases definitely diagnosed in this age group have mental disturbances of the functional type. The important conclusion is that psychoses in children under age fifteen are most likely to be due to organic disease and defect states.

In the next age group, fifteen to nineteen, first admissions to mental hospitals for both psychotic and nonpsychotic cases show a sharp rise, and there is also a marked change in the type of cases. The total number for the United States in 1945 was 5,610, or 6.4 percent of all first admissions. Of these, 83 percent were psychotic, and 17 percent were diagnosed as being without psychosis. The most important point is that schizophrenia accounts for 58 percent of the admissions of those with psychoses. Cyclothymic cases accounted for 8 percent, and neuroses 6 percent. If we add the cases of psychosis with psychopathic personality and of paranoid condition to the above groups, some 75 percent of those with psychosis have functional or psychogenic disorders. The other 25 percent belongs in the groups with recognized pathology, that is, associated with disease and defect states. Psychoses with mental deficiency are the most frequent, followed by those with convulsive disorders, and then neurosyphilis. Together, these three diagnoses account for nearly a fifth of the psychotic cases. Alcoholic and drug psychoses, psychoses with epidemic encephalitis, with metabolic diseases, and due to trauma, all show a marked increase by comparison with the group under fifteen years of age.

For all the functional cases and for those with mental deficiency and convulsive disorders it is reasonable to believe that there was maladjustment manifested by a variety of symptoms over a long period, perhaps most of the lifetime, before the onset of the psychosis. Certainly mental deficiency and epilepsy must have shown revelatory symptoms and signs long before the onset of the psychosis. The same is true of the functional cases, especially schizophrenia and the neuroses. Personality and behavior difficulties can usually be detected in the histories of these cases for a considerable time prior to the actual onset of the psychosis or the appearance of frank neurotic symptoms. With the cyclothymics, this is not so common. It seems clear, therefore, that here is a field of preventive psychiatry which has not yet been fully explored.

Among the nonpsychotic admissions, mental deficiency and epilepsy account for more than half the cases. The diagnosis of psychopathic personality was made in 25 percent of the cases, an enormous increase, both actually and proportionately, over the 6 percent of diagnoses in the under-fifteen-year-old group. At the same time, there is a sharp drop both absolutely and relatively in the diagnosis of primary behavior disorders, from 38 percent in the under-fifteen-year group to 13 percent in the fifteen to nineteen group.

Several interesting possibilities are found here. One is that there is some tendency in dealing with this age group to consider cases exhibiting behavior disorders as psychopathic in origin rather than as belonging with the primary behavior disorders. When the two groups are combined, the percentage of occurrence among the non-psychotic cases drops from 44 to 38 percent, not as sharp a difference as has been found in other years.

A second possibility seems to have some validity. This is that the diagnosis primary behavior disorder is used in actual practice chiefly for younger children. It may be that such disorders can be demonstrated clearly only in such children, being the precursors of more definite or at least more fixed aberrations which are diagnosed as such in adolescents. This is doubtful; it is far more likely that the variation is in the use of terms. In any case, the fact remains that for the United States there were 325 diagnoses of primary behavior disorder in people under twenty years of age, and only 200 for all other ages. This difference is especially important in view of the fact that there were nearly seven times as many nonpsychotic admissions age twenty and over as there were under age twenty. Primary behavior disorders constitute about 20 percent of the group under twenty and only one percent of the group age twenty and over.

Diagnoses of psychopathic personality and of primary behavior disorders occur in all age groupings. The highest percentage of primary behavior disorders occurred in the age group under fifteen years, while psychopathic personality was most frequent in the twenty to twenty-four-year age group. If the behavior disorders and the cases of psychopathic personality are combined, more than half the diagnoses occur in the age groups under thirty. Some 58 percent of the total diagnoses of psychopathic personality occur in age range fifteen to twenty-nine; of the cases of primary behavior disorder, 38 percent were under age fifteen, and 62 percent were under age twenty.

These figures are given somewhat *in extenso* because of the

points discussed elsewhere which seem to indicate that the psychopathic personalities are not dependent upon fixed, innate,
biological factors, but are rather the result of environmental factors
acting from early life and over a long period, until severe and fixed
internalized pathology results. A reciprocal relationship between
the diagnoses would be highly suggestive with regard to diagnostic
standards. Since no such relationship exists, it can only be hinted
that the abrupt drop in the use of the term primary behavior disorder for cases age twenty and over, and the sharp increase in the
use of the term psychopathic personality in the next two decades,
may have a relationship. In other words, when older persons continue to exhibit a juvenile sort of behavior pattern, it may indicate
to many that the maladjustment is fixed and therefore psychopathic
rather than situational.

EPILEPSY

The United States Census report for 1945 includes the cases of
epilepsy admitted to all institutions for mental defectives and
epileptics. It shows a total of 1,530 cases admitted during the year,
37 percent being under fifteen years of age, with more than half
of these under ten. The epilepsies are commonly reported to have
their onset before the age of ten in a considerable proportion of
cases; about three fourths are established before the age of twenty.
How many cases of epilepsy there may be in the community under
the age of fifteen, or even twenty, is a matter of conjecture. Since
many defectives have convulsions, or the presence of convulsions
in early life leads to a deteriorative process or to a cessation of intellectual development, the question of the incidence of early epilepsy
is still further confused.

If convulsions are frequent or particularly severe, or if there are
serious personality distortions and related behavior disorders, these
children are ordinarily excluded from school on a physician's certificate. They may thereupon become troublesome to the community, if not actually menacing in many ways. Aside from the

convulsions, these children are likely to display some or all of the characteristics of the so-called epileptic personality, such as explosive temper, overactivity, destructiveness, assaultiveness, and brutality during the explosions, or even as continuous behavior sets. They may be obsequious and arrogant by turns, distinctly egocentric and selfish. Intermittent bed-wetting and sleep disturbances are likely to occur, and when behavior of this sort is reported, other signs of epilepsy should be sought.

Prior to puberty the amount of socially disturbing behavior may not be extensive, though cruelty, bullying, temper outbursts, and episodes of impulsive, blind assaultiveness may occur. Following puberty, perverse sexual activity and sexual attacks may appear; the latter may be associated with murder or with marked and senseless brutality.

Epilepsy produces difficulties in learning, even in the absence of demonstrable deterioration, because of the recurrent disturbances of consciousness and memory. Hence, such children are frequently handicapped in regular school competition, even though intelligence tests may show high IQ. If the convulsions can be kept under control by medication, children may make average or better progress in regular schools. So far as is known, no public school system has established special classes for epileptics. If the disorder is severe, the children are unquestionably better off in an institution for epileptics. If the attacks are only of the petit mal type, or if the disorder can be held in check, then it would be best to keep the child at home and in a regular school; that is, if the attitudes at home or in the school are not inimical to the child's personality development.

The important points to bear in mind are the chronicity, the probable, but not certain, amenability to medical treatment, and that the epileptic child or adult is potentially a danger to himself and to others. Finally, if medical treatment has not been successful and the condition is at all severe, then placement in an appropriate institution is to the best interests of the child, the family, and the community.

MENTAL DEFICIENCY AND INFERIORITY

Public school provision for intelligence testing and for special classes for the mentally retarded has brought about a considerable change in ideas regarding the incidence of mental deficiency and its relationship to behavior disorders. Massachusetts has for over twenty years had a state-wide system of examining all children three or more years retarded in school progress. This procedure gives the state a continuing record of all defectives and of pupils with inferior intelligence, in addition to those who are certified to the state training schools.

It follows that during the school experience the best opportunities occur to ascertain which children are feebleminded or of borderline intelligence. From such knowledge comes the best planning for special training in public school or in specialized institutions, for needed assistance and supervision in the community, or for custodial institutional care. Massachusetts is a geographically compact state, comparatively densely populated, so that a state-wide program is easily possible. Such a state-operated service has the advantage of reaching all the local communities and rural areas which perhaps could not otherwise afford this service or might see no need for it, public knowledge of the causes for school retardation being what it is.

Generally speaking, psychological testing service is available only in large communities and in some wealthy suburbs of large cities. Special classes are usually established with financial aid from the state. The law providing for such aid specifies an upper IQ limit, usually 70; no special provisions are made for the inferior group with IQ 70–90. Ordinarily, also, children are not tested for IQ until they have reached third-grade age, when their school progress is already definitely retarded. No large school system is known to have an adequate register of its defective and inferior children, nor is any school system known to have enough special classes to care for all its defective children.

As a cause for behavior disorders and delinquency, feeblemindedness has loomed large in general thinking since the diagnosis came to have a quasi-exact status through the widespread use of intelligence tests. Idiots and low-grade imbeciles, for reasons obvious from the previous discussion of these conditions, are rarely regarded as behavior problem children. Their handicaps are so generalized and so obvious that they take precedence over any behavior disturbances, though these, and possibly convulsions, may be the factors which lead parents to seek institutional care. Most of the idiots and low-grade imbeciles are recognized early and are given some sort of special care. Not many are sent to school, and most of those who are sent are promptly rejected.

The situation is different with some higher-grade imbeciles, the large group of morons, and the still greater group with borderline or inferior intelligence. The largest group of feebleminded are high grade, whether children of school age or older people. Morons and, to a lesser extent, high-grade imbeciles, are not always quickly identified. The inferior group is much larger than the group of defectives. As previously noted, if the distribution of intelligence followed the binomial curve accurately, 25 percent of the population, children included, would fall below average. Whether being below average would constitute a pathological state, render the individual incapable of making social adjustments, maintaining himself, and managing his affairs with ordinary prudence would still be matters to be decided upon according to other criteria.

Inferior intelligence, including mental defect, operates in a number of ways to produce behavior disorders.

1. The intelligence may be so inferior that concepts of acceptable behavior cannot be formed. Ideas of right and wrong are hazy or nonexistent; in other words, ethical standards are nearly or definitely lacking. Especially among high-grade morons, this may not be so much an actual lack of capacity as it is lack of adequate training.

2. One third to at most one half of the cases of mental deficiency are familial. This means that standards of behavior and adjustment in the family are at a defective level. There is evidence that these

standards will to a considerable degree reflect the standards of the community in which the family lives and the treatment afforded the family by the community. That is, if a family lives in a delinquency area, delinquent behavior is to be expected. If they live in an area where delinquency is the exception rather than the rule, the defectives may be expected to conform more or less closely to community standards. This is particularly true if they have vocational and other opportunities in keeping with their abilities.

3. What has been said under item 2 is directly related to what is ordinarily called the heightened suggestibility or lessened will power of the intellectually inferior. As previously brought out, there is good reason to believe that this is not entirely due to suggestibility; rather it is the result of such defective reasoning and judgment that the individual, being unable to think through the issues for himself, apes the behavior of others. Even more important is the urge to secure the approval of the group or of particular members of it. This is emphasized many fold if the individual or the family develops emotional conflicts because of repeated failures in the many types of competition which must be sustained in the ordinary processes of living.

4. The mere inability to succeed in competitions tends to create feelings of personal inadequacy and personal insecurity in groups. These feelings are likely to be increased by the attitudes of the other children in the group, who are quick to seize upon any evidence of weakness and lack of ability. In ruthless protection of their own egos, children emphasize the inferiorities of others, and so tend to fix for the intellectually inferior both the feeling of personal inadequacy and the feeling of group insecurity. Lacking other avenues to success which might help to balance their feelings of inadequacy and insecurity, they resort to various types of socially inadequate and even delinquent behavior in an effort to acquire status in the group.

A number of studies have been made of the distribution of behavior problems in school populations. They uniformly show that there is a marked increase in behavior problems as intelligence levels diverge from the average. Thus, children showing either extreme of intelligence have a higher incidence of behavior problems than do those in the average group. This increase in incidence is greater for the inferior group than for the superior.

·Studies of the intelligence levels of children brought before juvenile courts show a definitely higher incidence of mental defect and inferior intelligence than among children of similar age levels in the general population. Various explanations have been advanced. One is the old familiar notion that the intellectually inferior are more prone to commit offenses because of an assumed inferiority of will power. For this idea there seems to be remarkably little real evidence. Another theory is that these individuals are defective in moral sensibilities. Suffice it to say at this point that some are, in a limited sense, but that the great majority are not. A third idea is that since they are stupid the inferior are more easily apprehended. In this theory there is considerable truth, but much more important are certain sociological facts. One is that since they belong to intellectually, socially, and economically disadvantaged groups, such children are more likely to land in court than are those from higher grade families. Having been brought to court, such inferior children have fewer familial resources to draw upon; there are fewer opportunities in general for the intellectually inferior to engage successfully in activities which would tend to keep them out of further trouble. There is evidence that low level families are more likely to turn to courts for help with their recalcitrant, incorrigible children than are families with higher standards. The latter are more likely to turn to pastor, doctor, teacher, behavior clinic, child study association, or social worker. Furthermore, in large cities the tendency is for disadvantaged families to live in the cheaper and more crowded sections, where delinquency rates tend to be high, where there are fewer playgrounds and recreation centers, and where the competition for mere breathing space is at a maximum. These facts help to account for the statistical frequency of inferiority factors in juvenile offenders.

It has been definitely shown that so far as intelligence levels obtained by standard tests are concerned, the incidence of feeblemindedness and inferior intelligence is about the same among older delinquents and criminals incarcerated in reformatories and prisons, as it was for the drafted men in the 1917–18 war, both with regard to totals and when the several nativity and racial groups are compared. An interesting exception is one large group of reformatory inmates which showed a higher proportion of superior and a lower proportion of inferior results from the test than did the army.

The discrepancy in findings on intelligence tests between the juvenile court cases and those in the late adolescent and adult delinquents may have several explanations. But the most plausible one, for which there is considerable direct and indirect evidence, is that delinquent or potentially delinquent younger feebleminded, when recognized as defective, were either committed to training schools for defectives or placed under prolonged social supervision. As a matter of direct observation it seems clear that special classes in the public schools have had a considerable effect in reducing delinquent behavior or the need for such behavior among those fortunate enough to be placed in special classes early in their school career. These classes offer a competitive situation in which the defective may achieve success and therefore develop feelings of personal adequacy and satisfying group relationships.

A group of defective delinquents has been legally recognized. Particularly in New York state, special laws for sentencing individuals in this group and specialized institutions for their custody and training have been provided. Inmates of such institutions are, in general, older individuals who are recidivists and the pattern of antisocial, delinquent behavior has become relatively fixed. Sentences are indeterminate, and release on parole is dependent upon psychiatric, psychological, and behavioristic observations. These are the defectives who have proven themselves unfit for community life and for whom no preventive program has been effective, if, indeed, one has been tried.

5. While it can definitely be shown that the behavior disorders

of the younger feebleminded are due to the interaction of environmental factors and the internal pathology, in this instance the basic defect, there are others who present abnormalities of personality and behavior which seem not to be adequately explained by feeblemindedness alone. They are sometimes called psychopathic defectives, which seems an entirely adequate descriptive term. It is generally believed that their emotional and instinctive defects, lack of inhibitions, impulsive reactions, and inability to learn suitable social behavior according to methods ordinarily effective with the more docile feebleminded, are due to the same sort of failure to develop that accounts for the defect in intelligence and in other mental characteristics in the usual feebleminded types. This may be true, but it seems unlikely that it is the only answer, for two reasons.

One of the reasons is that no *specific* pathology, either macroscopic or microscopic, has been found in the nervous systems of the high-grade feebleminded, who constitute the majority of cases showing reactions of this psychopathic type. In general physical appearance they usually resemble normal or average people; stigmata of degeneration, lack of co-ordination, and other signs of defective physical development are absent. Similarly, the brain is usually normal in size and modeling; there are no characteristic changes in the microscopic pictures, either in cellular arrangement or in the number and type of cells.

The second reason, brought out in Chapter XIV, is that the same types of antisocial, explosive, egocentric, cold-blooded, unstable, inadequate, and paranoid reactions are also encountered in persons of average and of superior intelligence. These higher-grade individuals are likewise unable to learn through experience and are not influenced by rewards and punishments which influence normal children and adults.

We shall, I think, have to depend upon further studies of fetal physiology to throw light upon the problem of constitution in these psychopathic defective states. Studies of the effects of grossly pathological environments will help to determine to what extent these states are reactive or psychogenic.

6. The social behavior of the constitutionally inferior, as previously defined, is inadequate, explosive, infantile, or otherwise indicative of general inferiority. They are usually not well received by their peers because the inadequacies are not acceptable. Motor inco-ordination, particularly, interferes with many types of competition important to children, as does inability to withstand frustration and the generally infantile attitudes. For such children, even more than for those of similar IQ who are physically average or superior and of good disposition, childhood competitions, especially in school, are continuous sources of frustration, resentment, and unhappiness. Provision of earlier motor-manual training than is now available—at least as early as the third grade—would lessen the incidence of minor and serious behavior problems in this group.

It is idle to speculate on the causation of these constitutionally inferior states. They are inborn, biological deviations. To call them hereditary is certainly stretching the meaning of the term heredity. In rare instances it is fairly convincing that some specific disease in the mother during pregnancy is the cause. In others, dysfunction of one or more endocrine glands in the mother may appear to have a specific relationship. It is possible that maternal dietary and vitamin deficiencies play a role. Evidence is, in general, to the effect that these inferior states tend to occur most frequently in families of low socio-economic status, but they do occur in all types of families.

PSYCHOPATHIC PERSONALITY

It has already been pointed out that the diagnosis of psychopathic personality is very rare among state hospital admissions under the age of fifteen and that there is a sharp increase in the fifteen to nineteen-year-old group. The definition and description of the young psychopath do not differ essentially from those given in the chapter on psychopathic personality.

In actual clinical practice the tendency is not to make such diagnoses for young children, but only for adolescents and older persons. This depends upon the important point that in younger children both environmental and internal factors can clearly be seen at work. Hence the reactive nature of much or all the behavior is more definitely in evidence. Furthermore, with regard to young children, all workers take an optimistic view respecting the effectiveness of treatment, since the personality is regarded as plastic and so more easily influenced. This optimism is hardly justified, for several reasons, among which two stand out. The first, and perhaps most significant, is that in the treatment of the young child the treatment of the mother or mother surrogate is much more important than direct treatment of the child. Indeed, it may be possible to treat the child effectively only by shifting the environment.

The most valuable element in direct treatment of the young is the quality of the child's relationship with the worker. It is essential that the therapist become the good, permissive, completely trustworthy parent image. After such a relationship is established, the child may express his aggressions, hostilities, curiosities, fears, and sexual and excretory interests without anticipation of reprisal, criticism, or punishment. But it is especially difficult for the young child to understand that this permissiveness applies only to the treatment setting. As a result the behavior is much more likely to be carried over into the home and create more difficulties between parent and child.

It follows, therefore, that effective work with the mother is absolutely essential. Advice or education about child development or any other type of intellectualization of the problems is not enough. It is essential that the mother acknowledge the need for and accept treatment of a disturbed mother-child relationship in which the mother has an active role. She must also accept the idea that attitudes derived from her own early experiences are present and must be corrected if the parent-child relationship is to assume normal proportions.

The second point which stands out with regard to the over-optimistic view of treatment possibilities for the young child is in relation to the extent of the milieu pathology. The infant who is either rejected from birth or treated as though he were rejected, will have acquired distinctly pathological modes of response to the environment by the time he reaches the age of three. This may be manifested either by retreat from the environment or by rebellious, overactive, attention-getting attempts to dominate all situations; or the two extremes of behavior may alternate. Nowhere does this stand out more clearly than in children reared in infants' homes. By the age of three there is a marked personality deviation shown by affect hunger, isolation, intense narcissism, inability to form substantial and permanent relationships with others, and incessant demands for affection and attention. At the same time, such children are unable to give affection or to show consideration for others; usually there is much destructive overactivity. The deviation tends to be permanently fixed, irrespective of the type of care and attention shown during the next several years.

The same general picture may be seen when there is a change in the home status or care of the infant during the second or third year. The symptoms are not usually so intense or so fixed if the emotional relationships prior to that time have been normal and healthy so that the child has had an opportunity to develop object relationships and has begun to express affection. Also, it is essential that another person or persons be available to continue the process of stimulating the development of relationships interrupted by, let us say, the death of the mother. Behavior manifestations such as these can be seen in the making and their pattern traced for years, up to and through adolescence, with little or no change in fundamental characteristics. It is accordingly extremely difficult to accept the idea of an innate, constitutionally deviate make-up as the essence of psychopathic personality with its concomitant conduct disturbances.

Without wishing to deny or minimize the existence of constitutional factors, on which many competent observers lay great stress, I must, nevertheless, point out that they have usually not had much direct experience with young children. The concept that there are constitutional factors has been derived by reconstruction from the history of older individuals. The interpretation is ordinarily based on a factual survey of the behavior itself, what efforts were made to correct it, and the results. It is still true that the majority of psychiatrists do not look for and cannot interpret the dynamic interplay between the child and the people in his environment, the mother especially, which determines the general trend of personality in its social aspects.

On the other hand, nothing is more certain than that there are marked physiological variations in infants. This is noticeable during the fetal period, as well as immediately after birth. A crude but effective evidence of this can be found in the amount of prenatal activity. Many mothers have said they were sure they would give birth to a boy because the fetus was so active in the last months *in utero*. Of course, many may have thought or said this and then given birth to a girl. Granted a normal birth process, such infants are active from the first. Many show evidence of being physiologically accelerated beyond the average for newborns by as much as three or four weeks, though they are not necessarily large babies.

In other cases, fetuses are relatively inactive *in utero*. After birth they are likely to be quiet, good babies, not overactive and demanding. They may show acceleration or the reverse with regard to the stage of their psychological development at birth, and there is again no special relationship to size at birth. It should be emphasized that in both these instances full-term births are being considered.

Whatever the level of activity and energy output shown prenatally, it is likely to be continued in postnatal life. The important point for our present purpose is that no data have yet been adduced to show any relationship between such widely varied types of activity at or before birth and the presence or absence of a later recognized psychopathic personality or any other specific type of mental abnormality.

This is, perhaps, a good place to emphasize the fact that the individual is born with innate capacities which are biologically determined and vary from person to person. It is possibly more accurate to say that they are born with potential capacities, including a physical and mental growth potential. Any factor or trait of human personality, intellectual, emotional, or instinctive, has its own natural range of variation, even though we may have no very precise way of measuring it.

What happens to a capacity, that is, whether it lies fallow, is developed in ordinary degree or to the fullest extent, or takes perverse routes for expression, depends upon environmental stimulation in terms of the general and specific experiences of living. The incidents and accidents of disease of one kind or another must, of course, be taken into account. It is the relatively great freedom to have capacities recognized and developed which is the most important and the most distinctive feature of American life. By comparison with most other countries, this is true even for the underprivileged and disadvantaged groups in the United States.

It seems, therefore, that data are still inadequate to weigh the relative significance of constitutional and environmental factors in the production of particular character sets or personality types and certain kinds of mental disorders. That all are due to *interaction* of the individual constitution and environmental experiences seems obvious—so obvious that the point has often been overlooked. So far as the psychopaths are concerned, the weight of evidence seems to indicate a preponderant influence of pathological experiences acting at an early age to produce an habitual pathological type of response. For some children, especially younger ones, successful response to treatment has been secured. For the majority, however, treatment has been totally ineffective.

The behavior disorders of psychopathic children run the gamut of socially disturbing behavior and include many sex offenses. The clinical types are the same as in adults, but many more show mixed reactions. Of particular interest and importance in children are the affect hunger, the isolation, and the insatiable, overactive types.

The 1937 census figures revealed that the psychoneuroses constituted 2.7 percent of first admissions with psychosis under age fifteen to state hospitals, and slightly more than one percent of all admissions in this age group. For the age group fifteen to nineteen there were a little more than 3 percent with psychosis and slightly over 2 percent of combined psychotic and nonpsychotic cases. Hence, of all admissions under age twenty, 2.4 percent were psychoneurotic. The figure for total admissions in all age groups is 2.7 percent, again being slightly higher if only admissions with psychosis are considered. At all ages these were presumably the more severe cases, which could not be successfully treated or cared for in the community, since only a small percentage of neurotics are admitted to state hospitals.

So far as those under age twenty are concerned, there is an unknown additional number of cases of primary behavior disorders with neurotic traits. Fully developed neurotic states are not common in young children, but typical hysterias or, more frequently, tics, habit spasms, sleep disturbances, stammering, phobias, and compulsions do occur as individual symptoms or in combination. In fact, any of the many behavior disorders of children may, on careful investigation, prove to have a neurotic basis.

Among adolescents, typical neuroses are encountered nearly as often as among adults. Normally, adolescence is a period of considerable psychological stress, due both to physiological changes and to the flowering of inner drives related to the social setting. This is the period for normal resolution of the Oedipus situation, consummation of the heterosexual stage of psychosexual integration, achievement of relative independence from the family, setting up of vocational and general social goals, physical sexual maturation, and maturation of ego and superego. Inner conflicts are therefore numerous, and conflicts which have previously been active but repressed, may break forth with renewed vigor or with different symptomatology. A careful history will reveal the previous existence of such conflicts and their symptoms.

All the classical neurotic pictures appear in this age period. Conversion symptoms are especially common; homosexual conflicts may be particularly pronounced. The use of alcohol increases sharply, as does other escape behavior. Hypochondriacal symptoms, usually as a transitory phase, may be conspicuous. Neurasthenic syndromes and anxiety states are relatively uncommon, but are markedly intractable to treatment. Psychasthenic phobias and compulsions are fairly common.

It is important to bear in mind that symptoms which appear to be neurotic may actually be only the prodromal symptoms of schizophrenia. Particularly, what appear to be phobias, obsessions, and anxiety states may stand in this relationship.

The treatment of the neuroses in this age range is essentially the same as for older patients. Symptomatic behavior may be more or less disregarded except when it is also a symptom of the neurosis. Of particular social importance is the occurrence of delinquent acts followed by amnesia for the period of the delinquency. By appropriate measures, such as hypnosis or free associations and analysis of dream material, the content of the amnesic intervals can usually be recovered.

CHAPTER XVII

REACTIVE BEHAVIOR DISORDERS

BEHAVIOR DISORDERS without concomitant inner pathology may be termed nonspecific, since disease and defect states are absent as etiological factors. Nonspecific problems are therefore of the type formally classified as primary behavior disorders, but the group is not so inclusive. According to my viewpoint, most of the primary behavior disorders with neurotic traits are to be classed with the neuroses, especially for treatment. The behavior problems to be discussed in this chapter comprise the reactive disorders, or, perhaps more precisely, the interactive maladjustments. In this category are the majority of problem children seen in child guidance clinics and in private practice.

Reactive behavior disorders occur chiefly in children whose personality structure and functional levels are essentially within normal limits of variation and who live in a setting which is also within normal limits of variation according to our rather crude standards. Maladjustment between the child and the dynamic environment is expressed in the child's problem behavior. We must remember that the child may not see any problems whatever in his own behavior, though he may complain of difficulties in his environment and interpersonal relationships.

The problem behavior encountered in this group of children, average to superior in one or in several ways, does not differ in essence from the problems shown by abnormal and inferior children. There is a difference, however, in the frequency of occurrence of the problems, and in their severity. In general terms, behavior problems of all types and degrees of severity occur in children and adults regardless of the physical condition; they occur at any intelligence level above that required to react socially, on all societal and economic levels, and in all racial and religious groups. Concerning social factors, it must be remembered that there are wide divergences in standards by which behavior is judged in different groups. Even in one family, the criteria for objectionable conduct vary from time to time and from child to child.

COMMON TYPES OF BEHAVIOR PROBLEMS

Children are referred to child guidance clinics for many patterns of behavior which are the subject of complaint at home, in school, or in the community at large. Numerous generalized statements have been made regarding the nature and origin of socially disturbing behavior, and a few elaborate statistical studies have appeared. No detailed analysis will be attempted in this chapter; instead, a few of the most common complaints will be analyzed to illustrate the complexity of causation and the principles of treatment.

In a series of 1,000 consecutive cases studied at the Institute for Child Guidance,* there were 635 boys and 365 girls, about the usual proportion of the sexes referred to behavior clinics. This suggests at once that the conduct of boys is regarded with more seriousness by parents and other adults or is somehow thought to be more menacing than that of girls. Otherwise the two sexes should be approximately equal in number among clinic cases. The age range in this study was from under three to over eighteen years. Half the boys were ages seven to twelve, inclusive; more than half the girls were eight to fourteen years. The peak age for boys was nine; for girls it was fourteen. More young boys than young girls were referred, while more of the older children were girls. The bulk of the cases were of grade school age.

The difference in age groupings of boys and girls is, perhaps, significant in relationship to social attitudes toward behavior, or

* All figures in this section are derived from unpublished tabulations made in 1932–1933 at the former Institute for Child Guidance, New York City.

possibly it represents a difference in the age at which aggressive behavior has its highest incidence in the two sexes. It is at least clear that girls are referred for behavior problems only about half as often as are boys and that the tendency is to refer girls at an older age. This, in turn, seems to imply that girls are regarded as more controllable than boys over a longer period of time.

Altogether, twenty-three problems were indexed; many of the headings used include manifestations referred to by various terms. "Negativism," for instance, is used to cover all complaints of disobedience, stubbornness, rebelliousness, as well as negativism itself. An average incidence of approximately 3.5 problems per case was found. The problems as stated by the referring source are presented in tabular form, in the order of total incidence.

Problems as Presented

	Boys	Girls	Combined
Negativism	257	144	401
Temper and tantrums	198	109	307
Lying	143	83	226
School failure	149	69	218
Nervousness	129	73	202
Enuresis	139	60	199
Fears	122	70	192
Excessive fantasy	114	65	179
Stealing	129	48	177
Sleep disturbances	112	60	172
Masturbation	129	33	162
Truancy, home and school	109	42	151
Food fads and refusal	80	66	146
Sensitiveness	70	46	116
Speech defects	82	32	114
Thumb sucking	55	49	104
Show-off behavior	49	33	82
Jealousy	52	21	73
Timidity	51	21	72
Sex activity	36	21	57
Reading disability	44	13	57
Bullying	42	8	50
Cruelty	8	3	11

Several points should be borne in mind respecting this tabulation. First, practically no cases with a court record are included, since the New York Children's Court has its own psychiatric clinic which effectively cares for the cases reaching it. It would therefore not be expected that the Institute list would contain many of the more serious types of antisocial behavior, and the few types included in the list had not yet reached the court.

Secondly, if the problems were of equal weight and importance in the two sexes, then girls should account for 36.5 percent of the occurrence of any problem, and boys 63.5 percent. These relationships are approximated in several groups, but deviate sharply in others. Proportional frequency of occurrence is practically the same, differing by not more than 3 percent for both sexes in the following nine problems: negativism, temper and tantrums, lying, nervousness, fears, excessive fantasy, sleep disturbances, sensitiveness, and sex activity. The percentages below indicate that the following three problems appear more frequently in boys: show-off behavior, 3.5 percent; food fads and refusal, 9 percent; thumb sucking, 10.6 percent. Boys show greater than expected occurrence by the noted percentages of the following eleven problems, girls showing an equivalent lesser incidence: school failure, 5 percent; enuresis, 6.4 percent; jealousy, 7.4 percent; timidity, 7.5 percent; speech defects, 8.5 percent; truancy, 9 percent; cruelty, 9.2 percent; stealing, 9.4 percent; reading disability, 13.7 percent; masturbation, 16 percent; bullying, 19.5 percent.

Rank order for problems varies somewhat with the sex. This is illustrated in the table (page 314) of the twelve most frequent problems, arranged according to the order for the *combined* groups. Note that problems of rank order 13 and 14 for the girls appear in this list, while thumb sucking and refusal of food do not. Both these problems are relatively more frequent among girls than among boys.

The tabulations present the problems concerning which complaints were made, usually by the parent during the intake interview. Very few of these cases were directly referred by social agencies or schools, and none was accepted without interviewing at least one parent, almost always the mother, or the parent substitute.

RANK ORDER OF THE MOST FREQUENT PROBLEMS

	RANK ORDER		
Problem	Combined Groups	Boys	Girls
Negativism	1	1	1
Temper	2	2	2
Lying	3	4	3
School failure	4	3	6
Nervousness	5	7	4
Enuresis	6	5	9
Fears	7	9	5
Excessive fantasy	8	10	8
Stealing	9	6	12
Sleep disturbances	10	11	10
Masturbation	11	8	14
Truancy	12	12	13

Among these cases relatively few were feebleminded or psychopathic. It was a part of Institute policy to exclude from its treatment service cases of these types which had already had a competent diagnosis and recommendation for treatment. A few cases were given diagnostic study only for the purpose of training workers; a few defective and more psychopathic children were accepted for treatment for research purposes.

The tabulations give a reasonably adequate picture of the behavior that adults find objectionable in otherwise reasonably normal children. The first three are specifically problems in interpersonal relationships which particularly insult the ego of the adult.

FACTORS IN CAUSATION

Since problems and causative factors are multiple for all cases, a diagnostic synthesis of findings was used. This was of especial value in the effort to determine treatment needs and possibilities and to focus treatment effort.

Among the various causative factors, certain ones showed up in surprisingly large numbers. For example, 707 of these children, 442 boys, 265 girls, were more than 10 percent underweight or overweight according to the standard height-weight tables. Nearly half the boys were underweight. If a boy is not too much underweight, it is not a serious handicap to him in his direct evaluation of himself, in his evaluation by other boys, or in the competitions which mean so much to boys. Slightly more than one quarter of the boys were overweight. This is likely to be a more serious problem than is underweight for a boy, because of the handicap it imposes in many athletic competitions. Extremely skinny and extremely fat boys are picked out for both friendly and hostile ridicule by other boys, as is shown by the nicknames applied to them. Either extreme may be a source of great pain and unhappiness.

About one third of the girls were overweight. In general this is a more serious problem for girls than it is for boys, especially for the older girls, among whom the greatest competitions revolve around securing the attention of boys. Another third of the girls were underweight, a condition which becomes troublesome for them only when it is extreme.

Approximately three fifths of the total group were more than 10 percent under or over average height for age. About one third of the boys were under average height, and another third were over. Being short is much more of a psychological problem for a boy than is being too tall, although either extreme is painful. The concepts of tallness, muscular strength, and ability to succeed in athletic competitions are equated with masculinity and superiority within masculine ranks in our culture. Some degree of an inferiority complex will usually be found in older boys and men who are much below average height. They are likely to overcompensate for this in some way or reveal an undercurrent of bitterness.

Among the girls, one third were under average height, and nearly one third were over. For a girl, being too tall is quite as much or more of a problem than is being short for a boy. Previous comments regarding extremes apply here also. It is true that the recent change in social evaluation, with praise for tall girls, is altering this picture somewhat, but the influence is not yet great. Too tall girls tend to show much compensatory behavior, such as stooping, wearing low heels, and low coiffures to reduce the impression of height, just as short boys wear cuban heels, pompadour their hair, and attempt to stretch themselves by posture and exercise. The figures given on height and weight must be interpreted with caution. It seems to be indicated that problem children tend to deviate with respect to these averages as well as others.

Chronic fatigue, which may be the proximate causative factor in cases showing overactivity, irritability, underweight, poor appetite, insomnia, scattered attention, and inability to concentrate, must always be borne in mind. Chronic fatigue may be due solely to emotional conflicts, it may have a physical background, or there may be a combination of the two.

Chronic disease operates to produce behavior problems in several ways. Associated with a chronic disease is always some limitation, mild to severe, in one or more capacities to react or perform, and such limitation may constitute a problem in and of itself. The disease may produce a chronic fatigue state, with its sequential symptoms. Because of shame, depression, or other unpleasant emotions the sufferer may develop a reaction of withdrawal and become unsocial. Children, however, are more likely to rebel against the restrictive inactivity imposed upon them. Often they consider it unjustifiable and engage in the forbidden activity to their own detriment. Or they engage in some delinquent or other difficult behavior designed to give them status with their peers, thereby creating difficult problems. If the chronic disorder leaves visible signs, such as crippling, the exposure of the disability to public view often operates to aggravate the mental conflict caused by being different, and the behavior problems resulting therefrom.

Conflict over difference is the nuclear emotional difficulty of the too-much-talked-about inferiority complex. This was found to be an important factor in the production of problems in about 10 percent of the Institute group, somewhat more frequently in boys than in girls. Girls complain much more about *feeling* self-conscious, ill at ease, and timid than do boys. On the other hand, casual observation indicates that boys show more self-consciousness and more often appear uneasy than do girls.

Feelings of inferiority may have a reality basis. In fact, it may be so pronounced and so permanent that the only alternative is to face it and find some type of compensation. The basis in reality may be found in any attribute concerning which the individual feels himself to be disadvantaged in any type of competition. Or it may be that the difference is constantly pointed out unfavorably by parents, siblings, teachers, or companions.

Without attempting to go into detail, some types of difference which produce conflicts serious enough to cause maladjustments are: color, race, religion, socio-economic status of family or individual, height, weight, any and all particular characteristics of physique and appearance, intellectual ability, manual ability, special talents (either their absence or their presence may be the source of conflict), athletic ability, vocation, income. Indeed, anything which singles out the individual, either as he sees himself or as he thinks others see him, may be a factor in the origin of such conflicts. Resentment is obviously also inevitable in producing this conflict. If there were no resentment and the difference, real or imagined, were acceptable or pleasant, then conflict would not result.

In the Institute series the most common behavior problems associated with conflict over difference were, in order of frequency of occurrence, for the boys: negativism, temper tantrums, enuresis, failure in school (a potent factor in causation), nervousness, truancy, excessive fantasy, lying, stealing, and masturbation. There are significant differences in the problems presented by the girls. The most frequent was fear, followed by sensitiveness, nervousness, negativism, sleep disturbance, temper tantrums, lying, sex activity, enuresis, and school failure. It is seen, therefore, that boys tend to react to their conflicts with external aggression, while girls more often show internal evidence of symptom formation.

Analysis of a number of other factors reveals that none more frequently produces conflict than the feeling of being "different." Parental attitudes and sibling rivalry operate to produce or to increase the conflicts. Especially disturbing is the child's feeling of being rejected. The behavior resulting from such unhappy mental states may be of any unfortunate type.

Examination of stealing and lying in relation to other behavior problems and to a variety of causative factors will serve as a paradigm for any type of delinquency. Stealing is much more common among boys than among girls. Complaints of stealing show that boys begin to steal at an earlier age than do girls. Stealing is universally regarded as an antisocial act of considerable consequence, but social standards vary greatly concerning it. These variations have to do with the age of the culprit, the educational and social levels, type of articles stolen and their value, from whom stolen, the abuse of confidence involved, and, to a lesser extent, ideas regarding the communal nature of property.

Social attitudes toward stealing are perhaps best seen in the nature of legal definitions and legal penalties. In England there was a time when the theft of articles valued at more than a few shillings was punishable by death. We are told that throngs flocked to see the hangings, while pickpockets busily plied their trade. In our own West, not so long ago, horse stealing was universally regarded as a capital crime, because a man's life might depend upon his possession of a horse. In more recent times stealing, robbery, burglary, and other crimes against property have received legal definitions which make many differentiations regarding the degree of offense and the severity of punishment. For present purposes the legal classes of petit larceny and grand larceny, depending upon the amount involved, will suffice for illustration. The first is a misdemeanor, sentences are light, and no loss of civil rights is involved. Grand larceny, however, is a felony, and conviction carries longer sentences in a penitentiary, with loss of civil rights and the social stigma of being regarded a criminal.

To appropriate or attempt to appropriate the possessions of others is a universal trait among small children who have not yet learned to differentiate between mine and thine. They react to the attractiveness of the objects, with no social concept of ownership. In later childhood and youth and even in adult life there is often a similar attitude toward impersonally owned property, as in schools and colleges, hotels, and Pullman cars. Masked under the name of souvenir hunting, it is nevertheless, by any definition, stealing. Yet the moral code of many people permits them to take such things with an easy conscience, whereas they would recoil in horror from a similar theft from an individual. Cheating of restaurants, stores, and public-service corporations is also frequently condoned.

Stealing is intimately linked up with all forms of evasion and dishonesty, such as lying, cheating, and swindling. Such acts vary in the degree of aggression involved, but all are to be classified among the acts of aggression against others, individually or collectively. Even defensive lying is an aggressive act, as is truancy; both represent rebellion and an attempt to escape unpleasant situations. It is not surprising, therefore, to find that lying is far and away the most frequent associated symptom in those who steal. It is a justifiable conclusion that the several forms of dishonesty are likely to appear in the same cases and to stem from the same roots.

Lying frequently occurs in association with stealing, truancy, negativism, masturbation, and enuresis, in that order. In fact, the group of liars contains 64 percent of all the stealers, 45 percent of the truants, 34 percent of the masturbators, 30 percent of the negativistic cases, 29 percent of the enuretics, 24 percent of those exhibiting temper tantrums, 24 percent of the school failures, 23 percent of those who have excessive fantasies, 22 percent of sleep disturbance, to mention the associated problems occurring in more than 20 percent of the cases. Surely there is here some justification for the stress parents put upon lying as indicative of a serious character disturbance, entirely aside from the obvious insult to the ego of a parent upon being lied to by a child.

The two factors in the family situation which stand out in this group as positively increased over the average rates are open maternal rejection and faulty discipline. Maternal overprotection and sibling jealousy are considerably below the average. The marked increase in faulty discipline and dislike by mother, combined with the marked reduction in maternal protectiveness, shows the relatively unfavorable position in the family of the child who lies.

The essential motivations of stealing and lying must be examined separately. It is true that there is a high incidence of association in these cases. In fact, in this series 48 percent of the stealers also lied, and 64 percent of the liars also stole. Of the 403 cases listed under lying and stealing, 26.8 percent did both. No other combination quite reaches these figures, not even negativism and temper tantrums, which comes nearest. Truancy is also closely associated with lying and stealing, but probably in a casual or permissive way. Statistics indicate that 90 percent of truants steal and lie, but if this were brought down to individual cases the percentage would certainly be lower. The fact is that many more children lie and steal than truant. It could be true that all truants lie and steal; all thieves could be liars, but not truants; and all liars could have temper tantrums and be negativistic, but not all could be thieves or truants. This is important in interpreting any multiple frequency table. All problems of lesser frequency could be associated with any problem of greater frequency, but the latter could not be completely matched by the former group. This makes rank orders and their shifts important in interpreting the occurrence of problems.

Lying of one or another type is of universal occurrence. If lying be strictly defined, then the omnipresent little white lies of social intercourse would be included. It is an interesting parlor game to get people to give reasons why it is justifiable to depart from the truth. Skillful evasion of the truth and the use of half-truths, concealment, bluffing, and so forth are all part of everyday life and are supposed to contribute to the techniques of diplomacy and tact. They deserve only this passing mention.

The several varieties of lying to be more closely examined are: imaginative, defensive, malicious, revengeful, and pathological. Parents are usually most concerned about the first two, with which they seem to have the most experience. Imaginative stories are a part, and an essential part, of the process of growing up and achieving a balanced sense of the real and the unreal. The essential relationship between dream-stuff and waking imagination has long been recognized. Throughout life the value of imagination and day-dreams is amply shown, not only for the individual but for society as well. Constructive imagination has resulted in the wealth of technological developments which have given our civilization its cast as well as the output of the creative arts and sciences.

Imagination is not always constructive; it has its dark, destructive side, both mechanically and psychologically. Under ordinary circumstances parents encourage their children when very young to display their imaginations, but when the imaginative stories begin to deal with things which parents regard as terrible, bloodthirsty, or trashy, they attempt to stop the process. It is only a step, then, to considering these fanciful stories as lies, especially if they seem to reflect in any way upon the parent. Repressive measures usually follow, without any effect upon the essential process, though they may result in causing the child to cease verbalizing his fantasies.

The essential issue is not to restrain the fantasy; rather it is to help the child, and the adult for that matter, keep a clear line of demarcation between fantasy and reality. It is important not to begin this process too early. When the child is first starting to investigate the world, it is a magic world. The child has no such conceptions of meanings and symbolisms as has the adult, and his conception of the world is extremely different. Only gradually does he develop the capacity to discriminate between good and bad, between the acceptable and the unacceptable, between the wholesome and the unwholesome. To determine the category into which anything will fit, he must make tests. For example, there is the period when everything is given the mouth test for consistency, taste, and other sensations. In a similar way, everything is subjected to sensory tests and to trials of usage. Words are merely sounds until they acquire meaning because of the reactions of others or possibly because of the feeling tone they inspire in the child. Long before words have acquired an auditory structure the infant is having the experience of emotional response to the feeling tone associated with sounds or words emitted by the adults. Throughout early life children react to the emotional climate expressed in facial and bodily postures and movements and to the loudness or softness of the voice, rather than to the words. Later, words as symbols come to be the major medium of expression and communication, though words do not constitute the whole of speech. In fact, many complex ideas are communicated in pantomime or by sign language. It is unfortunate, however, that so many adults lose the ability to interpret correctly the language of shifting bodily tensions and depend so nearly exclusively on words. The extreme of this seems to be the person who is pedantically literal in attaching meanings to words and overlooks all the other factors in communication.

Because the child does not have adult discriminatory capacity, he is not impressed by the blood and gore of nursery rhymes. Nor do these rhymes present to him any confusion or permanently affect his ability to discriminate between reality and unreality. It is just as magical that his father can step over a two-foot barrier as that a cow could jump over the moon. Both are unattainable to the small child, and the *degree* of unattainability or impossibility is of the utmost insignificance to him.

All sorts of words, concepts, and behavior of great significance to the adult have no meaning at all or very different meanings to the child. Death, dying, killing, stealing, lying—these are all merely words until his own experience or the emotional attitudes of adults endow them with an emotional importance which the child accepts. Anyone who has tried to answer all the "whys" about these and other concepts or has tried to explain to a child the limitations of time, space, human abilities, or the differences between various classes of objects and animals, will understand what is meant here. To the child, therefore, the world of make-believe is, at least in the beginning, no more unrealistic than the world in which he lives. Later he finds of great value, especially as solace, the imaginative world into which he may retreat at will. The chief difficulty for older people is not that of separating this dream world from the world of reality, but avoiding the pitfall of finding the dream world so attractive as compared with the grimness of the real world that he retreats into it more and more, until it is possible truly to live an illusion.

There are many practical devices by which one can avoid creating a dream world of one's own or can supplement defective imagination. Fiction, drama, movies, music, art, and other forms of recreation all present methods or mechanisms for temporary escape. Taken in judicious doses, they are extremely valuable as escape valves and balances. The grimmer the realities one faces, the greater the need to escape into the lighter diversions.

One point here is directly connected with this question of harnessing the imagination, with special reference to the so-called comic books and their effects on children and their parents. Aside from the fact that they are rarely comic, the effect of these productions is primarily to outrage the finer sensibilities of the parents, who do not see how *their* children could enjoy "such trash." They fear two things: that the child will model his future ideas of the world and his behavior upon the characters in the books, and that his standards in literature will be permanently impaired. These two concepts may be quickly disposed of in the light of what has already been said. The appeal of these booklets is primarily based on the vicarious sense of power and goodness they permit children to feel by identification with the hero or heroine. They fulfill, vicariously and harmlessly, many drives and needs of the child which are not, and in some cases cannot be, met in our ordinary routine of living. That they offer substitute outlets for aggression and feelings of hostility, or that their children are capable of feeling these emotions, may be horrifying to parents. Nevertheless, it is a healthy release for most children. How many children recently wanted to be Superman so that they could kill Hitler of Hirohito or Germans or Japs?

In the usual course of development the vast majority of children replace at least part of this kind of reading matter with other material more adapted to their emotional and intellectual levels of maturity. The average superior person continues throughout life to use literature for adventure, escape, movement, danger, and insecurity to enrich his ego; he is thrilled to find expressed what he himself has suppressed. The reading habits and capacities of people vary in the same way as other habits and capacities. "Picture reading" is far more ancient than is the alphabet. A great truth may be more effectively expressed in a picture with a brief legend than in a sentence, a paragraph, or a chapter of words. Because a certain medium is a valuable or perhaps the only medium for conveying concepts, especially concepts of behavior, at a given stage of development, it does not follow that the individual will always resort only to that medium. On the contrary, there is ample evidence not only against this conclusion but also in favor of the fact that attempts to force children to read literature beyond their level of emotional needs and intellectual comprehension usually results either in making them nonreaders or at least in making it impossible for them ever to reach the point of being able to read and appreciate what is classified as good literature.

What many parents and educators forget is that the ordinary social level of interest in reading is not high and that books which they regard as lurid and sensational, superromantic and supersentimental are obviously more closely geared to broader needs than are the classics, the great essays, or the great satires. Vocabulary limitation is a great barrier; public education has so far succeeded in producing for the masses only a state of semi-literacy. Exceptionally bright children may be left to make their own choice, but there must be *material* from which to make the choice. Again, there is no need to worry lest a particular book be too adult or too grimly realistic and hence too stimulating. The child, like the adult, will take from the book what he wants or needs, and the rest will be overlooked, denied, changed, or forgotten.

There is one point that requires caution: some children display an exaggerated reaction to certain types of books, movies, and radio programs. When it is found that horror stories, however presented, are affecting sleep or appetite or producing other evidences of anxiety, the child should be protected against repetitions until he has matured enough to withstand such impacts. If the symptoms are severe or there are many of them, they serve to indicate a need to investigate what is happening in the child's emotional life to cause these severe reactions. Often the anxiety is not really the child's; instead, the parents—one or the other or both—project their own anxiety on him.

Another unfavorable end result of overdevelopment in fantasy life is the passage, by imperceptible degrees, into the status of pathological lying, which has already been described with the psychopathic personalities. One often hears it said of a child that "he seems to prefer to tell a lie even when the truth would serve him better." Pathological lies, adhered to in the face of demonstrated falsity and to the detriment of the perpetrator, may spring directly from wishes and frustrations. In many cases the lies are obvious wish fulfillments, while in others they are symbolically expressive of disguised wishes. Most of these fantasies aggrandize the child in some way, perhaps by removing or circumventing an obstacle in his path. Either in the realistic experiences of the present or in the suppressed traumata of the past, the origin of this type of lying is usually readily discerned in the younger child. In the adolescent, as in the adult, the original factors are likely to be more deeply buried and even impenetrable. In some cases the fixity may be such that the fantasies acquire the status of delusions.

Defensive lying is the type which gives parents the greatest concern. Even if its function as defense is not clearly recognized, it is correctly seen as a reaction to something awry in what should be an open, trustful, confidential relationship between parent and child. The child has been punished, or there has been inconsistent handling of a situation, or because of an attitude or reaction of the parent, the child resorts to lying in order to escape unpleasant consequences or to secure some advantage or pleasure. Fear is therefore the chief motivation, and it is not infrequently copied from the behavior of adults or older siblings in the family.

Lying for revenge and malicious lying may be discussed together.

Each has the common thread of intentional injury to someone else, either to requite a real or fancied injury to the liar or to bolster his own ego at the expense of another, an act of malice. The origin of the malicious lying is complex, and it results in less satisfaction and less guilt; motivation is more indirect, often unconscious, and less of a direct reaction to an untoward event; therefore it is more difficult to analyze and to treat. Frequently the mechanism involved is that of symbolic revenge on parent or sibling for earlier traumatizing experiences.

To speak of such activity as lying seems to imply a conscious and deliberate perversion of the truth, but there are unconscious retaliatory drives. The individuals who are lied about in some way present characteristics or activities which stir up buried resentments. In order to help the liar, he must first be made fully aware of what he is doing, recognize that it is unjust, and develop feelings of guilt and anxiety about his own actions. Merely pointing out to him what he is doing will not help him achieve the necessary insight.

Stealing has many, often complex, motivations. In the literature much has been made of the relationship between repressed or distorted sexual impulses and stealing, which is often interpreted as a substitute sexual act. Such cases do occur, but not in sufficient numbers to explain any considerable proportion of stealing. In a way, stealing is a more or less universal phenomenon, but is only to be considered a problem when it is a persistent mode of reaction continued beyond the time when the indiscriminate collection of belongings should be replaced by clear-cut conceptions of ownership and property rights. In the country, orchards and melon patches are considered fair game. In the city, fruit stands, candy stores, and the five and dime stores replace the rural targets. The motivating force behind such stealing as this is desire. Satisfying the desire does not produce much feeling of guilt, both because of the impersonality of the act or the plentifulness of the supply of what is taken, on the one hand, and on the other, the fact that the stealing is usually done, or at least begun, in groups. The protective coloration of the group or gang is important to the novice, especially when leadership is vested in the older youths who appear glamorous and heroic to the beginner because of their bold and adventurous activities.

Experience in different clinics with children who steal seems to vary considerably, but it remains obscure whether this is due to actual differences in type of case, differences in the data sought, or differences in interpretation. Among children, at least, there appear to be three major motivations for stealing: (1) To satisfy an appetite or a desire for possession, with insufficient power of inhibition to restrain the act of gratification. (2) To secure status in the group by proving boldness and competence in thieving, or to purchase the favor of the group by sharing the spoils. This sort of splurge stealing is probably the commonest type referred to clinics for study. (3) The third is symbolic stealing, in which sexual symbolism is especially important, though other symbolisms are also frequent. It is particularly the cases in which symbolism is prominent that intensive psychotherapy is indicated.

In cases of splurge stealing, treatment must be directed toward removing the factors which produce the feelings of difference and insecurity with relation to the group and helping the child to achieve status and satisfactions by legitimate and healthy means. In all types of stealing, unsatisfying home relationships, especially during the early years, will be found to play a part. The difficulties in relationship run the gamut of inadequate home standards of social behavior, inadequate training or discipline, overprotection, rejection, and sibling rivalry. Overprotection is of particular interest in this connection, since one malign result is that the child is almost always protected from the consequences of his acts. Where such antisocial behavior as stealing is concerned, overprotection leads to an increase of the activity in a constantly widening sphere. Since no superego is developed, because the overprotecting parent assumes that role and accepts the punishment, the child feels little guilt and develops no inhibiting mechanisms. The result is the continuation of infantile, hedonistic attitudes, and the necessity for immediate gratification of impulses and desires. When well developed, these adverse mechanisms operate in all social situations; the individual takes whatever he wants materially, psychologically, and otherwise, but offers and gives little or nothing in return. There is no awareness on his part that there is anything abnormal in his attitudes and relationships or that his demands and takings are without adequate recompense on his part. This demanding, selfish, unrewarding attitude toward others is one of the most devastating and trying types of dependence. The resultant tyrannizing over people in the environment is quite as enervating and as difficult to combat as the tyranny of weakness that is imposed by the chronic neurotic invalid.

Stealing, then, has socio-economic as well as psychological and psychiatric factors. These combine in various ways to determine the extent and varieties of the activity. A revenge motivation against society in general or against particular groups or individuals is often found, and the grievances may be real or fancied. In any case, treatment for stealing must be based on a thorough understanding of the individual's background and personality. Especially for the cases with chronically exhibited antisocial behavior, it is not enough to view merely the external features of the environment, such as the economic situation, deprivations, and so forth, and assess the blame for the delinquent behavior to them. It is the person who commits the acts who must be examined; the acts result from factors within his personality. What is of the utmost importance is the structure of the personality, how that structure was evolved, and at what points the personality may be influenced for purposes of reconstruction. Ethics, morals, religion, and laws have not solved these problems of delinquency. The roots of the development of the attitudes which permit and perhaps encourage antisocial behavior are to be found in the early emotional relationships that determine the trends and the extent of development of certain fundamental attitudes toward the self and others. For neither the individual nor society can develop, mature, and endure without personal self-confidence and inner security, on the one side, and stability, order, and mutual respect, on the other.

As has already been brought out, negativism, which includes disobedience and stubbornness, is the most frequent problem in the Institute group, occurring in 40 percent of all cases. Its relation to the other problems is therefore of considerable interest. All problems occur in some of the cases showing negativism. Temper tantrums lead, occurring in two fifths of the cases; lying, enuresis, nervousness, and stealing follow. Not all of the less frequently occurring problems present significant differences in percentage when compared with the group as a whole. Temper tantrums, lying, stealing, and refusal of food show significant increases, while fears and school failure are decreased by significant differences. Half the boys and two thirds of the girls who exhibit show-off behavior also present negativism.

Rank orders of problems for boys and girls and for the total group show some interesting variations. They are given in the table on page 330, negativism being omitted from all columns. These are the problems which occur in over 15 percent of the negativistic cases. Show-off behavior does not appear in the above listing, chiefly because behavior of the show-off type in general occurs infrequently in our series; doubtless a great deal of extravagant, attention-getting behavior is designated by other and more interpretive titles.

It is significant that in this negativistic group there is an advance in the rank order of such problems as nervousness, enuresis, stealing, refusal of food, sleep disturbances, and truancy. All these represent aggressive reactions which may be motivated by a desire for revenge or centering the attention of others, usually the mother, on the self. Quite certainly they represent overt reactions to a disturbance in interpersonal relationships, in which there are both ego and libidinal frustrations. That there was less school failure in this group tends to emphasize the fact that the primary source of frustrations and therefore the stimulus to retaliatory behavior was in the home.

These children were reported to show significantly less inferiority feeling. This is to be expected in view of the nature of the behavior, since lay people usually do not see the interrelationship between feelings of insecurity and inadequacy and extravagant, rebellious, stubborn behavior.

RANK ORDER OF PROBLEMS

Problem	Associated with Negativism			For Group of 1,000 Negativism Excluded		
	Total	Boys	Girls	Total	Boys	Girls
Temper tantrums	1	1	1	1	1	1
Lying	2	2	2	2	3	2
Nervousness	3	5	4	4	5	3
Enuresis	4	4	6	5	4	8
Stealing	5	3	10	8	6	11
Refusal of food	6	11	3	12	13	6
Sleep disturbances	7	6	8	9	10	9
School failure	8	8	7	3	2	5
Truancy	9	9	11	11	11	13
Masturbation	10	7	15	10	7	14
Excess fantasy	11	12	5	7	9	9
Fears	12	10	12	6	8	4

Excess fantasy and fears also appear much less frequently than in the entire group. In cases presenting negativistic behavior as an outstanding mode of reaction to situations, it is well known that fears and fantasy formation may be present to an extreme degree. These may be masked both by verbal reticence and by the overt behavior, which often seems to express the exact opposite of fears and fantasies. If fantasies are expressed, they seem to be particularly bold, grandiose conceptions. On the other hand, fears and fantasies are integral parts of neurotic pictures, and the negativistic children do not present many symptoms of a neurotic nature. That is, their response is direct, not through the elaboration of inner symptoms and the presentation of conflicts in symbolic form.

In the family picture faulty discipline, unfavorable comparisons, nagging mothers, sibling jealousy, and protective fathers are all significantly greater than in the total group. The increase in paternal protectiveness is shown almost entirely with regard to boys. There is a similar increase in protectiveness by the mother for the girls. These two points throw important light on the family drama in these particular cases. They highlight the fact that there is dissension, perhaps not overt, between mother and father, and that each is protecting the self by protecting the child of the same sex.

A slight increase in the factor of maternal rejection is about equal for boys and girls. This and other points raise the question of the contribution of maternal dislike or rejection, a difficult factor to evaluate. It is more frequently masked by an overprotective attitude or expressed only in subtle bits of behavior than it is openly verbalized. Even a mother whose behavior toward a child is openly and perhaps even abusively rejecting will deny that she dislikes the child; what she does is "for his own good" or because he "is such a bad child."

OUTLINE OF THERAPY

Treatment methods for mental disorders in childhood and adolescence have been sufficiently discussed. Some elements of procedure in the reactive behavior disorders have also been indicated, so that a brief discussion of the essentials of therapy for behavior problems may help to focus the antecedent presentation of the psycho-social factors.

Therapeutic techniques may be classified according to several principles. From one basic point of view, all treatment procedures in this field may be sorted into direct and indirect approaches, in accordance with the special focus of therapeutic effort. Although some criticisms have been directed at this particular formulation, it actually offers a useful orientation concerning treatment in its manifold aspects.

In this method of distribution, the child and his problems become the focal point of treatment effort. All activities carried out with the child and designed to affect his attitudes and conflicts are classed as *direct therapy*. Medical treatment, individual and group psychotherapy, remedial tutoring, special educational measures, and planned recreation are examples of direct procedures. Some of

these techniques belong to fields which are not primarily therapeutic in intent, but the methods are effectively adaptable to
achieve therapeutic results in children who present particular
problems.

Efforts to modify the environment belong in the category of
indirect therapy, in which two major sorts of manipulation are
easily discernible. In one type the child may be moved bodily from
one set of surroundings to another, presumably more favorable.
Instances of this would be a change from his own home to another,
transfer to a hospital or other institution, transfer from one grade
to another in school or to a special type of class, placement in sum-
mer camp, and other changes in general or special settings. This
removal from one environment to another, chosen because it seems
to be better adapted to the needs of the individual, is the most
ancient and primitive of all methods so far devised for dealing with
maladjusted people. Banishment and imprisonment represent punitive measures adopted primarily for the protection of society
against the person and his depredations.

When social conscience regarding dependent, orphaned, and
homeless children became aroused in this country, the first move
was the establishment of institutional accommodations in the form
of orphan asylums. The use of adoptive and boarding or foster
homes was developed in conjunction with the orphanages, or as
an independent endeavor. Similarly, institutions were organized for
the special care and training of delinquent and incorrigible children
of both sexes. During the past twenty-five years in particular there
has been a pronounced shift away from the use of institutions in
favor of foster homes for dependent children. The character of the
training and supervision in the better correctional institutions has
undergone marked changes, with a more clinical approach based
upon individual differences. However, there are still many correctional schools which have not developed modern viewpoints and
methods. The development of behavior clinics has been paralleled
by the conviction that children with behavior problems should be
treated in their usual environments and that institutions are to be

used only for special cases or as a last resort. This has affected disposition of juvenile offenders by the courts, as shown by a steady drop in commitments to public institutions during recent years.

In the evolution of these ideas and procedures, many special community facilities have been developed by social agencies, schools, courts, religious bodies, health organizations, and in recreational programs. Many of the special provisions are designed to be both therapeutic with reference to existing problems and aimed to prevent more serious developments. In other instances the projects are intended to be broadly and constructively preventive. As such, they are applicable to large groups and utilize a minimum of therapeutic techniques, though to be most effective they must embody sound principles of mental hygiene.

The second general type of indirect treatment comprises all therapeutic activities with persons whose relationships with the child are important in the emergence of the problem behavior. While the focus of effort continues to be the problems of the child, work with people in the environment may quickly come to center on adjustment difficulties, on certain attitudes or emotional conflicts which interfere with the interpersonal relationships of a particular adult. To deal adequately with these personal problems requires direct psychotherapy, which often leads into areas of conflict and confusion that may seem to be somewhat remote from the child's problems. Nevertheless, these may be the most important points to be cleared up in the interest of more constructive relationships.

In the case of adults other than the parents who are important in the child's environment, a therapeutic procedure is frequently impractical, unnecessary, or impossible. In these instances one utilizes educational measures designed to increase the grasp of mental hygiene principles and their utilization with children in general and the problem child in particular. An example of this would be the training of teachers in mental hygiene and its application in the classroom. This activity is not aimed toward treatment as such, but rather to the production of an environmental climate most favorable to personality growth and integration, while minimizing those influences which tend to give rise to behavior and other individual problems. In the course of securing the necessary knowledge and adapting it to classroom and other situations involving groups of children, the adult should gain at least a certain degree of insight into himself in terms of behavior, biases, conflicts, and other aspects of his own personality structure and function. Such a training experience is therefore potentially or actually therapeutic in its effects, but this is not the primary result sought for the adult in training; nor is it a process planned to relieve or cure manifestations of a disease or his personality maladjustment.

We may therefore schematize the indirect treatment measures used with persons as being primarily (a) educational or (b) psychotherapeutic in intent and technique. Education with respect to individual differences and the influence of interpersonal relationships always carries the possibility of therapeutic effects. Sometimes, it must be added, education along these lines may release considerable anxiety and guilt, thus upsetting an existing compensation without providing a superior one. When this occurs it is an indication that definitive psychotherapy is necessary.

Psychotherapy, however it may be carried out, always entails some degree of education and re-education, but not in the sense of any formal pedagogical practices. To a considerable extent it is the emotions and their utilization or control which are influenced or disciplined through the educational aspect of the therapy. It is also true that in specific instances psychotherapy of adults may at times be favorably affected by formal courses dealing with behavior and personality, or by the use of carefully selected reading material. The same observation holds for the adjuvant effects of systematic or unsystematic occupational or avocational activities.

For the young child, individual psychotherapy is often contraindicated; the best results may be obtained through environmental manipulation, especially from therapy with the mother. For the adolescent it is frequently true that intensive direct therapy is essential to a successful result. In other instances indirect treatment is also necessary, and this may again involve work with one or both parents or even separation from the home.

In the great majority of cases, however, it seems clear that the most lasting effects, both as therapeutic results and in terms of prevention of further elaboration of inner maladjustments, are secured by judiciously blending direct and indirect approaches. In general, this means direct treatment of the child by the method most appropriate for his problems and stage of development, combined with treatment of the parent or other adult most deeply involved in the problems, plus manipulation of other environmental factors which play a part in the production or maintenance of the troublesome situation. While the intensity of effort in these three fields may vary from time to time in a particular case, they all require attention at some point in treatment, especially, perhaps, the first two. In my opinion it is a general principle of great import that the simplest therapy which will achieve the desired effect is the best. A corollary to this is the conviction that it is advisable not to upset a compensatory mechanism which is working reasonably well unless one is sure that a superior type can be developed. These points and some general principles of psychotherapy are further discussed in Chapter XIX.

CHAPTER XVIII

PROBLEMS OF REJECTEES AND VETERANS

DEALING WITH men who have been rejected or discharged from the armed services on neuropsychiatric grounds is an intricate problem. No more can be here attempted on the subject than to indicate some general principles of approach to the issues involved. According to the best information available, these men number several hundred thousand. Many interested groups, impressed by these huge figures, evolved numerous plans for their rehabilitation. One of the major difficulties about these plans, as attested by the experiences of psychiatrists and clinics, is that many of the men who need mental hygiene services will not accept them. Others who are eager for help become so involved in red tape that weeks or months pass before definite decisions are made regarding the disposition of their cases. In despair, they decide to get along as best they can without help. The number accepted for treatment by psychiatrists in private practice, for nominal fees or without charge, is so small that scarcely any impression is made on the great number of individuals who need and desire help.

Some of the rejected men were greatly upset when they were informed that they were psychoneurotic. Not having suspected the condition, they worried' about the significance of the term. A simple explanation satisfied many of them; a few undertook treatment. For the most part, however, the diagnosis was completely disregarded; many of the men were resentful and refused to have anything to do with psychiatrists or clinics. Numerous others were of the same opinion as were their civilian counterparts; what ailed them, they thought, was something they could straighten out by themselves—by a tonic, perhaps, or some other simple medication.

General medical attitudes are often factors in influencing people. There are still physicians who believe that psychiatric treatment is acceptable only for cases that are obviously psychotic. They will often assure the neurotic patient that there is nothing wrong with him and prescribe vitamins, sedatives, tonics or other medication, or give him a pep talk. Long after considerable damage has been done the patient may eventually find himself in the psychiatrist's office; he may then report that his physician's parting advice was, "Whatever else you do, don't go near a psychiatrist."

The families of service men influence them tremendously. A family is likely to believe that loving care and tender solicitude are sufficient to clear up the problem or, perhaps, that it is only necessary for their menfolk to return to work. Whether the patient has a normal desire to return to work, or having returned, he has the ability to continue is of little concern to the family. Public and private agencies of several types also exert a negative influence. They often see the patient's problems as lying entirely within the purview of the agency, disavowing any need for psychiatric advice or treatment. The misunderstanding by families and agencies of the patient's problems further confuses him so that he is embarrassed to seek psychiatric treatment even if he wants it.

It is true that psychiatric facilities for treatment are woefully inadequate, but they will be even more so if all discharged neuropsychiatric cases eventually accept treatment. Nineteen years after the First World War neuropsychiatric casualities were entering veterans' hospitals for the first time. There is no indication that the aftermath of the Second World War will be different. For reasons to be presented, it is my opinion that a large percentage of dischargees do *not* need psychiatric or mental hygiene treatment; also, that for many conditions to which the label "psychoneurosis" was applied, no effective treatment techniques are known.

This again brings up the vexing question of the use and misuse of terms. In 1914–15 the term "shell shock" was used to cover just about every mental disorder that occurred in combat troops. The term was based on the erroneous conception that the mental disturbances were organic in origin, related to brain injuries sustained in explosions. The term continued to be used long after it became clear that most of the disturbances were familiar and ordinary types of neurotic and psychotic reactions, precipitated by the trauma of battle situations. Even today, people talk of their shell-shocked relatives. Specialists substituted the term "war neurosis," thereby indicating both the actual nature of the disorder and the fact that its emergence was related to war experiences. This term is still in use and is valid when applied in accordance with precise criteria.

By the time the United States entered the First World War, the experience of the several combatant armies had clearly indicated the need for excluding from service the mentally, as well as the physically, handicapped. For that reason, and for the first time in world history, the American army draft was surveyed by psychiatrists and psychologists. As a result, many men were excluded from service, chiefly those who were obviously and severely handicapped. Some were accepted for limited service, such as in labor battalions.

Despite the screening, many men broke down both during training and later. Some had past histories of mental disturbance or of social maladjustment, but social histories were not available for the screening process. At that time very few psychiatric hospitals had social workers, and psychiatric social work as we know it today was only in its infancy. In fact, it was the war experience and its proof of the need for psychiatric aids that was directly responsible for the establishment of the Smith College School for Social Work.

Psychotics, epileptics, neurotics, and psychopaths posed special problems to the armed services during the war and to governmental agencies later. Among provisions to meet these problems, mental hospitals and wards were established both abroad and at home. Many psychotic patients were handled through station hospitals, and most of them were sooner or later transferred to hospitals in their home states.

Beginning in 1918–19, the Veterans Administration established its own mental hospitals. In 1937 these hospitals numbered twenty-six, caring for approximately 26,000 patients at the end of the year. Admissions during that year numbered over 10,000, of whom nearly 4,500 were *admitted for the first time*. Recall that this large number of new cases occurred nineteen years after the cessation of hostilities, when our armed forces were at a low point in numbers. There were practically no facilities for out-patient treatment. By 1945 the number of Veterans Administration neuropsychiatric hospitals had increased to thirty-three, with 25,500 patients and 5,197 admissions during the year, of which over 3,500 were first admissions. Additional hospitals have been established, and others are being planned. Extensive out-patient facilities already exist.

These figures should cause us to ponder past policies and consider carefully the potential future load. The recent war has seen three times as many men and women mobilized as were in the previous one. Advances in the science of medicine and surgery in the period between the two wars are responsible for keeping alive many of the wounded in the recent war who would otherwise have succumbed. These are the veterans who will undoubtedly sooner or later need some sort of professional help in civilian life. It is understandable that casualties of all types are far greater than they were in the earlier conflict. Severe and prolonged trauma often leaves its mark even on the strongest personality. Many individuals will require a mental hygiene approach for problems arising out of their physical disabilities.

Many more were rejected for neuropsychiatric disabilities in the Second World War than in the First, and the number rejected since 1945 is equally large. It is important in this connection that procedures for clearing names of draftees through the files of state departments of mental diseases, departments of correction, and through social service exchanges have been extensively used. In a number of areas social workers provided social histories for the use of local draft boards and their psychiatrists.

Directives regarding the diagnoses to be used in rejecting and discharging men have varied from time to time. This has produced considerable confusion in the minds of the men themselves and of civilian psychiatrists who have to deal with the men. Most of the diagnoses appear to have been "psychoneurosis, severe." However, as used in the services, the term has been variously applied to many conditions—the mild psychoses, psychopathic personality, homosexuality, and mild epilepsy, as well as to the neuroses. The diagnosis must therefore be carefully checked before treatment of the man as a neurotic is undertaken; that is, the real condition must first be determined.

The actually psychotic—at least the more seriously disturbed—have been sent to mental hospitals after separation from the services. Those whose rejection or discharge was due to overt homosexuality have not as a rule wanted treatment. This is equally true of the civilian homosexual. Most are satisfied with their sexual outlets and generally make an adequate adjustment socially and vocationally. It is when the homosexual becomes alcoholic or addicted to drugs or in some other way loses his sense of social discretion that difficulties arise which may lead to treatment. However, such unrestrained activities usually lead to confinement in penal institutions.

Many types of service may be needed by the neuropsychiatric casualties. They would include psychiatric exploration, advice, and treatment; group psychotherapy; medical treatment; vocational testing, counsel, and job placement; casework in relation to personal or family problems; group and recreational activities; educational and re-educational programs. The development of veterans' service centers, where the veteran may quickly ascertain what services and agencies are available to help him with his problems as he sees them, is important.

The actual approach, if it is to be effective, must be in terms of mental hygiene treatment. By this is meant that both internal and environmental factors, problems, and assets must be envisaged and treated or manipulated. This embodies the distinction I long ago made between mental hygiene treatment and psychiatric treatment. The latter may be successful through dealing only with the patient and is applicable in certain situations. But even in such individualized treatment the patients always bring out factors and problems in interpersonal relationships within the family and elsewhere, which must also be analyzed and treated.

In many treatment procedures for veterans the social worker plays the primary role. Many types of organization have been proposed, and there has been much discussion of where responsibility must lie. Eventually, it seems likely that the Veterans Administration will assume practically all responsibilities.

Because veterans tend to reject psychiatrists and psychiatry, they are more likely to be drawn into needed psychiatric treatment through the medium of clinics designed to help them with their readjustment to family and social life. Veterans' children and their problems seem to form a particularly fruitful avenue of approach to the veteran and his problems.

During actual service, many men with combat fatigue were successfully treated by several methods and were then returned to full or limited duty. These men had adequate and stable personality make-up, but succumbed temporarily to intolerable battle strain. More chronic conditions emerged, both in combat troops and in men stationed for long periods in isolated, inactive outposts. These cases present difficult problems; in many instances the lack of early recognition of the problem operates to produce a fixed abnormal state.

While in the service, many psychopaths got into difficulties which landed them in the brig, often with long sentences. Others were dishonorably discharged, while still others were discharged as neuropsychiatric cases. The latter group may profit from some sort of supervision, but how much they can accept and use is, of course, doubtful.

Some of the most difficult mental hygiene problems with which families, social workers, and other professional people are faced have to do with attitudes toward and treatment of the physically maimed. These cases call for careful understanding of their psychological problems, as well as earnest effort to reduce the incapacitation caused by loss of sight, limbs, and so forth. Some of the thrilling stories that have emerged about these casualties have to do with the marked developments in workable prosthetic devices and plastic surgery.

This war has given greater impetus to psychiatry than did the preceding one, chiefly because we have so many more treatment techniques, a far more dynamic approach, and a great deal more knowledge of preventive methods. To my mind, social work as therapy shares in these advances and should accordingly achieve far more significance than even the high estate it has held in the past. What the ultimate needs for social psychiatric treatment will be and how they will be met seems uncertain. Probably the most important point to be remembered is that the problems of dischargees and of veterans are the problems of human beings. Unless they are too ill to exercise independent judgment, they should be allowed to set their own pace in reconversion to civilian life. This includes the right to determine whether or not they wish treatment and the kind of treatment they can accept. The social worker should be in the front line in dealing with many problems of readjustment of these service men and women to civilian life.

CHAPTER XIX

THE SOCIAL WORKER AND TREATMENT

CASEWORK NEEDS

PSYCHIATRIC CASES always present social difficulties, and a great many of them require some sort of social action. It has already been noted that it is the disturbance in social behavior which determines the commitment of psychotic cases. The conduct disorders of the psychotic may have serious implications for the patient, the family, and society at large. Dementing processes interfere with normal self-maintenance, even though the patient does not himself disturb the peace. Mental deficiency, epilepsy, and psychopathic personality also interfere with social adaptation. Neurotics, however, do not usually present the serious conduct disorders or marked failures of self-maintenance which occur in other types of psychiatric case. The primary or reactive behavior maladjustments present a wide range of disturbances in social relationships. Delinquent and criminal activity may occur with any type of mental disturbance, as well as without evidence of personality maladjustment.

Numerous situations requiring social casework treatment are found among the families of psychiatric patients. Typical situations which may call for casework procedures are those in which measures must be taken to keep the family together when a key member becomes incapacitated, when there is need for temporary or permanent placement of children, when it is necessary to explain to the family the diagnosis and prognosis of the illness and to prepare them for the patient's return to the home. The patient himself habitually presents need for diversified casework services, a few instances of which are rehabilitation measures such as vocational training or placement, a supportive relationship with a worker, or general supervision for care in his own family or in the community. With some patients it may be necessary for the worker to provide a rather intensive therapeutic relationship. Where family conflict and domestic disharmony or the behavior problems of children constitute the focus of casework effort, other techniques may be necessary.

Social service with psychiatric cases which present gross mental deviations may be carried out under the aegis of the mental hospital or the psychiatric clinic. However, social work has a more prominent place and is better integrated in the child guidance and mental health clinics, whose work is usually community-wide and as a result closely correlated with the activities of the social agencies, health services, and the educational system of the particular area which all organizations serve in common. In one definition of psychiatric social work it is stated to be that branch of social casework which deals with psychiatric cases in a clinic or hospital, where the social work is co-ordinated with psychiatry and clinical psychology. Actually, however, the fundamental principles of psychiatric social work have increasingly proven to be essential elements in the training of all social workers. In fact, accumulated experience demonstrates that the basic concepts of generic casework and of psychiatric social work are nearly or completely identical, in part because the major goal of both is personal-social adjustment.

Training for social casework concentrates especially on treatment that is based upon adequate social diagnosis; skill is developed through closely supervised work. Because personality and its disorders enter so frequently and so largely into the production of the client's problems, casework has developed many methods of its own and adapted much from dynamic psychopathology. One result of the emphasis on treatment is that psychotherapeutic techniques are constantly employed, even though modified in detail and with regard to goals. The use of such techniques by case workers has led to considerable division of opinion with respect to whether they actually do or should practice psychotherapy, and what the dividing line between casework and psychotherapeutic techniques may be. This dispute, quite heated at times, seems to me merely a polemic and, as such, far from realistic. No hard and fast line of demarcation can be drawn between the two procedures, since there are many close parallels between casework treatment and psychotherapy. There is considerable overlapping in the nature of the problem situations which are presented by clients and in the techniques that are available to meet them. These points are thrown into clear relief by two of Mary Richmond's definitions of social casework. In one, she said it consists of "those processes which develop personality through adjustments consciously affected, individual by individual, between men and their social environment." The other statement was that social casework "may be defined as the art of doing different things for and with different people by cooperating with them to achieve at one and the same time their own and society's betterment."

These and later formulations of casework treatment and objectives stress personal-social adjustment, individualization and variable techniques, self-realization, release of the individual's capacities, economic and psychological self-help and self-determination, recognition and utilization of individual differences, mutiple goals, and personality development. These particular points are selected from a much greater number as examples of the emphasis laid on personal adjustment in the intricate processes of social rehabilitation. The personality of the client and the nuances of the family drama are of primary importance in relation to socially reconstructive procedures, while the casework relationship provides the medium through which treatment is effected.

PSYCHOTHERAPY

Therapy is literally defined as the treatment of disease; psychotherapy as "the mental treatment of illness, especially of nervous diseases and maladjustments, as by suggestion, psychoanalysis, or reeducation." Psychotherapy was formerly defined in identical

terms with "mental healing," a procedure which ignores diagnosis
and the nature and etiology of disease processes. Mental healing
belongs in the same general category with magical incantations,
exorcisms, and other superstitions. Psychotherapy, in the modern
sense of the term, is a legitimate branch of therapeutics having its
own sphere of applicability, and is comprised of a body of principles which are constantly being refined. It includes a number of
delimited techniques, and methods of transmission for training
purposes have been formulated. Psychotherapeutic techniques have
proven valuable in many difficulties other than the neuroses and
psychosomatic states, such as the personality disturbances which
occur in organic disease and in the nonspecific behavior disorders.
There are only a few clearly distinctive methodologies in psychotherapy, but there are numerous variations in emphasis, chiefly in
rather minor details. Many of these modifications have been described as though they were new or separate types of psychotherapy, embodying principles and technical procedures indige-
nous to the particular method, for which originality is claimed.
For example, some technical approaches have been elaborately
described and vigorously set forth as having no relationship to
psychoanalytic technique or as refuting the psychoanalytic approach. Yet even cursory examination often shows that both the
procedure and its theoretical basis are definitely psychoanalytic,
albeit fragmentary and inadequate or even distorted in some manner.

The general principles of psychotherapy may be formulated
with comparative ease, but their actual application in practice
presents several complications. One important point is that an
adequate knowledge of the various methods, and skill in their application, cannot be acquired by reading or from lectures. Actual
experience and practice *under supervision* are required. Certain
attitudes on the part of the therapist are important in the treatment
situation, especially since they frequently contrast sharply with
habitual reactions in everyday interpersonal relations. These therapeutically important attitudes are, perhaps, most easily acquired

by observing other therapists at work, but it is not a simple matter to arrange for continuous observation of an actual treatment situation during each step of its progress. However, through sitting in on interviews, listening to recordings, or observing through a one-way screen it is possible to make direct observations of technique and the interpersonal situation in therapy. An effective and more usual method is through supervisory conferences on cases being carried by the beginner, where interview content may be reviewed and interpreted, technical steps discussed, and errors analyzed. Valuable lessons may also be learned by discussing procedures used by supervisors in particular cases.

Any contact between two people may affect the attitudes, emotional tensions, personality integration, and the behavior of one or both, but it would stretch the concept beyond useful limits to classify as psychotherapy the results of incidental or casual contacts. In another area, the educational process should produce wholesome developments in personality integration, increase personal insight, improve social relationships, reduce unreasonable prejudices, release a certain amount of anxiety, and bring about other generally constructive effects. Educational procedures, however, are not planned to relieve symptoms, ventilate conflicts, clear up disturbed psychodynamics, or correct disorders of behavior. We may therefore make an initial distinction between technical procedures which are intended to promote healthy development, of which education is an example, and purposeful efforts to correct personality deviations and behavior problems. Only activities of the latter type are properly classified as psychotherapy, which connotes the use of definitive psychological techniques designed to relieve demonstrable disturbances in psycho-social adjustment.

Psychotherapy is intended to clear up conscious and unconscious complexes and conflicts, with their resultant effects as they appear in somatic symptoms, personality integration, and successful utilization of the self. It follows that adequate diagnostic formulation, with particular reference to the dynamisms involved, is essential in determining whether psychotherapy is indicated, if it is possible, and what technique is best suited to a particular case. Essential to our understanding in this connection is knowledge of the intact portions of the personality and some idea, however rough, of the level of personality integration we may hope to achieve through therapy. Data for the necessary diagnostic synthesis are derived in the first instance from the anamnesis, with particular attention to the immediate difficulties. Skillfully taken and adequately interpreted, a dynamic history provides the indications for those examinations of the patient which may be needed to clarify both diagnosis and choice of treatment procedure. Except in cases which are obviously unsuitable for a psychotherapeutic approach, emphasis in these interviews, which also serve the function of securing information, is on the dynamic aspects of the patient's thinking, feelings, and conduct. In the early period of contact, any treatment procedure chosen on the basis of the clinical picture revealed by the analytic synthesis should not be planned in too great detail, nor should it be rigidly applied. Allowance must be made for possible errors in observation and interpretation, and there must be flexibility in approach. The collection of data for diagnosis and the development of the therapeutic relationship proceed simultaneously, whether or not this is considered to be a desirable process. It is unnecessary and, indeed, impossible to divide the actual development of the therapeutic situation into a period of study, followed by treatment; nor is the establishment of a treatment relationship required before one "takes a history." Therapeutic interaction begins with the first contact. As it develops, it fluctuates in intensity and may vary from one emotional pole to another, which is essential if the interplay is to be therapeutic. Should the contact become static or deteriorate into superficial, personal, or social sessions, the relationship loses its treatment value.

Rapport is a convenient general term to apply to all phases and levels of the interaction of therapist and patient, and rapport is by far the most important single aspect of the therapeutic situation. It is difficult to reduce the complexity of rapport to its elements in detail, though its uses are clear and many factors which facilitate or inhibit its development are explicit. For present purposes, the two most important aspects of rapport appear in connection with (1) the current reality situation and (2) the phenomenon of transference. It is generally true that all reactions to current situations and objects are colored to a greater or less degree by transferences from earlier experiences, but it is possible to make valid and worthwhile distinctions between these two levels or types of rapport.

The first feature which characterizes a therapeutic situation, as distinct from a casual contact, and injects a stimulating or restraining dynamic influence on the evolution of the relationship, is simple and obvious. Two persons are involved and have a particular objective, that of assisting one of them toward the solution of a personal problem. This orientation of purpose between two people clearly presents possibilities which positively or negatively influence the development of that rapport which is necessary to advance treatment. For example, a person's defenses against admitting to himself and to others a weakness or defective self-sufficiency are threatened or broached by a need to seek assistance. Therefore the patient's statement of his problems as he sees them constitutes the springboard for the beginning of treatment. The therapist may see other and deeper problems than the patient outlines; or he may be more impressed than the patient is with the gravity of the situation, but he usually finds it best not to arouse further defenses by announcing his views at the start. Instead, he must bear in mind the fact that a primary objective in therapy is the creation of an emotional climate which fosters the expression by the patient of his inner thoughts and feelings. Attainment of this objective may be hampered by any words or actions of the therapist which seem to be critical or condemnatory, or appear to emphasize a superiority-inferiority status which the patient already feels.

The development of an interrelationship conducive to effective treatment depends to a considerable degree upon the therapist. His attitudes and many other aspects of his own personality and adjustment are important determinants of his adequacy in the therapeutic role. Ability to control emotional reactions toward the patient and his problems is essential to the establishment and maintenance of the necessary rapport. Open-mindedness, permissiveness, and objectivity permit the therapist to sustain the patient's variable dependency, hostility, and other attitudes. The therapist must also realize the nature and extent of his own drives to coerce, punish, or be passive. There are, of course, limitations which pertain to the therapeutic situation, just as there are limits of one or another sort in every circumstance of living. Such items as the office setting, the definite time for appointments, their spacing and their length, the material available for play and activity sessions with children, and the determination of proper treatment techniques constitute limitations which in part establish the external framework within which therapy is carried on. These examples of universal or impersonal limitations imposed from without apply to therapist and patient alike; they do not vary according to whim or expediency, but are important rules of procedure.

Certain general conditions under which treatment is conducted also have considerable influence on the selection of technique and on the course of therapy. Variations notably occur according to whether treatment is conducted in wards of general or mental hospitals, in an out-patient clinic, in a community clinic, in a social agency or through a group closely connected with one, or in private practice. An organizational setting, be it hospital, extramural clinic, or social agency, presents many advantages in meeting the inclusive needs of patients, but there are handicaps, some of which are rather difficult to counteract. Four issues are distinctly important in this connection: (1) the selection of cases in accordance with function and equipment of the agency; (2) size of case loads and the extent of waiting lists; (3) the issue which frequently arises of transferring cases from one therapist to another; (4) the numerous questions which occur in connection with properly safeguarding the patient's interests in organizations in which a major function is teaching and clinical training and where much of the direct work with patients is carried on by students.

Organizations are commonly limited in scope because of specialization of function, the particular auspices and directives under which they operate, the specified area they serve, or a combination of these factors. Thus, hospitals are general or special, public or private, teaching or nonteaching, and are available only to residents of a particular area. Most hospitals provide experience for internes; many have multi-service out-patient departments; some are connected with medical schools and participate in the clinical training of medical students; a few are purely research institutions. An increasing number of general hospitals have in-service facilities for psychiatric cases, but there are still too few of them. Hospitals vary just about as much regarding the types of disorder they will not admit because they are not equipped for them, as they do about the types they will accept. The amount and the nature of social work available in hospitals and utilized by the medical staff also varies widely, so that patients who require extensive social services are usually referred to appropriate agencies.

The same sort of analysis applies to social agencies—they are general or special, public or private, may be districted, and may or may not be centers for field training. Even in the same general field agencies differ in philosophy of operation, in the variety of services offered, with respect to the caliber of staff, and therefore in the quality of services they render. Some social agencies employ psychiatrists and psychologists as consultants, or have a full clinic unit attached to the staff, while other agencies deny that there is need for any such services, even as auxiliaries.

If treatment is focused on a particular pathological state, such as pneumonia, a broken leg, or a psychosis, it is possibly true that the interpersonal relationship is of secondary importance. This is also possible with many accidental, external circumstances of living which require immediate, though temporary, social agency assistance. Any such relegation of relationship to a minor role is unthinkable in chronic disease or disability, in repetitive failure of self-maintenance, or with the many people whose personal-social or somatic difficulties are based on neurotic mechanisms. Since people whose difficulties fall into these categories constitute our major interest, the relationship basic to psychotherapy is of primary importance, and any extraneous factors which interfere with its establishment and maintenance are matters of concern. Serious consideration must therefore be given to the possible effects of organizational functions and policies, and efforts must be made to minimize any blocking tendencies which appear.

One of the elements essential for psychotherapy is the freedom of the psychotherapist to give undivided attention for an adequate period of time to the individual patient. Especially for neurotics, a common and most frustrating experience is the difficulty of finding someone who is interested and takes the time to listen intelligently and with understanding to the story of their difficulties. Large case loads, with the many attendant details, may make it impossible for workers to give sufficient time and to display the degree of interest which a patient urgently needs. It should be apparent to a patient that time spent with him belongs to him alone, and attention should be closely focused on him throughout.

It is well recognized that the first and potentially the most significant step in treatment is the patient's decision to seek assistance. To be put on a waiting list for weeks or months or to find intake closed can be distressing to a person to whom making the decision to seek help was crucial. The result of such frustration is often loss of impetus to proceed. Certainly many situations viewed as emergencies by the prospective patient clarify themselves during a period of waiting, and he withdraws his application. The first or intake interview is an important one, and many organizations try to have the applicant receive enough counsel or other assistance in it so that his purpose will be sustained during any necessary waiting period. This is valuable practice, since no matter how long a disturbing situation has been in existence, it looms up as an acutely distressing emergency to the patient when he finally does seek treatment.

The shifting of patients from one therapist to another occurs especially in training programs. Separate intake personnel or changes in and absences of staff for whatever reason often lead the patient to doubt that he and his problems are regarded as important. There are safeguards against unfavorable results in such situations; it is important to utilize and develop both the patient's capacity to adapt and the cross-identifications he makes of personnel through the medium of the agency. The latter tendency will best be fostered if, from the beginning, the patient blends the person of the therapist with the chief of service or some other key staff member. These variable identifications are peculiarly a part of the transference situation and, as such, can be manipulated in the interests of treatment if the therapist is alert to them and sufficiently objective to be able to use them. Shifting the patient from worker to worker is part of the current reality situation and definitely constitutes a limiting factor with reference to the treatment relationship. Perhaps enough has been said to make it clear that to practice psychotherapy it is necessary to bear in mind the limitations imposed by the particular setting, as well as the limitations imposed by the equipment and potentialities of the therapist. The patient, his difficulties, and his attitudes also present limitations for therapeutic possibilities. These, however, are subjected to diagnostic survey and for the most part constitute objectives for therapy.

One point deserves mention here. While sensitiveness in the neurotic patient is outstanding, there is evidence that it is frequently overweighted by the therapist. The neurotic almost invariably believes that his case is unique and that he is the only person who has such shameful thoughts and wishes. In accordance with these ideas and emotions, the neurotic fears exposure and censure. He is usually relieved to learn that others have similar problems and weaknesses, emotions, and conflicts. The resulting dilution of guilt and anxiety from the realization that he is not unique often turns out to be a potent force in alleviating neurotic symptoms. Experience with group therapy for both children and adults amply proves that treatment is often facilitated when the neurotic has an opportunity, under guidance, to share experiences with other sufferers. Small children whose lives have been spent in groups are usually much freer to express themselves to an adult when in the company of other children than they are when alone with a strange adult. Many neurotic adults react in much the same way, apparently needing and being able to use the support and protective coloration of a group of their own kind.

The extent of the neurotic difficulties quite obviously varies from time to time, so that in many instances what seems to be spontaneous recovery takes place. In such cases it will usually be found that the conflict represents a reaction to some temporary, though severe, stress and strain, or that the general tendency toward integration is sufficient to overcome the conflict. It may happen that a person important to the patient unwittingly plays the role of therapist, perhaps by serving as the repository of the unpleasant emotions aired in the patient's cathartic unburdening. Also, some other sort of substitute outlet for the conflict may appear spontaneously and more or less accidentally.

In this connection, it must be recorded that advocates of quite diverse theoretical formulations of psychopathology obtain good results in therapy, despite their different postulates. That this is primarily related to the rapport developed by the individual therapist can clearly be shown in the analysis of records. It is also indicated by the fact that the originators of a particular set of theories and operational techniques based thereon are more successful in therapy than are their disciples. This is related to differences in conviction or perhaps the strength of bias in favor of a particular procedure, a point which will be further discussed in another connection.

Types of Psychotherapy

Among the procedures traditionally classified as specialized methods of psychotherapy are persuasion and suggestion, but today these are regarded as minor measures. Useful to influence behavior reactions and to relieve symptoms, they are not sufficiently comprehensive to assist in understanding and correcting essential causes of disorder. Both persuasion and suggestion are common in general social intercourse, but this is different from professional usage.

Persuasion is essentially argument, based on an intellectual analysis of symptoms or behavior, intended to produce a rationalized voluntary attempt by the patient to control his impulses and regulate his behavior. Self-criticism is invoked, but there is no attempt to probe the dynamic factors involved. Without penetration into origins, reasoning and intellectual understanding alone are notoriously inadequate to effect reintegration of personality and reaction patterns.

Suggestion is much more widely applied in therapy than is persuasion, either directly or by subtle, indirect means. When used with electricity, placebos, massage, or other auxiliaries, alleviation of the immediate disturbance may be adequate and is often dramatic, but such results are not to be credited to psychotherapy. The use of any accessory measure permits the patient to ascribe the disappearance of symptoms to instrumentalities outside himself and it follows that he would consider the causes also to be external. Such ideas contravene certain essential aims of psychotherapy, which should help the patient to realize that the relief of symptoms is due to his own efforts and to the understanding he develops of the unrealistic nature and purpose of the disturbance. The use of medicines, electricity, or other external apparatus may be advantageous with some acute phenomena, such as occur in conversion hysteria, where the major purpose would be to terminate the symptoms abruptly and dramatically. Without psychotherapy to follow up on the spectacular result, however, the same symptoms will reappear or new ones will evolve. This is inevitable, since the symptoms are only substitute expressions of the repressed basic conflict which remains untouched by this sort of staged show. Since the inner needs are not met by such an exhibition, the mechanism of repetition-compulsion continues to operate in the production of irrational and overdetermined activity in the form of symptoms.

Suggestion is properly a psychological measure used independently of extraneous agencies, and as such it requires the exhibition by the therapist of professional confidence and authority, combined with convincing evidence of his sympathetic and clear understanding of the patient's difficulty. Such an attitude enhances the patient's confidence in the therapist and in his knowledge, and promotes belief that results will occur as predicted. This disposition on the part of the patient is commonly called a state of heightened suggestibility; it will be seen that it is related to a narrowing of the field of attention and a diminution of critical faculties. Suggestibility is prominent in hysteria; it is particularly when the symptoms are manifestations of hysteria, yet comparatively recent and superficial in origin, that suggestion is most successful as therapy. However, suggestion not only fails to assist the patient to understand the psychodynamics of his difficulties but also increases his impressibility and limits insight. For more permanent results, therefore, re-educational procedures, which are also essential features of psychotherapy, must be employed.

It is important that the therapist should not appear to believe that the patient is exaggerating his disability or feigning symptoms. He must do or say nothing which savors of an attack on the patient's self-respect. The patient must be convinced of the meaning of his symptoms and convinced also that they have persisted because he believed his disabilities were real. He must be brought to believe that function can be restored to normal and that he is the agent responsible for its restitution.

Hypnosis is a special form of suggestion, in which there is a marked narrowing of consciousness such that the patient is in a somnolent state and remains in direct communication only with the hypnotist. During the hypnotic trance suppressed memories of past traumatic experiences may be explored and abreacted. Suggestions are made to the patient to be acted on at the termination of the session or even at a later time. Hypnosis requires a special technique and has a number of disadvantages, particularly the extent of the dependence which is likely to develop, together with an inadequacy on the part of the patient to solve his own problems. It is usually necessary to supplement hypnosis by re-educational measures and by methods designed to develop insight into underlying causes.

Hypnoanalysis is a development which combines technical principles from both hypnosis and psychoanalysis. Free association is employed as the main procedure, while hypnosis is used to uncover quickly the origin of resistances. Material thus brought out is carried on into the waking state and dealt with as though secured through free association. The usual analytic processes for handling the transference and its dissolution are followed.

Relaxation and the freeing of communication may also be produced by certain hypnotic drugs. Used for diagnostic purposes, the procedure is known as *narcoanalysis*. The method is also therapeutically useful to reduce anxiety and to facilitate the transference in certain cases, when it is called *narcosynthesis*.

It is clear that the central feature of methods which do not involve the use of drugs lies in the confidence the patient reposes in the therapist and his skill, which to a considerable extent is a reflection of the therapist's own belief in his knowledge and ability. This attitude is a phase or aspect of rapport, demonstrating certain peculiarities which tend to influence strongly any therapeutic relationship. The position of authority as a professional person is not merely assumed by the therapist; for the most part it is an investment consciously or unconsciously bestowed upon him by the patient. In these less extensive and more direct aspects of relationship it is important to realize that people are generally conditioned to respond to certain professions in accordance with long-existing traditions. Some of these traditions are distorted or outmoded, and some professions have not yet attained popular recognition for their knowledge and authority in their particular fields. In a psychiatric or mental hygiene clinic the professional authority of the physician is likely to receive the most unquestioning recognition, while the other members of the clinical team gain status only as their contributions to therapy evolve and their relationship to the total treatment program becomes clear to the patient and to others.

Several features, in addition to rapport, are common to a number of otherwise different technical approaches in therapy. One is the phenomenon of unburdening or ventilation, commonly known as *catharsis*. In this process the patient reveals guilt, anxiety, hostility, and traumatic experiences to the therapist. Unconscious material emerges, and some cause-effect sequences tend to become clarified to the patient in the course of his disclosures. Emotional reactions are reproduced, and other forms of acting out occur. During this process *insight* or reorientation develops, emotional tensions are released, and free-floating emotions tend to be reattached to their original objects. Probably most of the procedures which have been delimited as *insight therapies* depend largely on the cathartic process which, as may readily be seen, is fostered by the passive, permissive, relatively impersonal attitude of the therapist.

The attainment of insight into the subtleties of repressed material and the mechanisms through which conflicts come to expression in emotional or other disturbances is an essential aspect of treatment. In many instances the development of insight leads to marked improvement, which may, however, not be permanent. Too long continuance of the therapist's passive or neutral role often leads to difficulties, since the patient becomes involved in a transference conflict. Intellectual understanding is not sufficient to bring about marked alteration in reactions; there must be emotional reorientation or insight as well. Insight therapy as usually described seems to depend very largely on a form of educational or re-educational procedure which does not necessarily reach very deeply into emotional processes. However, educational procedures are certainly an integral part of all psychotherapy.

A few other aspects common to most therapeutic processes will be mentioned briefly. There is a marked tendency for the patient to identify with the therapist, revealed in a variety of imitations of the therapist's dress, speech, and other actions. The patient also strives to please the therapist and to maintain the cherished permissive atmosphere by doing and saying things he believes the therapist will approve. In some instances the patient may seek attention by the exhibition of unpleasant or unfriendly behavior. More often than not the mischievous behavior is an attempt to test the limits of the therapist's tolerance, which is really an attempt to define limitations for the patient's own ego. For this reason, clearly established limits have therapeutic value, since this process relieves anxiety and avoids confusion. Identification, striving to please, or even unpleasant behavior are indications of the patient's use of the therapist as a supportive ego and as a source of ego ideals. He also uses the therapist as an object on whom to project or displace various conflicts and responsibilities, thus to some extent alleviating troublesome emotions. As part of a relationship concerned chiefly with current realities and expressly intended to permit maximum growth and self-realization, all these processes have definite therapeutic value.

In both normal and abnormal psychological states there is a tendency for mental processes to stabilize. Also, the individual tends to seek group approval in accordance with general, but not universal, mores. These points correlate somewhat with certain aspects of the patient's drives in the therapeutic situation. Thus, there is a desire or drive to be well or recover, which is opposed by an unconscious drive to maintain the *status quo* because of secondary gains which are derived from the illness. This ambivalence and other factors introduce complications into the treatment situation which are constant sources of difficulty.

Variants of basic therapeutic techniques have been called attitude, relationship, and nondirective, therapy. For the most part these deal with the patient's current situation and have catharsis and self-determination as their major roots. All the valuable elements in the procedures fit into the generalized outline of psychotherapeutic process given above.

Play techniques are widely used, especially with children. Any manipulative materials may be used, and activity with the materials may be free or directed. Various types of dolls are employed; amputation dolls, from which head and limbs may be removed and replaced at will, and families of dolls are especially useful. Finger painting, drawing, water, fire, weapons, tools for expressing hostile aggression, and many other materials and toys have their place, as do puppets and puppet shows, pictures, and other methods of dramatizing persons or events. The important fact about all the play techniques is that they reveal underlying conflicts, anxiety, guilt, hostility and the like, and drain off thwarting emotions through the play and accompanying verbalizations. One form of treatment through play activities is called *release therapy*.

Group therapy in terms of specific techniques is a comparatively recent development, though the effects of groups and group life have been studied and used in haphazard fashion for a long time. The first medically oriented groups, definitely organized for therapeutic purposes, seem to have been established as "health classes" for cardiacs, rheumatics, and cases of tuberculosis. These appear to have been planned to permit the physician in charge to check on, educate, and reassure ambulatory patients. The reports on these early endeavors reveal very clearly the important group effects in therapy, which nevertheless did not seem particularly to impress the doctors as factors in the therapeutic results. Of course, group life in mental hospitals has long been known to have its effect on the patients, but until recently there was little systematic study of the dynamics and results of interaction in such groups.

For present purposes it will suffice to indicate that there are two major types of group therapy, which are quite different in orientation and operation. The first is *activity* group therapy, which is a major treatment technique for children, especially for ages about six to fourteen. In a permissive atmosphere, activities of diverse types, utilizing a wide variety of materials, are carried on. Interaction between members of the group is the essential factor in therapy; the therapist is not the central focus of the lines of relationship and therapeutic influence, but is one of the group in a peripheral relation.

Groups must be carefully set up to maintain an effective balance between aggressive, submissive, and neutral types. Within such a group, almost anything may happen and the therapist must be prepared to take it all in his stride, while maintaining his permissive neutrality. The make-up of groups, types of activity, cases not suitable for group therapy, details of procedure, training of therapists, and other factors in the process have all been the subject of careful study. It is necessary to emphasize the fact that not everyone possesses the qualities necessary to conduct therapy groups successfully, but the techniques can be acquired by those who have aptitude and interest. A therapy group cannot emerge from a number of individuals indiscriminately combined. Properly grouped, about 85 percent of the children brought to behavior clinics for treatment will profit far more from group therapy than from individual therapy.

Interview group therapy is the second major type. Especially suitable for adolescents and adults, the early orientation of interrelationships is from patients to therapist. As treatment progresses, and often very early, the lines of influence tend to develop more and more between patients. In the end, the tendency is for the therapist to be in a peripheral position as a member of the group, and not the dominating personality. Here again there has been intensive study of all the factors making for success and failure of this type of treatment. Training and operational procedures are now pretty well established. Groups have been conducted according to psychoanalytic rules of procedure, with interesting theoretical and practical results. The proportion of adults needing treatment who can accept and profit from group therapy is perhaps 15–20 percent. Nevertheless, the interview type of group therapy has been successfully employed with selected psychotics and neurotics, and its use is destined to increase.

Therapeutic principles have been systematically injected into the entire organization of a few institutions, with notable results. This organizational group treatment is, of course, supplemented by special group therapy sessions and, when indicated, individual sessions as well. Developments of this sort are to be welcomed, but they require much further careful study to determine the limits of applicability and controversial issues as to procedure.

Most of the subdivisions of psychotherapy discussed up to this point are dynamic procedures whose effectiveness is dependent on the relationship and the way in which it is manipulated by the therapist. These procedures, whether major or minor, are based upon and greatly influenced by the knowledge of psychodynamics derived from two sources: (1) the reconstructions and theoretical formulations of psychoanalysis and (2) direct clinical observations of children and their problems as they develop in the nexus of the family and in other settings. Psychoanalytic findings and orthopsychiatric observations thus complement each other very nicely. Little has been said about environmental manipulation, chiefly because the primary problems in the environment are the people in it, and the principles of treatment apply to them as well as to the patient. The lessening of general pressures and the mitigation of grinding realities involve other aspects of environmental manipulation, which enter so indirectly into the present discussion that they are omitted at this point.

Practically all the types of psychotherapy so far outlined can be carried out by properly trained and supervised workers of several professional disciplines. The data on which theory and practice are based are derived primarily from psychiatry, medicine, social work, and clinical psychology, especially as these disciplines are co-ordinated in the orthopsychiatric team and supplemented by contributions from such fields as social anthropology, education, child development, experimental psychology, and other organized approaches concerned with the human being in social and personal activities.

Psychoanalysis represents the most fundamental and the most penetrating of all psychotherapeutic techniques. Its findings and

postulates have profoundly altered all our concepts of psychotherapy and have illuminated every aspect of the intricate problems
of human nature and behavior. Special training and experience,
including a personal analysis, are prerequisite for analytic work,
which should not be attempted without such preparation. At the
same time, psychoanalytic orientation is necessary for practically
all constructive endeavors with people in trouble. Knowledge of
unconscious drives and of mental dynamisms is essential if one is
to understand conscious drives and motivations of behavior.

By contrast with the therapeutic procedures previously mentioned, psychoanalysis probes deeply into the unconscious, thereby
revealing the continuity of mental life. In this process old emotional conflicts are reprecipitated and isolated so they no longer
pervade the activities of the individual. This leads to reconstruction
of the personality, thus freeing it to function at its maximum potential. The major points in the technique are the use of free association, the interpretation of dreams and fantasies (which are comparable in many ways to the revealing play activities of the child),
and the manipulation of the transference. The phenomenon of
transference requires some discussion, because it is a process which
affects all personal contacts. It assumes basic importance in every
therapeutic situation, while its proper management and resolution
are essential in psychoanalysis. A detailed presentation of the technique of psychoanalysis is not within the scope of this book, though
several phases of the procedure necessarily emerge in discussing the
transference.

When treatment effort is focused primarily on current realities,
as it is in casework, in general medicine, and in some psychotherapeutic procedures, the therapist ordinarily retains his identity both
as an individual and as a professional person. These two aspects of
his personality are more or less thoroughly blended in the patient's
mind, with the result that he maintains the therapist in a professional role. The patient reacts directly to the professional person as
such and also to the mental image conceived by the patient in terms
of the dependency attitude evoked by tradition and by personal

or vicarious experience with the profession represented by the therapist. However, the extent to which the patient is able to accept and develop a therapeutic relationship of this sort is influenced by a variety of factors, most of which are unconscious. Many seem to be minor when finally brought to light and subjected to careful scrutiny; nevertheless, they largely determine the facility with which effective rapport may be established. These dynamisms are emotional in nature and represent carryovers from earlier experience. Derived by transference of emotions from a previous objective, they define and color the patient's mental picture of the therapist. Transposals of this sort influence our first reactions to every new acquaintance and new situation, no matter how we rationalize our emotional responses to them. Such transferences are, accordingly, a matter of constant occurrence in everyday life; everyone is familiar with them in drama and fiction, if not aware of them in his own experience. But transference is more significant and far more intense in a therapeutic relationship than in other contacts.

In psychoanalysis the transference is intensified and takes on characteristics that differ from those so far mentioned. For the patient, the analyst is largely obscured, both as an individual and as a professional person. He loses his individual identity and becomes a shadow, a blank screen against and upon which the analysand projects his own conflicting emotions and drives. During the analytic session the analyst is in effect a puppet, cast in the role which the patient's needs of the moment dictate. The figure of the analyst becomes the substitute or symbolic representative for any individual or even for any event of especial significance in the analysand's emotional life. The emotions provoked by earlier experiences, and then repressed, are brought out and forcefully projected upon the analyst, who therefore plays many roles, none of which he selects for himself. At one time or another he represents father, mother, siblings, lover, spouse, or others important to the patient. Love, hate, anger, dependence, domination, and other emotions involving regression are vented on the analyst according to the figure he momentarily represents. As a result of all this, the patient may become confused, develop a sense of unreality related to the exhibition of feelings toward the analyst, or show curious blind spots and areas of amnesia.

If these transference reactions are to be manipulated in the interests of therapy, they must continually be analyzed so that the emotions expressed are attached to the original source of provocation. It is necessary to keep this in the foreground, lest the patient mistakenly regard the therapist as the actual objective of his reactions. Should this sort of fixation occur, therapy is blocked by the false attachment of the intense emotional state.

The patient not only identifies the therapist with important images from the past, but may directly identify the therapist with himself and so enter into shadowy, but troublesome, competition. The tendency is to identify the therapist as the good, permissive, and forgiving parent who does not, however, overindulge or encourage too much submissiveness or dependency.

In transference the patient is not aware of the character of the relationship or the origin of his emotional reactions and behavior, which are beyond his control. Through the transference he becomes free to talk of matters he would not usually discuss and to display behavior he would ordinarily conceal. The reactions transposed to the therapist as substitute object shift between positive and negative—that is, between love and hostility. Both polarities are proper subjects for interpretation, since insight and reintegration of personality depend upon adequate understanding of the influence which these repressed emotions exert upon conscious processes, including behavior.

It will be seen, therefore, that transference phenomena do not represent the attitudes of the patient toward the analyst as a person, but are instead repetitive of earlier situations, the analyst being used as a substitute. His own recognition of this fact is the chief protection the analyst has against reacting personally to the emotion discharged upon him. This does not mean that he does not react to his patient, nor is the therapist necessarily free from transference feelings. It is well known that such *counter-transference* occurs, and every therapist must be aware at all times of his own attitudes and keep them under control. The chief requirement, perhaps, is that he be constantly on the alert for his own blind spots and for reactions toward the patient which are excessive or inappropriate. Counter-transference may express itself in a host of ways, among them overidentification, minimizing or completely overlooking important elements in the patient's problems, being too permissive or too punitive, or even too passive. Like transference, counter-transferences are both negative and positive. As is true of the patient's transference behavior, the therapist must also be aware of his own counter-transference if treatment is not to be impeded.

We may conclude that all relationships have transference elements and that they are especially strong and particularly complex in the therapeutic situation, reaching their maximum during psychoanalysis. The reactions of both patient and therapist require study and interpretation. The knowledge that the patient's transference reactions are projected upon the therapist as a substitute provides some protection against direct counter-reaction. The continuous analysis of transference manifestations and of the therapeutic situation fosters the patient's development of insight, releases repressed emotions which had been escaping into distorted behavior, and results in the reintegration of personality. It is the relationship and its manipulation which constitute the core of psychotherapy, not in the sense of direct, uncontrolled, and uninterpreted emotional reactions of one person to another, but chiefly in terms of the influence of transference and its continuing interpretation.

SELECTED READING LIST

PSYCHIATRY, PSYCHOANALYSIS, AND MENTAL HYGIENE

Adler, Alfred. The Practice and Theory of Individual Psychology; trans. by P. Radin. New York, Harcourt, Brace, 1924.

Aichhorn, August. Wayward Youth. New York, Viking Press, 1936.

Alexander, Franz. Our Age of Unreason. Philadelphia, Lippincott, 1942.

—— Fundamentals of Psychoanalysis. New York, Norton, 1948.

Alexander, Franz, and Thomas E. French, eds. Studies in Psychosomatic Medicine. New York, Ronald Press, 1948.

Allen, Frederick H. Psychotherapy with Children. New York, Norton, 1942.

American Psychiatry, 1844–1944. New York, published for the American Psychiatric Association by Columbia University Press, 1944.

Barker, Lewellys F. Psychotherapy. New York, Appleton-Century, 1940.

Beers, Clifford. A Mind That Found Itself. New York, Doubleday, Doran, 1940.

Bleuler, Eugen. Textbook of Psychiatry; trans. by A. A. Brill. New York, Macmillan, 1924.

Brill, A. A. Freud's Contribution to Psychiatry. New York, Norton, 1944.

—— Basic Principles of Psychoanalysis. New York, Doubleday, 1949.

Bromberg, Walter. The Mind of Man. New York, Harper, 1937.

Brown III, Sanger, and Howard W. Potter. Psychiatric Study of Problem Children. Utica, N.Y., State Hospital Press, 1930.

Cleckley, Hervey. The Mask of Sanity. St. Louis, Mosby, 1941.

Deutsch, Albert. The Mentally Ill in America. New York, Doubleday, Doran, 1937. New Printing, New York, Columbia University Press, 1948.

English, O. S., and G. H. J. Pearson. Common Neuroses of Children and Adults. New York, Norton, 1937.

—— Emotional Problems of Living. New York, Norton, 1945.

Fenichel, Otto. Problems of Psychoanalytic Therapy. New York, Psychoanalytic Quarterly, 1941.

—— Psychoanalytic Theory of Neurosis. New York, Norton, 1945.

Flügel, J. C. The Psycho-analytic Study of the Family. New York and London, Hogarth Press, 1935.

Freud, Anna. The Technique of Child Analysis. New York, Nervous and Mental Disease Monographs, 1928.

—— The Ego and the Methods of Defense. New York, International Universities Press, 1946.

Freud, Sigmund. General Introduction to Psychoanalysis. New York, Liveright, 1920.

—— Collected Papers. 4 vols. New York and London, Hogarth Press, 1925.

Healy, Bronner, and others. The Structure and Meaning of Psychoanalysis. New York, Knopf, 1930.

Hinzie, Leland E. Concepts and Problems of Psychotherapy. New York, Columbia University Press, 1937.

Hutchings, Richard H. A Psychiatric Word Book. Utica, N.Y., State Hospital Press, 1943.

Isaacs, Susan. Social Development in Young Children. New York, Harcourt, Brace, 1933.

Jung, C. G. Psychological Types; trans. by H. G. Baynes. New York, Harcourt, Brace, 1926.

Karpman, Benjamin. The Alcoholic Woman. Washington, D.C., Washington Institute for Medicine, 1949.

Lawton, George. Aging Successfully. New York, Columbia University Press, 1946.

Lennox, William G. Science and Seizures. New York, Harper, 1946.

Levine, Maurice. Psychotherapy in Medical Practice. New York, Macmillan, 1942.

Levy, David. Maternal Overprotection. New York, Columbia University Press, 1943.

—— New Fields in Psychiatry. New York, Norton, 1947.

Lewis, N. D. C. Outlines for Psychiatric Examinations. 3d ed. Utica, N.Y., State Hospital Press, 1943.

Lindner, Robert M. Rebel without a Cause. New York, Grune & Stratton, 1944.

Lorand, Sandor, ed. Psychoanalysis Today. New York, International Universities Press, 1944.

—— Technique of Psychoanalytic Therapy. New York, International Universities Press, 1946.

Menninger, Karl A. The Human Mind. 3d ed. New York, Knopf, 1945.

—— Love against Hate. New York, Harcourt, Brace, 1942.

Noyes, Arthur P. Modern Clinical Psychiatry. 3d ed. Philadelphia, Saunders, 1948.

Orthopsychiatry, 1923–1948: Retrospect and Prospect; ed. by Lawson G. Lowrey and Victoria Sloane. New York, American Orthopsychiatric Association, 1948.

Philosophy of Insanity; introduction by Frieda Fromm-Reichman. New York, Greenberg, 1947.

Preston, George H. The Substance of Mental Health. New York, Farrar & Rinehart, 1943.

Rank, Otto. Beyond Psychology. Philadelphia, privately printed, 1941.
—— Will Therapy *and* Truth and Reality; trans. by Jessie Taft. New York, Knopf, 1945.

Saul, Leon J. Emotional Maturity. Philadelphia, Lippincott, 1947.

Schilder, Paul. Goals and Desires of Man. New York, Columbia University Press, 1942.

Slavson, S. R. An Introduction to Group Therapy. New York, Commonwealth Fund, 1943.

Stekel, Wilhelm. Technique of Analytical Psychotherapy; trans. by Eden and Cedar Paul. New York, Norton, 1940.

Sterba, Richard. Introduction to the Psychoanalytic Theory of the Libido. New York, Nervous & Mental Disease Monographs, 1944.

Temporary Commission on State Hospital Problems. Report on Insulin Shock Therapy. New York, 1944.

Tredgold, A. F. Mental Deficiency. 7th ed. Baltimore, Williams & Wilkins, 1948.

Weiss, Edward, and O. S. English. Psychosomatic Medicine. Philadelphia, Saunders, 1943.

White, William Alanson. An Introduction to the Study of the Mind. New York, Nervous & Mental Disease Monographs, 1935.
—— Outlines of Psychiatry. 14th ed. New York, Nervous & Mental Disease Monographs, 1935.
—— Forty Years of Psychiatry. New York, Nervous & Mental Disease Monographs, 1935.

Zilboorg, Gregory. A History of Medical Psychology. New York, Norton, 1941.

PSYCHOLOGY

Alschuler, Rose H., and LaBerta Hattwick. Painting and Personality. 2 vols. Chicago, University of Chicago Press, 1947.

Beck, S. J. Rorschach's Test. 2 vols. New York, Grune & Stratton, 1944-45. I: Basic Processes; II: A Variety of Personality Pictures.

Bell, John E. Projective Techniques. Philadelphia, Longmans, Green, 1948.

Bender, Lauretta. A Visual Motor Gestalt Test and Its Clinical Use. New York, American Orthopsychiatric Association, 1938.

Gesell, Arnold. The First Five Years of Life. New York, Harper, 1940.
—— The Embryology of Behavior. New York, Harper, 1945.

Gesell, Arnold, and Frances L. Ilg. The Child from Five to Ten. New York, Harper, 1946.

Gesell, Arnold, and others. Developmental Diagnosis. New York, Harper, 1941.

Hunt, J. McV., ed. Personality and the Behavior Disorders. New York, Ronald Press, 1944.

Klopfer, Bruno, and D. M. Kelly. The Rorschach Technique. Yonkers, N.Y., World Book Company, 1942.

Landis, Carney, and M. Marjorie Bolles. Textbook of Abnormal Psychology. New York, Macmillan, 1946.

Louttit, C. M. Clinical Psychology of Children's Behavior Disorders. New York, Harper, 1947.

Monroe, Marian. Children Who Cannot Read. Chicago, University of Chicago Press, 1932.

Pennington, L. A., and I. A. Berg. An Introduction to Clinical Psychology. New York, Ronald Press, 1948.

Rapaport, David, Merton M. Gill, and Roy Shafer. Diagnostic Psychological Testing. 2 vols. Chicago, Year Book Publishers, 1947.

Stoddard, G. The Meaning of Intelligence. New York, Macmillan, 1943.

Terman, L. M., and Maude A. Merrill. Measuring Intelligence. New York, Houghton Mifflin, 1937.

Tomkins, Sylvan. The Thematic Apperception Test. New York, Grune & Stratton, 1947.

Tulchin, Simon H. Intelligence and Crime. Chicago, University of Chicago Press, 1939.

Watson, Robert I., ed. Readings in the Clinical Method in Psychology. New York, Harper, 1949.

Wechsler, David. The Measurement of Adult Intelligence. Baltimore, Williams & Wilkins, 1944.

Wickman, E. K. Teachers and Behavior Problems. New York, Commonwealth Fund, 1938.

Wolff, Werner. What Is Psychology? New York, Grune & Stratton, 1947.

SOCIAL WORK

Cannon, Antoinette, and Philip Klein, eds. Social Case Work. New York, Columbia University Press, 1933.

Crutcher, Hester B. Guide for the Development of Psychiatric Social Work in State Hospitals. Utica, N.Y., State Hospital Press.

French, Lois M. Psychiatric Social Work. New York, Commonwealth Fund, 1940.

Hamilton, Gordon. Theory and Practice of Social Case Work. New York, Columbia University Press, 1940.

—— Psychotherapy in Child Guidance. New York, Columbia University Press, 1947.

Lee, Porter R., and Marion E. Kenworthy. Mental Hygiene and Social Work. New York, Commonwealth Fund, 1929.

Queen, S. A., and D. M. Mann. Social Pathology. New York, Crowell, 1925.

Reynolds, Bertha C. Learning and Teaching in the Practice of Social Work. New York, Farrar & Rinehart, 1942.

Richmond, Mary E. Social Diagnosis. New York, Russell Sage Foundation, 1917.

—— What Is Social Work? New York, Russell Sage Foundation, 1922.

Robinson, Virginia. A Changing Psychology in Social Case Work. Chapel Hill, University of North Carolina Press, 1930.

Social Work Year Book. New York, Russell Sage Foundation, 1947.

Southard, E. E., and Mary C. Jarrett. The Kingdom of Evils. New York, Macmillan, 1922.

Sterba, Richard, B. H. Lundon, and Anna Katz. Transference in Casework. New York, Family Service Association, 1948.

Thomas, W. I., and Dorothy S. Thomas. The Child in America. New York, Knopf, 1928.

Towle, Charlotte. Social Case Records from Psychiatric Clinics. University of Chicago Press, 1941.

PERIODICALS

Relevant articles may be found in the following periodicals.

American Journal of Orthopsychiatry.
American Journal of Psychotherapy.
The Quarterly Journal of Child Behavior.
Psychiatry.
Journal of Abnormal and Social Psychology.
Journal of Clinical Psychopathology.
Mental Hygiene.
Survey.
Journal of Social Casework.
Journal of Psychiatric Social Work.

The National Committee for Mental Hygiene, 1790 Broadway, New York 19, supplies reprints of many articles on important psychiatric and mental hygiene topics, and will send a list of available titles on request.

INDEX